Pharmacology of Endogenous Neurotoxins

A Handbook

Edited by
Andreas Moser

Springer Science+Business Media, LLC

Editor:
Andreas Moser
Department of Neurology
Medical University of Lübeck
Lübeck, Germany

Library of Congress Cataloging-in-Publication Data

Pharmacology of endogenous neurotoxins / [edited by] Andreas Moser.
    p.   cm.
   Includes bibliographical references and index.
   ISBN 978-0-8176-3993-8   ISB 978-1-4612-2000-8 (eBook)
   DOI 10.1007/978-1-4612-2000-8
   1. Neurotoxicology.   2. Neurotoxins—Metabolism.   3. Neurotoxins—
Pathophysiology.   4. Neuropharmacology.   I. Moser, Andreas, 1960–   .
   [DNLM: 1. Neurotoxins—pharmacology.   QW 630.5.N4 P536 1997]
   RC347.5.P48   1998
   616.8′047—DC21
   DNLM/DLC
   for Library of Congress   98-12361
                                     CIP

Printed on acid-free paper.

©1998 Springer Science+Business Media New York
Originally published by Birkhäuser Boston in 1998

ISBN 978-0-8176-3993-8
Typeset by Braun-Brumfield, Inc.

9 8 7 6 5 4 3 2 1

List of contributors

Gerhard Bringmann, Institute of Organic Chemistry, University of Würzburg, Am Hubland, D-97074 Würzburg, Germany

Hans-Willi Clement, Institute of Physiological Chemistry, Department of Neurochemistry, University of Marburg, Hans-Meerwein-Straße, D-35033 Marburg, Germany

Michael A. Collins, Department of Molecular & Cellular Biochemistry, Loyola University Medical Center, 2160 South First Avenue, Maywood, Illinois 60153, USA

Philippe Dostert, Pharmacia-Upjohn, I-20159 Milan, Italy

Glenn Dryhurst, Department of Chemistry and Biochemistry, University of Oklahoma, 620 Parrington Oval, Room 208, Norman, Oklahoma 73019-0370, USA

Doris Feineis, Institute of Organic Chemistry, University of Würzburg, Am Hubland, D-97074 Würzburg, Germany

Ralf God, Institute of Organic Chemistry, University of Würzburg, Am Hubland, D-97074 Würzburg, Germany

Christoph Grote, Institute of Physiological Chemistry, Department of Neurochemistry, University of Marburg, Hans-Meerwein-Straße, D-35033 Marburg, Germany

Hanka Haber, Research Institute for Molecular Pharmacology, A.-Kowalke-Straße 4, D-10315 Berlin, Germany

Yoko Hirata, Laboratory for Genes and Motor Systems, Bio-mimetic Control Research Center, Institute of Physical and Chemical Research, Shimoshidami, Moriyama, Nagoya 463, Japan

Bernd Janetzky, University Hospital Carl Gustav Carus, Department of Neurology, University of Dresden, Fetscherstraße 74, D-01307 Dresden, Germany

Mitsuharu Kajita, Department of Pediatrics, Nagoya University School of Medicine, 65 Tsuruma-cho, Showa-ku, Nagoya 466, Japan

Wakako Maruyama, Laboratory of Biochemistry and Metabolism, Department of Basic Gerontology, National Institute for Longevity Sciences, Obu, Japan

Kazuo Matsubara, Department of Hospital Pharmacy and Pharmacology, Asahikawa Medical College, A Schikawa 078, Japan

Matthias F. Melzig, Institute of Pharmacy, Humboldt University, Goethestr. 54, D-13086 Berlin, Germany

Andreas Moser (Editor), Department of Neurology, Medical University of Lübeck, Ratzeburger Allee 160, D-23538 Lübeck, Germany

Toshiharu Nagatsu, Division of Molecular Genetics (II) Neurochemistry, Institute for Comprehensive Medical Science, School of Medicine, Fujita Health University, Toyoake, Aichi 470-11, Japan

Makoto Naoi, Department of Biosciences, Nagoya Institute of Technology, Gokiso-cho, Showa-ku, Nagoya 466, Japan

Edward J. Neafsey, Department of Cell Biology, Neurobiology & Anatomy, Stritch School of Medicine, Loyola University Chicago, 2160 South First Avenue, Maywood, Illinois 60153, USA

Clemens Neusch, Department of Neurology, Medical University of Lübeck, Ratzeburger Allee 160, D-23538 Lübeck, Germany

Toshimitsu Niwa, Department of Preventive Clinical Medicine, Nagoya University Daiko Medical Center, 1-1-20, Daiko-minami, Higashi-ku, Nagoya 461, Japan

George D. Prell, Department of Pharmacology, (box 1215) Mount Sinai School of Medicine of the City University of New York, 1 Gustave L. Levy Place, New York, New York 10029-6574, USA

Ingo Putscher, Research Institute for Molecular Pharmacology, A.-Kowalke-Straße 4, D-10315 Berlin, Germany

Wolf-Dieter Rausch, Institute of Medical Chemistry, University of Veterinary Medicine Vienna, Josef-Baumanngasse 1, A-1210 Vienna, Austria

Heinz Reichmann, University Hospital Carl Gustav Carus, Department of Neurology, University of Dresden, Fetschenstraße 74, D-01307 Dresden, Germany

Peter Riederer, Clinical Neurochemistry, Department of Psychiatry, University of Würzburg, Fuchsleinstraße 15, D-97080 Würzburg, Germany

Matthias Rottmann, Research Institute for Molecular Pharmacology, A.-Kowalke-Straße 4, D-10315 Berlin, Germany

Joachim Scholz, Department of Neurology, Medical University of Lübeck, Ratzeburger Allee 160, D-23538 Lübeck, Germany

Karl-Heinz Sontag, Max Planck Institute for Experimental Medicine, Hermann-Rein-Straße 3, D-37075 Göttingen. Germany

Wolfgang Wesemann, Institute of Physiological Chemistry, Department of Neurochemistry, University of Marburg, Hans-Meerwein-Straße, D-35033 Marburg, Germany

Josef Zipper, Research Institute for Molecular Pharmacology, A.-Kowalke-Straße 4, D-10315 Berlin, Germany

Contents in Brief

Table of Contents

Foreword

It is a great pleasure to write the foreword to this important volume for several reasons. First: As far as we know, already primitive societies had to cope with environmental toxins of many kinds and set up regulations to limit their effects on food and drug use. Modern science, synthesizing tens of millions of new compounds has incredibly magnified this challenge. Today, xenobiotic metabolism has become a crucial task for humans and many other species alike.

Second: When reading this book, one is impressed by the extraordinary speed at which neurotoxicology has advanced. Obviously, processing (and endogenous formation) of toxins has become an extremely relevant topic. When I had the chance, almost three decades ago, to work in chemical pharmacology with Bernard B. Brodie at NIH, the drug metabolizing system of the liver had just been recognized and characterized. We had just started to work on the biogenic amines, newly discovered cyclic nucleotides in rat brain, human cerebrospinal fluid, and on the effects of toxic drugs like amphetamines. Today, *bio*chemical *neuro*pharmacology is a mature field of neuroscience.

Third: As a clinical neurologist, I may underline the great importance of several contributions in the book for a new understanding of neurological diseases. The elucidation of endogenous neurotoxin formation, influenced by overcharge, genotoxicity, drug interactions, abuse and other factors, is promising to provide new insight into the origin and mechanism of neurodegenerative diseases, and, of interest to a wider audience, into normal and abnormal aging. Since the editor's background also includes clinical neurology, these aspects are dealt sufficiently with in the book. I am sure that this volume will be acclaimed—both as a timely review and as an extremely helpful handbook and reference source for the researcher in the field.

Hinrich Cramer
Professor of Neurology and Neurochemistry
University of Freiburg
Germany

Preface

"Since the discovery of MPTP . . . ." These introductory words appear at the beginning of a voluminous literature published by neuroscientists who are dealing with MPTP and the neurotoxicological aspects in pathogenesis of Parkinson's disease. Although many biochemical parallels do exist between Parkinson's disease and MPTP-induced parkinsonism, it should be clear that patients with idiopathic Parkinson's disease had never ingested MPTP in their lifetime. However, the nucleus of MPTP responsible for its toxicity is a common chemical moiety and thus, may occur in many other substances.

The search for environmental toxins that are related to neurodegenerative disorders has so far been unrewarding. There may be significant factors associated with industrialization, agrochemicals, or early exposure to a rural environment, including the use of well water for drinking.

The impact of these factors has, however, been relatively small and inconsistent in the studies undertaken. The potential involvement of MPTP-like compounds in Parkinson's disease may not be restricted only to those found in the environment, but may also involve endogenous neurotoxins. Thus, the aim of this book is to survey some of the important areas of neurotoxicological research together with the impact of potentially endogenously synthesized heterocyclic neurotoxins on normal and pathophysiological regulation in the central nervous system, and also on a number of specific organs and diseases.

The first part of the book deals with the chemical and biochemical aspects of the origin, formation and degradation, and biochemical pathways, of those heterocyclic compounds, including tetrahydroisoquinolines, β-carbolines, methylimidazoles, and tryptamines and their association to alkaloids. Heterocyclicants are then considered as potentially endogenously synthesized substances from catecholamines or other transmitter metabolites in mammals (including humans). The role of these substances in the understanding of disease processes is discussed by experts as the most intriguing problem. In the second part of the book, physiological, biochemical, and neuropharmacological aspects of enzymatic systems, including their interaction with heterocyclic neurotoxins, are treated, showing that the unraveling of the roles played by neurotoxins, may well become a key point in the understanding of the metabolism in the central nervous system.

Altogether, though many unresolved and challenging problems are stated and discussed in the text, this volume describes all of the potentially endogenously formed neurotoxins and relevant enzyme systems known to date. In this capacity, we hope, it may be widely used as a handbook by the researchers in the field and by the clinical neurologists with a special interest in neurodegenerative diseases.

Andreas Moser
Medical University of Lübeck
Germany

Part A

NEUROTOXINS

Chapter *1*

Isoquinoline Derivatives

*Toshimitsu Niwa, Mitsuharu Kajita and
Toshiharu Nagatsu*

Contents in Brief

1. Introduction

Since the discovery of 1-methyl-4-phenyl-1,2,3,6-tetrahydropyridine (MPTP) as a highly selective, irreversible dopaminergic neurotoxin, which produces parkinsonism in humans, monkeys and mice (Burns et al., 1983; Langston et al., 1983; Heikkila et al., 1984), other endogenous or environmental neurotoxins, structurally similar to MPTP, and also potentially causing Parkinson's disease (PD) have been examined. The neurotoxicity of MPTP is dependent on the conversion of MPTP by monoamine oxidase (MAO) (*EC 1.4.3.4*), type B, to the 1-methyl-4-phenylpyridinium ion (MPP[+]) in the brain (Markey et al., 1984; Naoi and Maruyama, 1993) (Fig. 1). The results of screening various MPTP- or MPP[+]-related compounds have implicated isoquinoline derivatives such as 1,2,3,4-tetrahydroisoquinoline (TIQ) as strong candidates for neurotoxins which may produce PD.

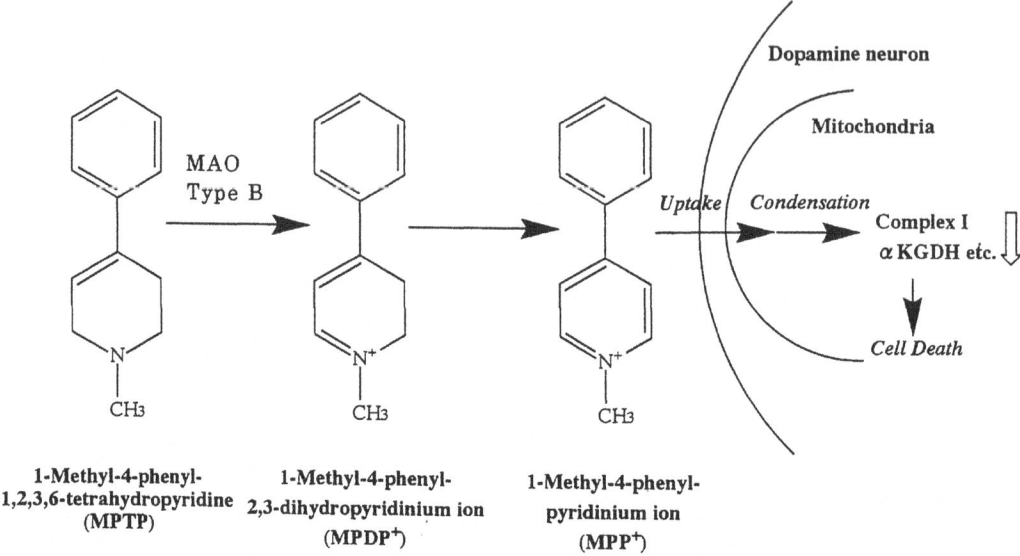

Fig. 1 Metabolism of 1-methyl-4-phenyl-1,2,3,6-tetrahydropyridine (MPTP) in the brain.

2. Tetrahydroisoquinoline (TIQ)

2.1. Presence of TIQ in nature and in food

Various TIQ alkaloids such as morphine have been found in plants. In the early 1970s, some TIQ alkaloids were found in the mammalian brain (Sandler et al., 1973). TIQs are thought to be synthesized from phenylethylamine (PEA) derivatives and aldehydes by the Pictet-Spengler condensation reaction which is a method of TIQ formation from β-aromatic ethylamines and aldehydes under acid catalysis (Cohen and Collins, 1970; Collins, 1980).

TIQ is commonly present in various foods and beverages (Makino et al., 1988; Niwa et al., 1989b) and may accumulate in the human brain over a long period of time, eventually causing PD. The concentrations of TIQ in various foods are shown in Table 1. TIQ is present in particularly high concentrations in cheese, milk, boiled eggs, and bananas. In

Table 1. Concentrations of TIQ in foods.

Sample	Concentration of TIQ (ng/g)	Sample	Concentration of TIQ (ng/g or ng/ml)
Cheese	5.2	Yolk of boiled egg	1.8
Banana	2.2	White of boiled egg	2.2
Broiled sardine	0.96	Wine	0.56
Broiled beef	1.3	Beer	0.36
Flour	0.52	Whisky	0.73
		Milk	3.3

(Niwa T. et al., 1989b)

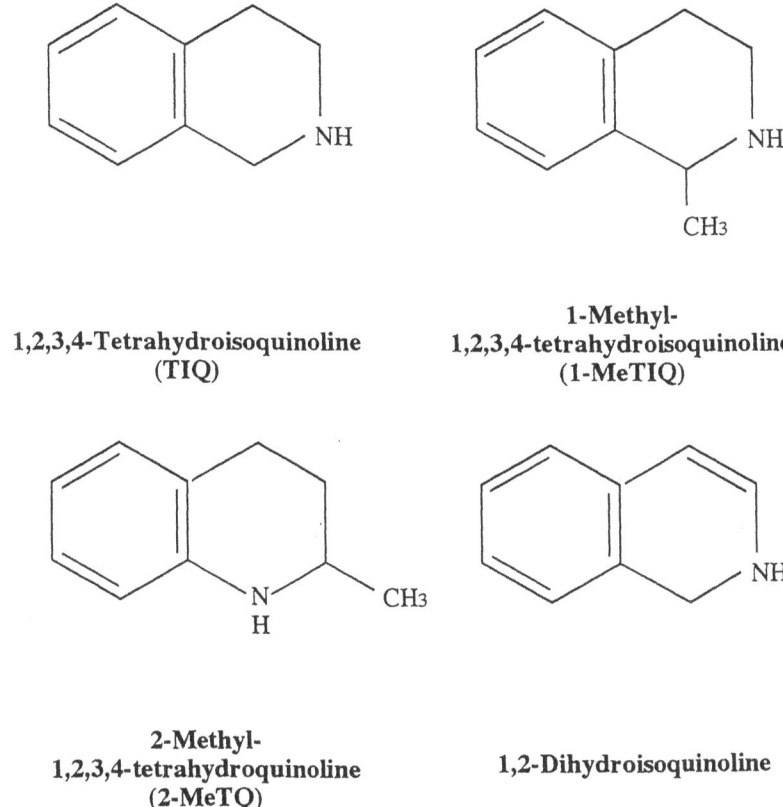

Fig. 2 Chemical structures of 1,2,3,4-tetrahydroisoquinoline (TIQ) and its related compounds.

addition to TIQ, 1-methyl-1,2,3,4-tetrahydroisoquinoline (1-MeTIQ) was also detected in foods such as white wine, cocoa, and cheese (Makino et al., 1988). The S-enantiomer of 1-MeTIQ is predominantly present in wine and cocoa (Makino et al., 1990).

Figure 2 shows the chemical structures of TIQ and its related compounds.

2.2. Methods for identification and measurement of TIQ

TIQ could be extracted from the brain, as described by Kohno et al. (1986), and then derivatized with heptafluorobutyric anhydride (HFBA) (Niwa et al., 1987, 1989a). HFB-derivatized TIQ was then detected by gas chromatography/mass spectrometry (GC/MS).

The R- and S-enantiomers of 1-MeTIQ were analyzed with a chiral derivatization agent and gas chromatography/negative-ion chemical ionization mass spectrometry (Makino et al., 1990).

2.3. Presence of TIQ in tissues

TIQ was discovered in parkinsonian human brains by GC/MS (Niwa et al., 1987, 1989a, 1995; Ohta et al., 1987). In rats, the concentration of TIQ was about 6 ng/g wet tissue in the spinal cord and about 2 ng/g in the brain, whereas in lung, intestine, and liver, it amounted to about 1 ng/g or less.

The S-enantiomer of 1-methyl-TIQ was predominantly present in mouse (R/S = 0.60) and human (R/S = 0.27) brains (Makino et al., 1990).

An analogue of TIQ, 1-MeTIQ, was also found in rat and human brains. The 1-MeTIQ content was markedly reduced in the parkinsonian brain, particularly in the frontal lobe. The level of 1-MeTIQ was also shown to decrease with aging (Kohno et al., 1986; Ohta et al., 1987).

Table 2 shows the reported concentrations of these TIQs in human and rat brains.

2.4. Endogenous synthesis of TIQ

TIQ and 1-MeTIQ may be formed by the condensation of PEA with formaldehyde and acetaldehyde, respectively (Ohta et al., 1987) (Fig. 3). The results of the R- and S-enantiomer analysis of 1-MeTIQ suggest that some enzymatic synthesis of TIQs may be present and, thus, may be related to the pathogenesis of PD.

2.5. Parkinsonism caused by TIQ

TIQ selectively inhibited the activity of NADH-ubiquinone reductase (complex I; EC 1.6.99.3) in mitochondria isolated from mouse brains (Suzuki et al., 1989). The biochemical properties of TIQ in this study were quite similar to those of the dopaminergic neurotoxin MPP^+.

A daily injection of TIQ (50 mg/kg per day, s.c. for 11 days) induced parkinsonism in marmosets, which was accompanied by a reduction in dopamine and biopterin concentrations and in tyrosine hydroxylase (EC 1.14.16.2, TH) activity in the nigrostriatal regions (Nagatsu and Yoshida, 1988; Yoshida et al., 1990) and by accumulation of TIQ in the brain.

Table 2.   Concentrations of TIQ alkaloids in human and rat brains.

	Concentrations of TIQ alkaloids in brains (ng/g)		
	TIQ	1-MeTIQ	References
Human Control			
Frontal lobe	1		*
	0.86 ± 0.23#	0.75 ± 0.25#	**
Caudate nucleus	0.64 ± 0.24#	0.52 ± 0.15#	**
Parkinsonian			
Frontal lobe	7–10		*
	0.58 ± 0.20#	0.05 ± 0.02#	**
Caudate nucleus	0.25 ± 0.08#	0.12 ± 0.03#	**
Rat	4.7–5.8	1.6–2.6	***

(#: mean ±S.D.; *Niwa T. et al., 1987; **Ohta S. et al., 1987; ***Kohno M. et al., 1986)

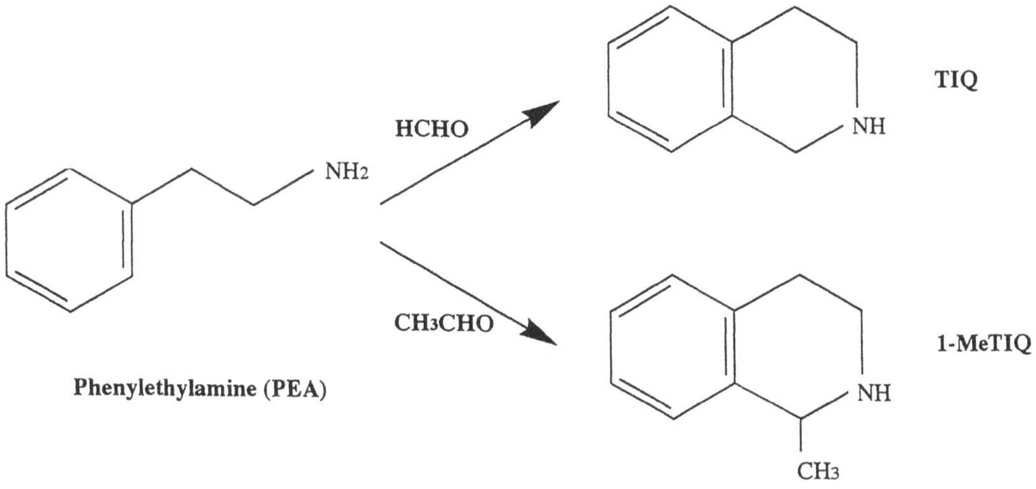

Fig. 3 Proposed mechanism of TIQ and 1-MeTIQ formation.

TIQ can thus pass easily through the blood-brain barrier (Niwa et al., 1988). A similar administration of TIQ (50 mg/kg per day, s.c. for 70 days) to mice induced a marked decrease in the number of TH-positive neurons in the *substantia nigra,* but no evidence of cell death in these neurons could be observed (Yoshida et al., 1990). This may have been due to the age of the animals and to the less specific neurotoxicity of TIQ toward dopaminergic neurons.

It is noteworthy that 1-MeTIQ pretreatment could prevent parkinsonism in mice treated with MPTP or TIQ (Tasaki et al., 1991).

2.6. Metabolism of TIQ in the brain

In addition to TIQ, N-methyl-TIQ (NMTIQ) also appears to be a neurotoxin based on the screening of various compounds structurally related to MPTP for neurotoxicity. NMTIQ is oxidized to the N-methylisoquinolinium ion (NMIQ$^+$) by monoamine oxidase in human brain synaptosomal mitochondria (Naoi et al., 1989a).

NMIQ$^+$ was found to inhibit tyrosine hydroxylase in rat striatal slices (Hirata et al., 1985), monoamine oxidase (Naoi et al., 1987), and aromatic L-amino acid decarboxylase (EC 4.1.1.28, DDC) (Naoi et al., 1989b). Intrastriatal microdialysis of NMIQ$^+$ in rat brain induced a massive release of dopamine, as was also noted following perfusion with MPP$^+$ (Booth et al., 1989). NMIQ$^+$ showed about 10% of the potency of MPP$^+$ in an intrastriatal dialysis assay; TIQ and NMTIQ were found to be MAO-B substrates, both oxidized at about 3% of the rate for MPTP. NMIQ$^+$ would thus appear to be a potent endogenous neurotoxin similar to MPP$^+$, an oxidation product of MPTP formed by monoamine oxidase.

NMTIQ may be an intermediate in the biosynthesis of NMIQ$^+$ from TIQ in the brain, and the N-methylation of TIQ to NMTIQ has been shown to occur *in vitro* by the action of an N-methyltransferase in the human brain (Naoi et al., 1989c). The reaction required S-adenosyl-L-methionine (SAM) as a methyl donor. The endogenous synthesis of NMTIQ from TIQ was found to occur *in vivo* by GC/MS analysis of the brain of a TIQ-injected marmoset. The concentration of NMTIQ was approximately 1% of that of TIQ in the brains of TIQ-injected marmosets (Niwa et al., 1990). Behavioral scores of NMTIQ-treated monkeys showed slight motor disturbances after 100 days' administration of NMTIQ, but neuropathological examinations of the substantia nigra revealed no differences between the NMTIQ-treated and the control monkeys (Yoshida et al., 1991).

Figure 4 shows the metabolic pathway of TIQ in the brain.

3. 1,2-Dihydroisoquinoline

1,2-Dihydroisoquinoline (Fig. 2) was found in an extract from the brain of a TIQ-injected marmoset. 1,2-Dihydroisoquinoline appeared to be an oxidized metabolite of TIQ, probably by monoamine oxidase, since it could not be found in the extract from the brain of the saline-injected control monkey (Niwa et al., 1993).

4. 4-Hydroxy-TIQ

4-Hydroxy-TIQ was detected as a metabolite of TIQ in liver microsomes and urine of a TIQ-administered rat (Ohta et al., 1990). The 4-hydroxylation of TIQ is a cytochrome P-450-dependent reaction in the liver, and it accelerates the excretion of TIQ into urine for the detoxification (Fig. 5). In female DA rats, an animal model of a poor debrisoquine metabolizer, metabolic detoxification is depressed and TIQ accumulation in the brain is enhanced. This may be related to the early onset of Parkinson's disease in poor metabolizers of debrisoquine (Barbeau et al., 1985).

5. 1-Benzyl-TIQ

1-Benzyl-1,2,3,4-tetrahydroisoquinoline (BnTIQ) was detected as a novel endogenous amine in mouse brain and parkinsonian cerebrospinal fluid (CSF) by the gas chromatography-selected ion monitoring (GC/SIM) method (Kotake et al., 1995). BnTIQ could be formed from PEA and phenylacetaldehyde, a metabolite of PEA generated by MAO-B (Fig. 6).

The level of BnTIQ was very high in the CSF of some parkinsonian patients compared

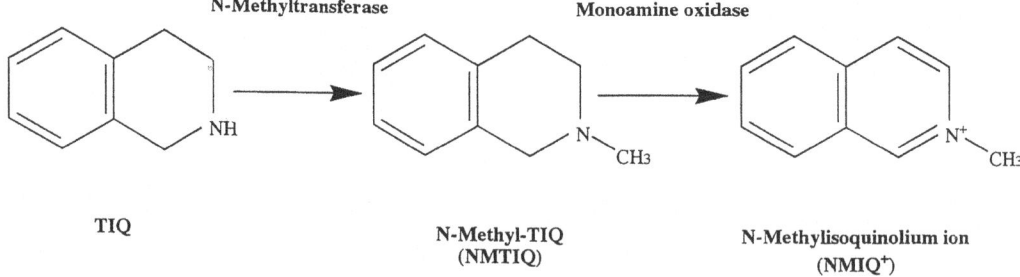

Fig. 4   Metabolic pathway of TIQ in the brain.

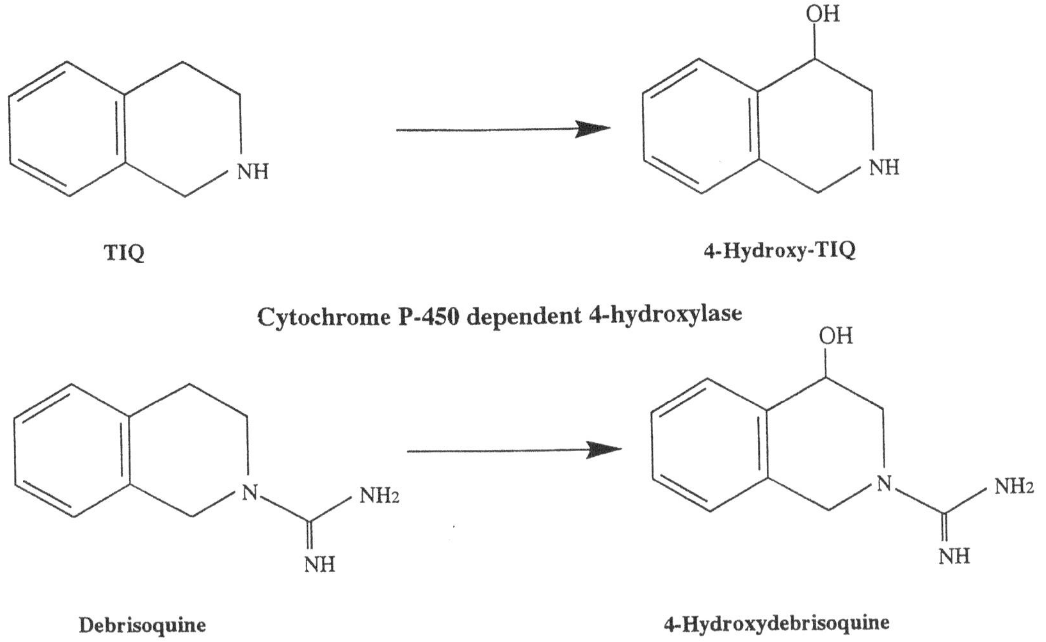

Cytochrome P-450 dependent 4-hydroxylase

Fig. 5 4-Hydroxylation of TIQ and debrisoquine.

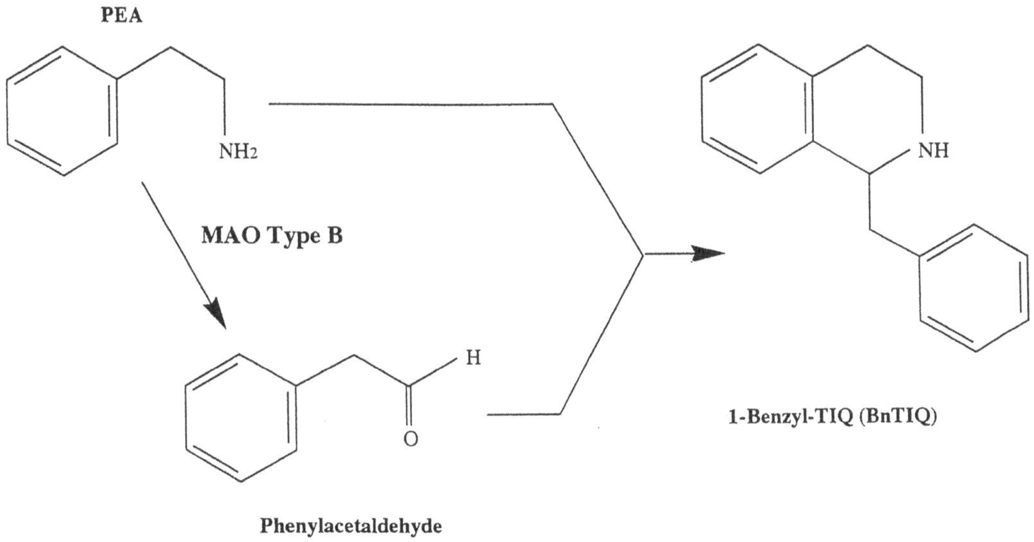

Fig. 6 Proposed biosynthetic pathway of 1-benzyl-TIQ (BnTIQ).

with that of controls suffering from other neurological diseases, the mean value being three times higher (parkinsonians: 1.17 ± 0.35 ng/ml of CSF, n = 18; *vs.* controls: 0.40 ± 0.10 ng/ml of CSF, n = 11; mean $\pm$ SEM, not significantly different).

By use of the pole test, it was shown that repeated intraperitoneal injection of BnTIQ in mice induced bradykinesia, a typical symptom of PD, which pretreatment with 1-methyl-TIQ could prevent.

6. 1-Phenyl-N-methyl-TIQ and 1-phenyl-TIQ

1-Phenyl-N-methyl-1,2,3,4-tetrahydroisoquinoline (PnNMTIQ) and 1-phenyl-1,2,3,4-tetrahydroisoquinoline (PnTIQ) were detected in the parkinsonian human brain by gas chromatography/tandem mass spectrometry (GC/MS/MS) (Kajita et al, 1995). Figure 7 shows the chemical structures of MPTP, PnNMTIQ, and PnTIQ. PnTIQ was detected only in the brains from two patients with PD (approximately 14 and 43 pg/g wet tissue), but not in the brain of a control patient. However, Pn-NMTIQ was detected in both diseased and normal brains (PD, 34 and 12; control, 19 pg/g wet tissue).

7. Salsolinol (SAL)

7.1   Presence of SAL in tissue and nature

Salsolinol (SAL), 1-methyl-6,7-dihydroxy-1,2,3,4-tetrahydroisoquinoline (Fig. 8), was first detected in the urine of parkinsonian patients on L-dopa medication (Sandler et al., 1973). Later on, SAL was found in human brain (Sjöquist et al., 1982, Sasaoka et al, 1988), urine and CSF (Sjöquist et al., 1981). SAL was increased in the urine and in CSF of alcoholics (Collins et al., 1979), and in the urine of patients with phenylketonuria (Lasala et al., 1979).

SAL is present in various foods and beverages such as bananas, soy sauce, wine, and beer (Smythe and Duncan, 1985). The R-enantiomer of SAL (R-SAL) predominates in human urine, and the S-enantiomer (S-SAL), in port wine. The R/S ratio is almost 1 in dried banana, a food rich in SAL (Strolin Benedetti et al., 1989; Dostert et al., 1989, 1990).

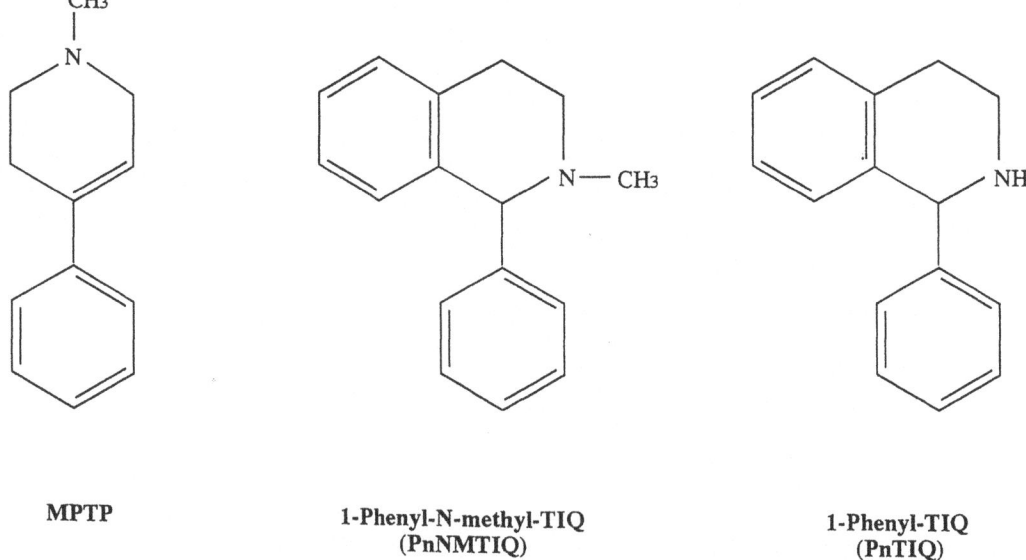

   MPTP   **1-Phenyl-N-methyl-TIQ**   **1-Phenyl-TIQ**
                                  (PnNMTIQ)   **(PnTIQ)**

Fig. 7   Chemical structures of MPTP, 1-phenyl-N-methyl-TIQ (PnNMTIQ) and 1-phenyl-TIQ (PnTIQ).

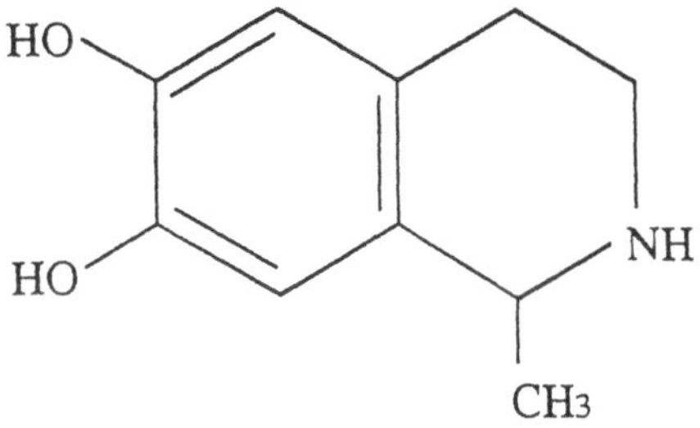

Salsolinol (SAL) 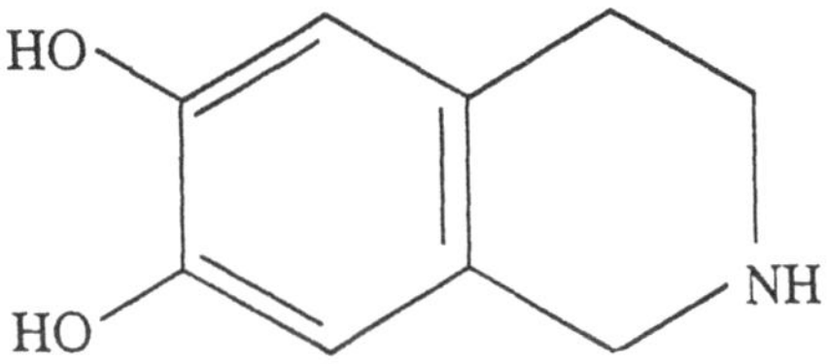　　　　　　　　　　**Norsalsolinol (NSAL)**

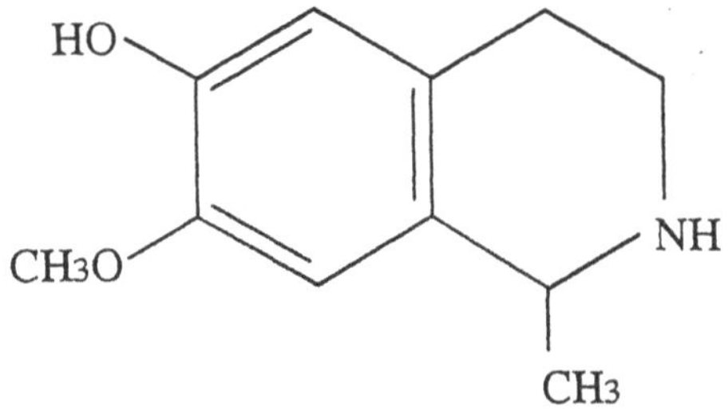

Salsoline 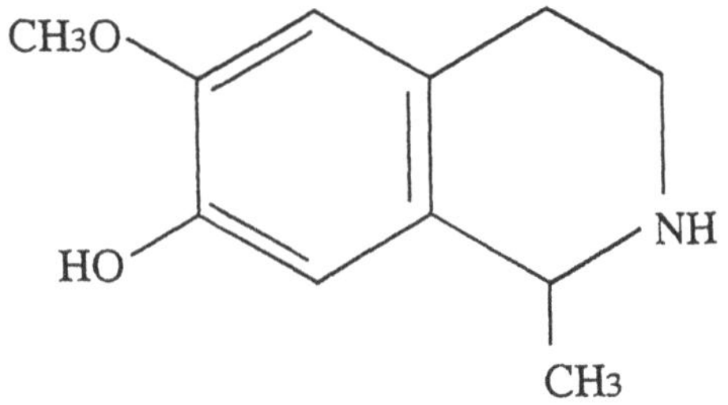　　　　　　　　　　　　**Isosalsoline**

Fig. 8　Chemical structures of salsolinol (SAL), norsalsolinol (NSAL), salsoline and isosalsoline.

7.2　Biosynthetic pathway of SAL

One biosynthetic pathway of SAL is non-enzymatic condensation of dopamine with acetaldehyde to yield the racemic mixture of both enantiomers (pathway A). Another pathway is the condensation of dopamine with pyruvic acid, followed by enzymatic decarboxylation and reduction (pathway B; Fig. 9) (Sjöquist et al., 1985; Ung-Chhun et al., 1985; Dostert et al., 1990). Recently, it was suggested that R-SAL might be formed enzymatically by stereospecific condensation of dopamine with pyruvic acid (Naoi et al., 1995b).

7.3　Neurotoxicity of SAL

SAL is accumulated and stored in rat brain synaptosomes. SAL inhibits the uptake of catecholamines, causes the release of stored catecholamines (Heikkila et al., 1971), inhibits tyrosine hydroxylase (Weiner et al., 1978) and monoamine oxidase activities (Meyerson et al., 1976). S-SAL was found to be a more effective inhibitor of dopamine accumulation in rat brain slices than the R-enantiomer (Cohen et al., 1974). However, an induction of

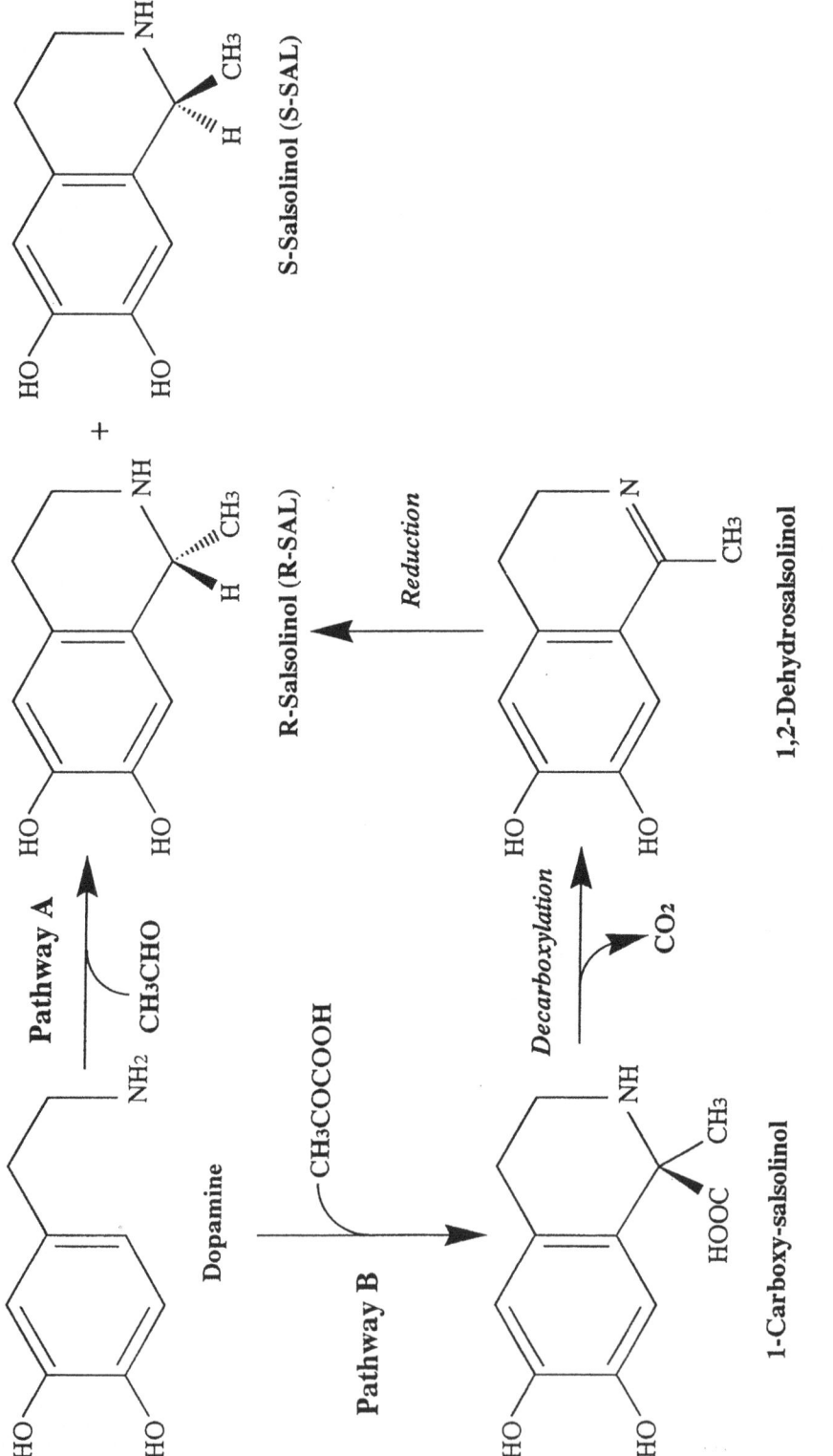

Fig. 9 Proposed biosynthetic pathway of SAL.

parkinsonism by administration of SAL has never been reported in mammals, which may be due to the fact that SAL cannot pass through the blood-brain barrier (Origitano et al., 1981), and that its cytotoxicity is not potent enough to cause the death of dopamine neurons (Naoi et al., 1993).

7.4 Metabolism of SAL

Salsoline (1-methyl-7-methoxy-6-hydroxy-1,2,3,4-tetrahydroisoquinoline) and isosalsoline (1-methyl-6-methoxy-7-hydroxy-1,2,3,4,-tetrahydroisoquinoline) are mono-O-methylated metabolites of SAL (Fig. 8). Catecholamine-derived 6,7-dihydroxy-TIQs, such as SAL, serve as substrates for catechol-O-methyltransferase (COMT, EC 2.1.1.6). SAL is O-methylated primarily *in vivo* at the 7-position, to form salsoline (Collins and Origitano, 1983), whereas catecholamines are O-methylated *in vivo* at the 3-position. The O-methylation of catecholamines causes elimination of their physiological properties, whereas 7-O-methylated TIQs such as salsoline can still be accumulated and stored in catecholamine nerve terminals of the brain where they may act as false or surrogate neurotransmitters (Cohen and Mytilineou, 1982).

The concentrations of salsoline in rat brains and livers following the intraperitoneal administration of SAL were quantitated by GC/MS, and salsoline levels in the brains and livers were found to increase following the administration of SAL (Sjöquist and Magnuson, 1980).

8. Norsalsolinol

Norsalsolinol (NSAL), 6,7-dihydroxy-1,2,3,4-tetrahydroisoquinoline, (Fig. 8) has been detected in normal rat brain by GC/MS (Barker et al., 1981). The level of NSAL was calculated to be about 10 ng/g wet weight of brain tissue. NSAL is formed non-enzymatically *in vivo* by Pictet-Spengler condensation of dopamine and formaldehyde. Formaldehyde is 15 times as reactive as acetaldehyde in the Pictet-Spengler reaction with dopamine. The brain level of NSAL may be of interest in alcoholism, where, particularly during withdrawal, the levels of methanol, formaldehyde, and formate increase significantly.

9. N-Methyl-salsolinol and N-methyl-norsalsolinol

6,7-Dihydroxy-TIQ derivatives such as N-methyl-salsolinol (1,2-dimethyl-6,7-dihydroxy-1,2,3,4-tetrahydroisoquinoline; NMSAL) and N-methyl-norsalsolinol (2-methyl-6,7-dihydroxy-1,2,3,4-tetrahydroisoquinoline; NMNSAL) were found and considered to be endogenously synthesized from dopamine. Figure 10 shows the chemical structures of NMNSAL and NMSAL.

NMSAL and NMNSAL were identified by the selective ion monitoring method (SIM) of GC/MS as novel endogenous amines in parkinsonian and normal human brains (Niwa et al., 1991). NMNSAL was also detected in the CSF of patients with Parkinson's disease (Moser and Kömpf, 1992). Moser et al. (1995) demonstrated that the level of NMNSAL was negatively correlated with the disease duration and that NMNSAL indicates an increased dopamine turnover in patients with PD. The enhanced metabolism at the beginning of the

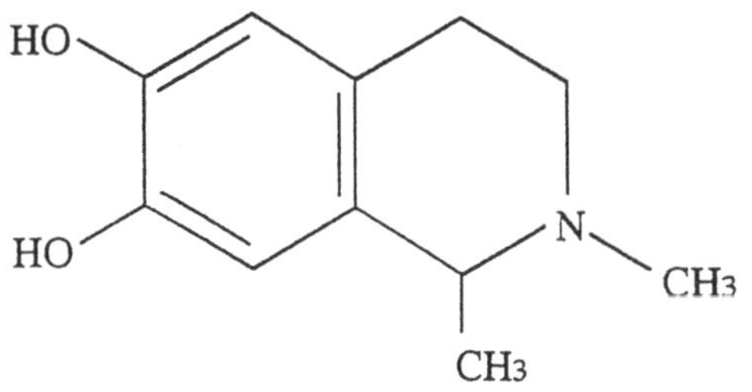

N-Methyl-salsolinol
(NMSAL)

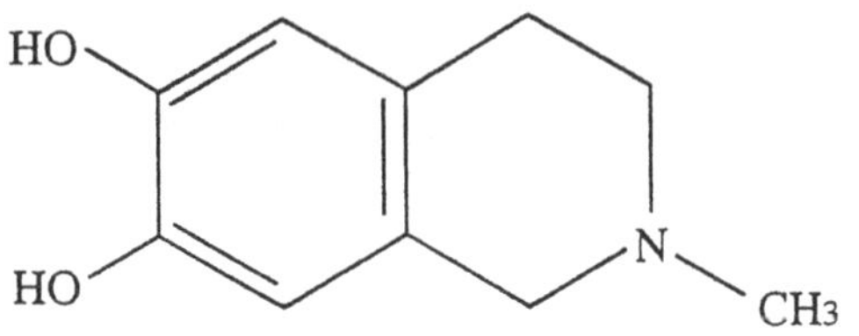

N-Methyl-norsalsolinol
(NMNSAL)

Fig. 10.   Chemical structures of N-methyl-salsolinol (NMSAL) and N-methyl-norsalsolinol (NMNSAL).

disease is not due to the presence of NMNSAL, since it inhibits dopamine metabolism. Thus, NMNSAL, potentially endogenously synthesized from dopamine, appears as a result of a compensatively activated dopaminergic system.

NMSAL is produced in the brain by N-methylation of SAL, which is formed from dopamine, and this production was confirmed by *in vivo* microdialysis in the rat brain (Maruyama et al., 1992; Niwa et al., 1992). The *in vitro* experiment suggested that NMSAL and NMNSAL could also be synthesized from N-methyldopamine (epinine) with formaldehyde and acetaldehyde, respectively, by the Pictet-Spengler reaction. Epinine was detected in human brains by GC/MS (Kajita et al., 1993). NMNSAL was identified in the rat brain dialysate after epinine perfusion in an *in vivo* microdialysis study (Kajita et al., 1994). Deng et al. reported that only the R-enantiomers of SAL and NMSAL were detected in human brain samples and suggested that the enzymatic pathway of R-SAL is the major pathway for NM-R-SAL production in the human brain (Deng et al., 1995) (Fig. 11).

Recently, NM-R-SAL was found to be enzymatically oxidized to 1,2-dimethyl-6,7-dihydroxyisoquinolinium ion (DMDHIQ$^+$) by an enzyme sample prepared from human brain cortex (Naoi et al., 1995a). The enzyme was not inhibited by the monoamine oxidase inhibitors, but it was sensitive to semicarbazide.

DMDHIQ$^+$ was found to be a potent inhibitor of type A monoamine oxidase and a much weaker inhibitor of type B (Naoi et al., 1994). Catechol structure was found to increase the inhibition selectivity of type A. The injection of NM-R-SAL into the rat brain caused behavioral changes similar to those seen in patients with PD, whereas R-SAL, S-SAL, and N-methyl-S-salsolinol (NM-S-SAL) injections did not. DMDHIQ$^+$ was also found to cause a syndrome similar to parkinsonism in rodents (Naoi et al., 1995b).

10. 1,2,3,4-Tetrahydro-2-methyl-4,6,7-isoquinolinetriol (TMIQ)

1,2,3,4-Tetrahydro-2-methyl-4,6,7-isoquinolinetriol (TMIQ) can be formed from epinephrine and formaldehyde by the Pictet-Spengler reaction (Bates, 1981) (Fig. 12). After intraventricular infusion in the rat brain, TMIQ caused a reduction in dopamine concentrations

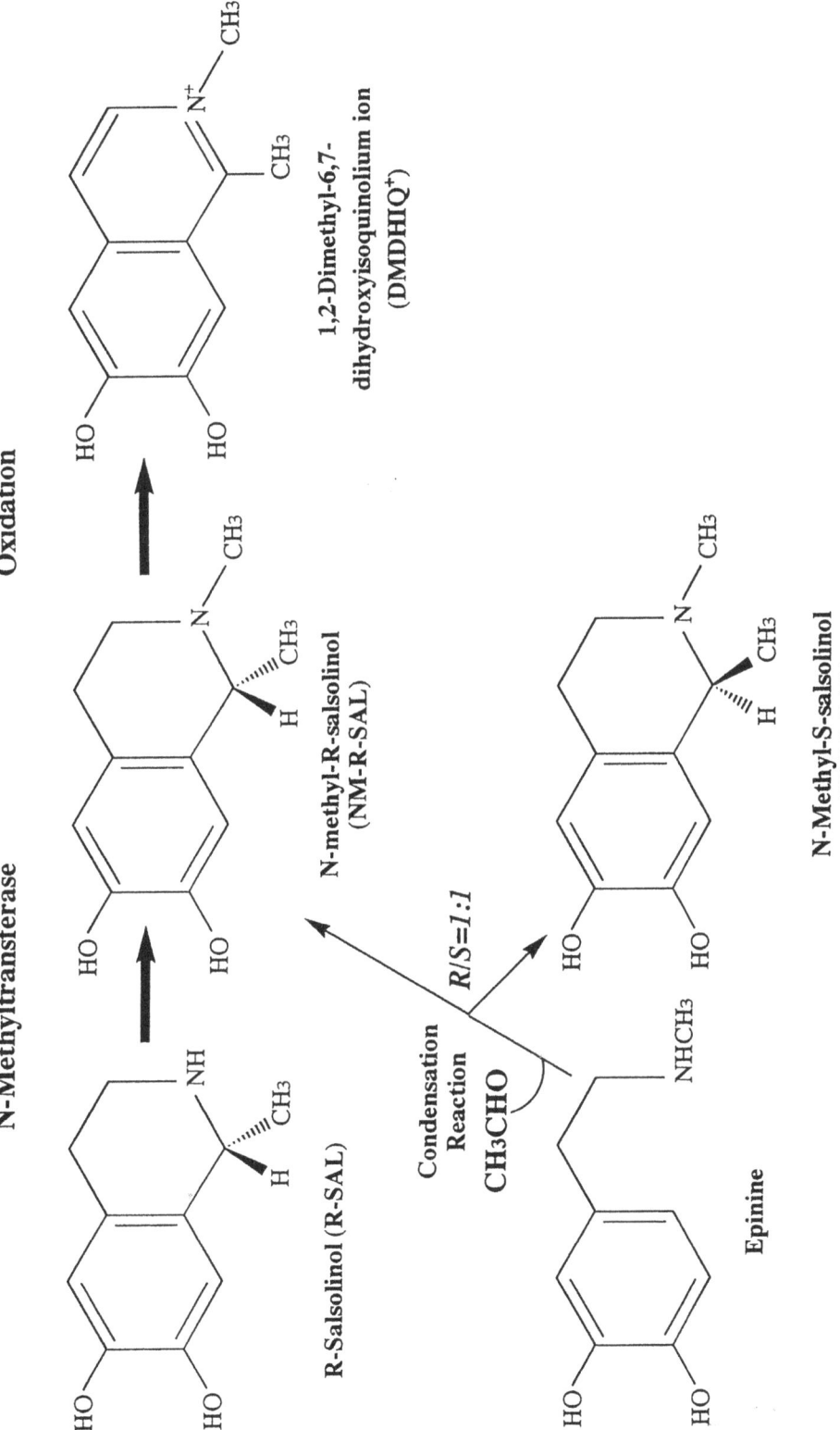

Fig. 11 Biosynthetic pathway of N-methyl-R-salsolinol (NM-R-SAL) in the brain.

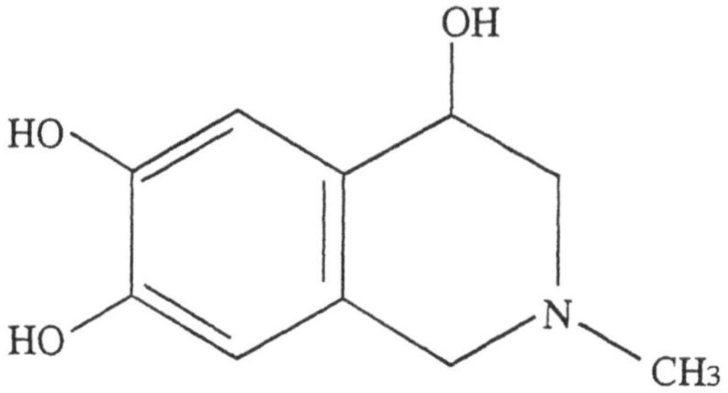

**1,2,3,4-Tetrahydro-2-methyl-
4,6,7-isoquinolinetriol
(TMIQ)**

Fig. 12   Chemical structure of 1,2,3,4-tetrahydro-2-methyl-4,6,7-isoquinolinetriol (TMIQ).

in *substantia nigra, corpus striatum, hypothalamus* and *dorsal raphe,* and a reduction in noradrenaline concentrations in the *locus coeruleus.* TMIQ also reduced the 5-hydroxy-tryptamine concentration in the *dorsal raphe* and *substantia nigra,* although with a lower potency. TMIQ and MPTP were approximately equipotent in depleting dopamine. Direct unilateral intrastriatal injection of TMIQ induced marked ipsilateral reductions in striatal dopamine, correlating with a behavioral response consisting of turning towards the injected side (Liptrot et al., 1993). The presence of endogenous TMIQ in human tissues has not been observed yet.

11. Methods for Identification and Measurement of Catecholic TIQs

For the extraction of catecholic TIQs from biological samples, such cleanup methods for catecholamine detection, as absorption on alumina combined with solid-phase extraction, are usually used. After extraction, the compounds are directly measured by high-performance liquid chromatography (HPLC) with electrochemical detection (ECD) or are derivatized for GC with electron capture detection or GC/MS detection (Harber et al., 1995a).

Baum et al. (1994) reported a sensitive method using HPLC-ECD with a cyclodextrin-OH-phase column for the determination of total dopamine, R-SAL, and S-SAL. It allowed the detection of these compounds in human plasma at concentrations as low as 0.02 ng/ml.

For selective liquid-solid extraction of catecholic TIQs, we used a phenylboronic acid cartridge (Niwa et al., 1992). These compounds were trimethylsilylated with N,O-bis(trimethylsilyl)-trifluoroacetamide (BSTFA), containing 1% trimethylchlorosilane (TMCS), and then analyzed by GC/MS.

Harber et al. (1995a) reported a new rapid method involving extraction and derivatization in one step by the Schotten-Baumann two-phase reaction with pentafluorobenzoylchloride for extraction, as well as for derivatization and analysis of the derivatives by

GC/MS. The detection limit for the analysis of SAL and salsoline in urine was 10 fmol/ml sample volume.

Several catecholic TIQ enantiomers were transformed into diastereomers by a two-step derivatization with N-methyl-N-trimethylsilyltrifluoroacetamide (MSTFA) and R-(-)-2-phenylbutyryl chloride and were analyzed by GC/MS (Harber et al., 1995b). SAL was extracted from biological materials with phenylboronic phase cartridges and transformed into diastereomers. The detection limit of quantification was found to be 100 pg/ml for each enantiomer.

12. The Sites of Toxicological Activity

12.1 Inhibition of mitochondrial respiratory enzymes

It has been reported that MPP^+ inhibits complex I activity (Mizuno et al., 1987) and adenosine triphosphate (ATP) in mouse brain (Mizuno et al., 1988). Mitochondrial respiratory failure, secondary to complex I inhibition, may contribute to the neurodegenerative process underlying nigral cell death in PD. McNaught et al. (1995a) examined the effects of 22 isoquinoline derivatives and MPP^+ on the enzymes of the respiratory chain in mitochondrial fragments from rat forebrain. All compounds, other than NSAL and N-n-propylisoquinolinium, inhibited complex I. Several isoquinoline derivatives were more potent inhibitors of complex I than MPP^+, the most active being N-methyl-6-methoxy-TIQ and 6-methoxy-TIQ. TIQ was the least potent complex I inhibitor. At 10 mM, only isoquinoline, 6,7-dimethoxyisoquinoline, and NMSAL inhibited succinate cytochrome C reductase (complex II-III; EC 1.8.3.1), but none of the isoquinoline derivatives inhibited cytochrome C oxidase (complex IV; EC 1.9.3.1). There were no clear structure-activity relationships among isoquinoline derivatives, but lipophilicity appears to be important for complex I inhibition.

A decrease in the activity of the α-ketoglutarate dehydrogenase (α-KGDH) complex of the TCA cycle occurs in the *substantia nigra* in PD (Mizuno et al., 1994). McNaught et al. (1995b) demonstrated, that six isoquinoline derivatives (isoquinoline, N-methylisoquinolinium, N-n-propylisoquinolinium, TIQ, NMTIQ, and SAL) and MPP^+, inhibited KGDH activity in mitochondrial fragments from rat forebrain. These findings may represent an additional mechanism contributing to mitochondrial dysfunction and cell death in PD.

12.2 Hydroxyl radical formation

It was suggested that oxidative stress such as dopamine auto-oxidation and hydroxyl radical generation may be involved in dopamine cell death in normal aging and PD (Chiueh et al., 1993).

NM-R-SAL was found to be oxidized into $DMDHIQ^+$ with concomitant formation of hydroxyl radicals. The oxidation and the radical production were completely inhibited by antioxidants, such as ascorbic acid and reduced glutathione, and the radical formation was enhanced by Fe (II) and, to a lesser extent, by Fe(III) *in vitro* (Maruyama et al., 1995a).

Using an *in vivo* microdialysis method, Maruyama et al. (1995b) measured hydroxyl radical levels in the rat striatum by HPLC after derivatization to 2,3-dihydroxybenzoic acid with salicylic acid. R-SAL, $DMDHIQ^+$ (40 and 200 μM), and NM-R-SAL (200 μM) reduced *in vivo* radical formation, along with the reduction of dopamine catabolism. R-SAL and DMDHIQ$^+$ reduced *in vitro* hydroxyl radical production from dopamine auto-oxidation. On the other hand, 40 µM NM-R-SAL increased the hydroxyl radical level in the *corpus striatum,* and the radical production by its auto-oxidation was confirmed *in vitro.* NM-R-SAL affected neither *in vivo* dopamine catabolism nor *in vitro* production of hydroxyl radicals from dopamine. These results show that R-SAL and NM-R-SAL may be neuroprotective and neurotoxic, respectively.

Various isoquinoline derivatives have been discovered as potent dopaminergic neuro-toxins, similar to MPTP and MPP$^+$ in human brains. However, a single toxin is not likely to cause parkinsonism in humans. The interaction between these compounds and/or the tendency of individuals with poor metabolism of TIQ to accumulate TIQs in their brains should be further studied to determine the role of these compounds in the pathogenesis of PD.

References

Barbeau A., Cloutier T., Roy M., Plasse L., Paris S., and Poirier J. (1985) Ecogenetics of Parkinson's disease: 4-hydroxylation of debrisoquine. Lancet 2, 1213–1216.

Barker S.A., Monti J.A., Tolbert L.C., Brown G.B., and Christian S.T. (1981) Gas chromatographic/mass spectrometric evidence for the identification of 6,7-dihydroxy-1,2,3,4-tetrahydroisoquinoline as a normal constituent of rat brain. Biochem. Pharmacol. 30:2461–2468.

Bates H.A. (1981) Pictet-Spengler reactions of epinephrine with formaldehyde and acetaldehyde. J. Org. Chem. 46:4931–4935.

Baum S.S. and Rommelspacher H. (1994) Determination of total dopamine, R- and S-salsolinol in human plasma by cyclodextrin bonded-phase liquid chromatography with electrochemical detection. J. Chromatogr. 660:235–241.

Booth R.G., Castagnoli N., Jr., and Rollema H. (1989) Intracerebral microdialysis neurotoxicity studies of quinoline and isoquinoline derivatives related to MPTP/MPP$^+$. Neurosci. Lett. 100:306–312.

Burns R.S., Chiueh C.C., Markey S.P., Ebert M.H., Jacobowitz D.M., and Kopin I.J. (1983) A primate model of parkinsonism: selective destruction of dopaminergic neurons in the pars compacta of the substantia nigra by N-methyl-4-phenyl-1,2,3,6-tetrahydropyridine. Proc. Natl. Acad. Sci. USA 80:4546–4550.

Chiueh C.C., Miyake H., and Peng M-T. (1993) Role of dopamine autoxidation, hydroxyl radical generation, and calcium overload in underlying mechanisms involved in MPTP-induced parkinsonism. Adv. Neurol. 60:251–258.

Cohen G., and Collins M.A. (1970) Alkaloids from catecholamines in adrenal tissue: Possible role in alcoholism. Science 167:1749–1751.

Cohen G., Heikkila R.E., Dembiec D., Sang D., Teitel S., and Brossi A. (1974) Pharmacologic activity of stereoisomers of 1-substituted 6,7-dihydroxy-1,2,3,4-tetrahydroisoquinolines: inhibition of ^{3}H-dopamine accumulation by rat brain slices and lipolytic activity with isolated mouse fat cells. Eur. J. Pharmacol. 29:292–297.

Cohen G., and Myiilineou C. (1982) Pharmacological properties of catecholamine-derived TIQs and 7-O-methylated metabolites in neuronal systems. In: Beta-Carbolines and Tetrahydroisoquinolines, pp. 265–274. Alan R. Liss, New York.

Collins M.A., Nijim W.P., Borge G.F., Teas G., and Goldfarb C. (1979) Dopamine-related tetrahydroisoquinolines: significant urinary excretion by alcoholics after alcohol consumption. Science 206:1184–1186.

Collins M.A. (1980) Neuroamine condensations in human subjects. Adv. Exp. Med. Biol. 126:87–102.

Collins M.A., and Origitano T.C. (1983) Catecholamine-derived tetrahydroisoquinolines: O-methylation patterns and regional brain distribution following intraventricular administration in rats. J. Neurochem. 41:1569–1575.

Deng Y., Maruyama W., Dostert P., Takahashi T., Kawai M., and Naoi M. (1995) Determination of the (R)- and (S)-enantiomers of salsolinol and N-methylsalsolinol by use of a chiral high-performance liquid chromatographic column. J. Chromatogr. 670: 47–54.

Dostert P., Strolin Benedetti M., Dordain G., and Vernay D. (1989) Enantiomeric composition of urinary salsolinol in Parkinsonian patients after Madopar. J. Neural Transm. [P-D Sect] 1:269–278.

Dostert P., Strolin Benedetti M., Bellotti V., Allievi C., and Dordain G. (1990) Biosynthesis of salsolinol, a tetrahydroisoquinoline alkaloid, in healthy subjects. J. Neural Transm. 81:215–223.

Haber H., Haber H.M., and Melzig M.F. (1995a) A new rapid method for the analysis of catecholic tetrahydroisoquinolines from biological samples by gas chromatography/mass spectrometry. Anal. Biochem. 224:256–262.

Haber H., Henklein P., Georgi M., and Melzig M.F. (1995b) Resolution of catecholic tetrahydroisoquinoline enantiomers and the determination of R- and S-salsolinol in biological samples by gas chromatography-mass spectrometry. J. Chromatogr. 672: 179–187.

Heikkila R., Cohen G., and Dembiec D. (1971) Tetrahydroisoquinoline alkaloids: uptake by rat brain homogenates and inhibition of catecholamine uptake. J. Pharmacol. Exp. Ther. 179:250–258.

Heikkila R.E., Hess A., and Duvoisin R.C. (1984) Dopaminergic neurotoxicity of 1-methyl-4-phenyl-1,2,5,6-tetrahydropyridine in mice. Science 224:1451–1453.

Hirata Y., and Nagatsu T. (1985) Inhibition of tyrosine hydroxylation in rat striatal tissue slices by 1-methyl-4-phenyl-pyridinium ion. Neurosci. Lett. 57:301–305.

Kajita M., Niwa T., Takeda N., Yoshizumi H., Tatematsu A., Watanabe K., and Nagatsu T. (1993) Presence of N-methyldopamine in parkinsonian and normal human brains. J. Chromatogr. 613:1–8.

Kajita M., Niwa T., Maruyama W., Nakahara D., Takeda N., Yoshizumi H., Tatematsu A., Watanabe K., Naoi M., and Nagatsu T. (1994) Endogenous synthesis of N-methylnorsalsolinol in rat brain during *in vivo* microdialysis with epinine. J. Chromatogr. 654: 263–269.

Kajita M., Niwa T., Fujisaki M., Ueki M., Niimura K., Sato M., Egami K., Naoi M., Yoshida M., and Nagatsu T. (1995) Detection of 1-phenyl-N-methyl-1,2,3,4-tetrahydroisoquinoline and 1-phenyl-1,2,3,4-tetrahydroisoquinoline in human brain by gas chromatography-tandem mass spectrometry. J. Chromatogr. 669:345–351.

Kohno M., Ohta S., and Hirobe M. (1986) Tetrahydroisoquinoline and 1-methyl-tetrahydroisoquinoline as novel endogenous amines in rat brain. Biochem. Biophys. Res. Commun. 140:448–454.

Kotake Y., Tasaki Y., Makino Y., Ohta S., and Hirobe M. (1995) 1-Benzyl-1,2,3,4-tetrahydroisoquinoline as a parkinsonism-inducing agent: a novel endogenous amine in mouse brain and parkinsonian CSF. J. Neurochem., 65:2633–2638.

Langston J.W., Ballard P., Tetrud J.W., and Irwin I. (1983) Chronic parkinsonism in humans due to a product of meperidine-analogue synthesis. Science 219:979–980.

Lasala J.M. and Coscia C.J. (1979) Accumulation of a tetrahydroisoquinoline in phenylke-tonuria. Science 203:283–284.

Liptrot J., Holdup D., and Phillipson O. (1993) 1,2,3,4-Tetrahydro-2-methyl-4,6,7-iso-quinolinetriol depletes catecholamines in rat brain. J. Neurochem. 61:2199–2206.

Makino Y., Ohta S., Tachikawa O., and Hirobe M. (1988) Presence of tetrahydroisoquino-line and 1-methyl-tetrahydroisoquinoline in foods: compounds related to Parkinson's disease. Life Sci. 43:373–378.

Makino Y., Tasaki Y., Ohta S., and Hirobe M. (1990) Confirmation of the enantiomers of 1-methyl-1,2,3,4-tetrahydroisoquinoline in the mouse brain and foods applying gas chro-matography/mass spectrometry with negative chemical ionization. Biomed. Environ. Mass Spectrom. 19:415–419.

Markey S.P., Johannessen J.N., Chiueh C.C., Burns R.S., and Herkenham M.A. (1984) Intraneuronal generation of a pyridinium metabolite may cause drug-induced parkin-sonism. Nature 311:464–467.

Maruyama W., Nakahara D., Ota M., Takahashi T., Takahashi A., Nagatsu T., and Naoi M. (1992) N-Methylation of dopamine-derived 6,7-dihydroxy-1,2,3,4-tetrahydroiso-quinoline, (R)-salsolinol, in rat brains: *in vivo* microdialysis study. J. Neurochem, 59:395–400.

Maruyama W., Dostert P., Matsubara K., and Naoi M. (1995a) N-Methyl(R)salsinol pro-duces hydroxyl radicals: involvement in neurotoxicity. Free Radic. Biol. Med. 19:67–75.

Maruyama W., Dostert P., and Naoi M. (1995b) Dopamine-derived 1-methyl-6,7-dihydroxy-isoquinolines as hydroxyl radical promoters and scavengers in the rat brain: *in vivo* and *in vitro* studies. J. Neurochem. 64:2635–2643.

McNaught K.S., Thull U., Carrupt PA., Altomare C., Cellamare S., Carotti A., Testa B., Jen-ner P., and Marsden C.D. (1995a) Inhibition of complex I by isoquinoline derivatives structurally related to 1-methyl-4-phenyl-1,2,3,6-tetrahydropyridine (MPTP). Bio-chem Pharmacol. 50:1903–1911.

McNaught K.S., Altomare C., Cellamare S., Carotti A., Thull U., Carrupt PA., Testa B., Jen-ner P., and Marsden C.D. (1995b) Inhibition of α-ketoglutarate dehydrogenase by iso-quinoline derivatives structurally related to 1-methyl-4-phenyl-1,2,3,6-tetrahydropyri-dine (MPTP). Neuroreport. 6:1105–1108.

Meyerson L.R., McMurtrey K.D., and Davis V.E. (1976) Neuroamine-derived alkaloids: substrate-preferred inhibitors of rat brain monoamine oxidase *in vitro*. Biochem. Phar-macol. 25:1013–1020.

Mizuno Y., Saitoh T., and Sone N. (1987) Inhibition of mitochondrial NADH-ubiquinone oxidoreductase activity by 1-methyl-4-phenylpyridinium ion. Biochem. Biophys. Res. Commun. 143:294–299.

Mizuno Y., Suzuki K., Sone N., and Saitoh T. (1988) Inhibition of ATP synthesis by 1-methyl-4-phenylpyridinium ion (MPP$^+$) in isolated mitochondria from mouse brains. Neurosci. Lett. 91:349–353.

Mizuno Y., Matsuda S, Yoshino H., Mori H., Hattori N., and Ikebe S. (1994) An immuno-histochemical study on α-ketoglutarate dehydrogenase complex in Parkinson's dis-ease. Ann. Neurol. 35:204–210.

Moser A., and Kömpf D. (1992) Presence of methyl-6,7-dihydroxy-1,2,3,4-tetrahydroiso-quinolines, derivatives of the neurotoxin isoquinoline, in parkinsonian lumbar CSF. Life Sci. 50:1885–1891.

Moser A., Scholz J., Nobbe F., Vieregge P., Böhme V., and Bamberg H. (1995) Presence of N-methyl-norsalsolinol in the CSF: correlations with dopamine metabolites of patients with Parkinson's disease. J. Neurol. Sci. 131:183–189.

Nagatsu T., and Yoshida M. (1988) An endogenous substance of the brain, tetrahydroisoquinoline, produces parkinsonism in primates with decreased dopamine, tyrosine hydroxylase and biopterine in the nigrostriatal regions. Neurosci. Lett. 87:178–182.

Naoi M., Hirata Y., and Nagatsu T. (1987) Inhibition of monoamine oxidase by N-methylisoquinolinium ion. J. Neurochem. 48:709–712.

Naoi M., Matsuura S., Parvez H., Takahashi T., Hirata Y., Minami M., and Nagatsu T. (1989a) Oxidation of N-methyl-1,2,3,4-tetrahydroisoquinoline into the N-methyl-isoquinolinium ion by monoamine oxidase. J. Neurochem. 52:653–655.

Naoi M., Takahashi T., Parvez H., Kabeya R., Taguchi E., Yamaguchi K., Hirata Y., Minami M., and Nagatsu T. (1989b) N-Methylisoquinolinium ion as an inhibitor of tyrosine hydroxylase, aromatic L-amino acid decarboxylase and monoamine oxidase. Neurochem. Int. 15:315–320.

Naoi M., Matsuura S., Takahashi T., and Nagatsu T. (1989c) A N-methyltransferase in human brain catalyses N-methylation of 1,2,3,4-tetrahydroisoquinoline into N-methyl-1,2,3,4-tetrahydroisoquinoline, a precursor of a dopaminergic neurotoxin, N-methylisoquinolinium ion. Biochem. Biophys. Res. Commun. 161:1213–1219.

Naoi M., and Maruyama W. (1993) Type B monoamine oxidase and neurotoxins. Eur. Neurol. 33 Suppl 1:31–37.

Naoi M., Maruyama W., Sasuga S., Deng Y., Dostert P., Ohta S., and Takahashi T. (1994) Inhibition of type A monoamine oxidase by 2(N)-methyl-6,7-dihydroxyisoquinolinium ions. Neurochem. Int. 25:475–481.

Naoi M., Maruyama W., Zhang J.H., Takahashi T., Deng Y., and Dostert P. (1995a) Enzymatic oxidation of the dopaminergic neurotoxin, 1(R),2(N)-dimethyl-6,7-dihydroxy-1,2,3,4-tetrahydroisoquinoline, into 1,2(N)-dimethyl-6,7-dihydroxyisoquinolinium ion. Life Sci. 57:1061–1066.

Naoi M., Maruyama W., and Dostert P. (1995b) Dopamine-derived 6,7-dihydroxy-1,2,3,4-tetrahydroisoquinolines; oxidations and neurotoxicity. Prog. Brain Res. 106:227–239.

Niwa T., Takeda N., Kaneda N., Hashizume Y., and Nagatsu T. (1987) Presence of tetrahydroisoquinoline and 2-methyltetrahydroquinoline in parkinsonian and normal human brains. Biochem. Biophys. Res. Commun. 144:1084–1089.

Niwa T., Takeda N., Tatematsu A., Matsuura S., Yoshida M., and Nagatsu T. (1988) Migration of tetrahydroisoquinoline, a possible parkinsonian neurotoxin, into monkey brain from blood as proved by gas chromatography-mass spectrometry. J. Chromatogr. 452:85–91.

Niwa T., Takeda N., Sasaoka T., Kaneda N., Hashizume Y., Yoshizumi H., Tatematsu A., and Nagatsu T. (1989a) Detection of tetrahydroisoquinoline in parkinsonian brain as an endogenous amine by use of gas chromatography-mass spectrometry. J. Chromatogr. 491:397–403.

Niwa T., Yoshizumi H., Tatematsu A., Matsuura S., and Nagatsu T. (1989b) Presence of tetrahydroisoquinoline, a parkinsonism-related compound, in foods. J. Chromatogr. 493:347–352.

Niwa T., Yoshizumi H., Tatematsu A., Matsuura S., Yoshida M., Kawachi M., Naoi M., and Nagatsu T. (1990) Endogenous synthesis of N-methyl-1,2,3,4-tetrahydroisoquinoline, a precursor of N-methylisoquinolinium ion, in the brains of primates with parkinsonism after systemic administration of 1,2,3,4-tetrahydroisoquinoline. J. Chromatogr. 533:145–151.

Niwa T., Takeda N., Yoshizumi H., Tatematsu A., Yoshida M., Dostert P., Naoi M., and Nagatsu T. (1991) Presence of 2-methyl-6,7-dihydroxy-1,2,3,4-tetrahydroisoquinoline and 1,2-dimethyl-6,7-dihydroxy-1,2,3,4-tetrahydroisoquinoline, novel endogenous amines, in parkinsonian and normal human brains. Biochem. Biophys. Res. Commun. 177:603–609.

Niwa T., Maruyama W., Nakahara D., Takeda N., Yoshizumi H., Tatematsu A., Takahashi A., Dostert P., Naoi M., and Nagatsu T. (1992) Endogenous synthesis of N-methylsalsolinol, an analogue of 1-methyl-4-phenyl-1,2,3,6-tetrahydropyridine, in rat brain during *in vivo* microdialysis with salsolinol, as demonstrated by gas chromatography-mass spectrometry. J. Chromatogr. 578:109–115.

Niwa T., Naoi M., Yoshida M., and Nagatsu T. (1993) Analysis of tetrahydroisoquinolines in the brain by gas chromatography/mass spectrometry. In: Methods in Neurotransmitter and Neuropeptide Research (Pravez S.H., Naoi M., Nagatsu T. and Pravez S. eds.), pp. 255–278. Elsevier Science B.V., Netherlands.

Niwa T. (1995) Mass spectrometry in Parkinson's disease. Clin. Chim. Acta 241/242: 223–250.

Ohta S., Kohno M., Makino Y., Tachikawa O., and Hirobe M. (1987) Tetrahydroisoquinoline and 1-methyl-tetrahydroisoquinoline are present in the human brain: relation to Parkinson's disease. Biomed. Res. 8:453–456.

Ohta S., Tachikawa O., Makino Y., Tasaki Y., and Hirobe M. (1990) Metabolism and brain accumulation of tetrahydroisoquinoline (TIQ), a possible parkinsonism inducing substance, in an animal model of a poor debrisoquine metabolizer. Life Sci. 46:599–605.

Origitano T., Hannigan J., and Collins M.A. (1981) Rat brain salsolinol and blood-brain barrier. Brain Res. 224:446–451.

Sandler M., Carter S.B., Hunter K.R., and Stern G.M. (1973) Tetrahydroisoquinoline alkaloids: *in vivo* metabolites of L-dopa in man. Nature 241:439–443.

Sasaoka T., Kaneda N., Niwa T., Hashizume Y., and Nagatsu T. (1988) Analysis of salsolinol in human brain using high-performance liquid chromatography with electrochemical detection. J. Chromatogr. 428:152–155.

Sjöquist B., and Magnuson E. (1980) Analysis of salsolinol and salsoline in biological samples using deuterium-labelled internal standards and gas chromatography-mass spectrometry. J. Chromatogr. 183:17–24.

Sjöquist B., Borg S. and Kvande H. (1981) Salsolinol and methylated salsolinol in urine and cerebrospinal fluid in human volunteers. Subst. Alc. Act. Musse. 2:73.

Sjöquist B., Eriksson A., and Winblad B. (1982a) Brain salsolinol levels in alcoholism. Lancet 1, 675–676.

Sjöquist B., and Ljungquist C. (1985) Identification and quantification of 1-carboxysalsolinol and salsolinol in biological samples by gas chromatography-mass spectrometry. J. Chromatogr. 343:1–8.

Smythe G.A., and Duncan M.W. (1985) Precise GC/MS assays for salsolinol and tetrahydropapaveroline: the question of artifacts and dietary sources and the influence of alcohol. In: Aldehyde Adducts in Alcoholism, pp. 77–84. Alan R. Liss, New York.

Strolin Benedetti M., Dostert P., and Canninati P. (1989) Influence of food intake on the enantiomeric composition of urinary salsolinol in man. J. Neural Transm. 78: 43–51.

Suzuki K., Mizuno Y., and Yoshida M. (1989) Selective inhibition of complex I of the brain electron transport system by tetrahydroisoquinoline. Biochem. Biophys. Res. Commun. 162:1541–1545.

Tasaki Y., Makino Y., Ohta S., and Horibe M. (1991) 1-Methyl-1,2,3,4-tetrahydroisoquino-line, decreasing in 1-methyl-4-phenyl-1,2,3,6-tetrahydropyridine-treated mouse, prevents parkinsonism-like abnormalities. J. Neurochem. 57:1940–1943.

Ung-Chhun N., Cheng B.Y., Pronger D.A., Serrano P., Chavez B., Fernandez Perrez M., Morales J., and Collins M.A. (1985) Alkaloid adducts in human brain: coexistence of 1-carboxylated and noncarboxylated isoquinolines and β-carbolines in alcoholics and nonalcoholics. Prog. Clin. Biol. Res. 183:125–136.

Weiner C.D., and Collins M.A. (1978) Tetrahydroisoquinolines derived from catecholamines or DOPA: effects on brain tyrosine hydroxylase activity. Biochem. Pharmacol. 27:2699–2703.

Yoshida M., Niwa T., and Nagatsu T. (1990) Parkinsonism in monkeys produced by chronic administration of an endogenous substance of the brain, tetrahydroisoquinoline: the behavioral and biochemical changes. Neurosci. Lett. 119:109–113.

Yoshida M., Ogawa M., and Nagatsu T. (1991) Can tetrahydroisoquinoline (TIQ) or N-methyl-TIQ produce parkinsonism? In: Parkinson's Disease. From Clinical Aspects to Molecular Basis (Nagatsu T. et al., eds.) pp85–94. Springer-Verlag, Vienna-New York.

Chapter *2*

TIQ Derivatives in the Human Central Nervous System

Andreas Moser

Contents in Brief

As described in Chapter 1, in addition to the main metabolic pathway of dopamine in mammals, in which the oxidative deamination by monoamine oxidase (MAO, EC 1.4.3.4) and methylation of one of the hydroxyl groups of the catechol ring by catechol-O-methyltransferase (COMT) play primary roles (Kaakula and Wurtman, 1993; Naoi et al, 1994), the reactions of dopamine with aldehydes or 2-oxoacids leading to 1,2,3,4-tetrahydroisoquinoline (TIQ) derivatives are also possible (Dostert et al., 1990; Minami et al., 1993). From many studies it is well known that 1-methyl-4-phenyl-1,2,3,6-tetrahydropyridine (MPTP), after oxidation to its pyridinium ion MPP^+ by MAO, is toxic for the dopaminergic system and produces a Parkinson-like syndrome in humans and other primates (Burns et al., 1983; Langston et al., 1984). Since TIQ derivatives, especially N-methyl-norsalsolinol (2-methyl-6,7-dihydroxy-1,2,3,4-tetrahydroisoquinoline, 2-MDTIQ) and salsolinol (1-methyl-6,7-dihydroxy-1,2,3,4-tetrahydroisoquinoline) are MPTP-like compounds, the question is raised whether they are present in the human central nervous system and potentially associated with Parkinson's disease. Figure 1 shows the chemical structures of dopamine, N-methyl-norsalsolinol, salsolinol, and 1-methyl-4-phenyl-1,2,3,6-tetrahydropyridine (MPTP).

1. How the Presence of TIQ Derivatives in Humans Was Discovered

The presence of dopamine-derived TIQ derivatives in humans was reported for the first time in 1973 by Sandler et al. who found salsolinol (1-methyl-6,7-dihydroxy-1,2,3,4-tetrahy-

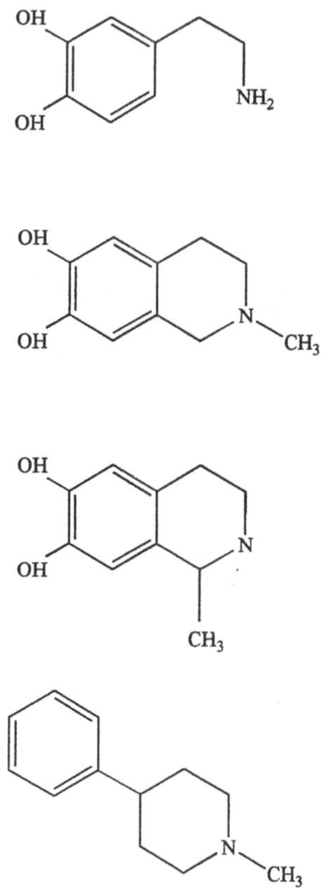

Fig. 1 Chemical structures of dopamine, N-methyl-norsalsolinol (2-MDTIQ), salsolinol (1-MDTIQ), and 1-methyl-4-phenyl-1,2,3,6-tetrahydropyridine (MPTP).

droisoquinoline) and tetrahydropapaveroline (1-[(3,4-dihydroxyphenyl)methyl]-1,2,3,4-tetrahydro-6,7-isoquinolinediol) in urine of parkinsonian patients on L-dopa medication by gas chromatography with mass spectrometry. These compounds were also detected in the brain and urine of mammals with administered alcohol, L-dopa, or pyrogallol. In 1977, Coscia et al. reported a new class of TIQs, norlaudanosolinecarboxylic acids, in the urine of parkinsonian patients on L-dopa with or without carbidopa (L-dopa decarboxylase inhibitor), that were detected by gas-liquid chromatography combined with mass spectrometry.

2. Analytical Methods

There are two major methods to detect 6,7-dihydroxylated TIQ derivatives in organ homogenates (e.g. brain homogenates), cerebrospinal fluid (CSF), plasma, and urine. Gas chromatography combined with mass spectrometry is the most sensitive method, while the handling of reversed phase high performance liquid chromatography with electrochemical detection is easier and can be used to measure hydroxylated tetrahydroisoquinolines, such as salsolinol or N-methyl-norsalsolinol. Since hydroxylated TIQ derivatives are probably in part conjugated (C-6 or/and C-7 position), hydrolysis with arylsulfatase and β-glucuronidase should be performed prior to analysis. In the case of plasma or urine analysis, an affinity chromatography (e.g., with boronate or alumina columns) is useful to reduce high amounts of metabolites which are not needed.

Determination of free salsolinol concentrations was described by Allievi et al. (1991) and Dostert et al. (1993): Salsolinol levels were measured using gas chromatography/mass spectrometry with electron-capture negative-ion chemical ionization after derivatization with pentafluoropropionyl anhydride. Deuterated salsolinol was used as a standard, and the limit of quantification was approximately 0.6 pmol/ml.

The following section gives a detailed description for analytical procedures to measure N-methyl-norsalsolinol in the CSF or salsolinol in the urine of humans by means of reversed phase high performance liquid chromatography with electrochemical detection.

2.1   Cerebrospinal fluid (CSF)

2.1.1 Lumbar puncture: CSF (cerebrospinal fluid) is collected via lumbar puncture. In earlier studies, in patients who were treated for Parkinson's disease, the interval between the last medication intake and puncture was approximately 2 h. In all cases, fluid used for measurement was taken from the first 10 ml of CSF drawn and was immediately frozen and stored at –40°C until analysis.

2.1.2 High performance liquid chromatography: According to previous studies of Moser and Kömpf (1992) and Moser et al. (1995a), the analytical assay of N-methyl-norsalsolinol (2-MDTIQ) was performed by means of reversed phase high performance liquid chromatography with electrochemical detection (HPLC-ECD, e.g. Waters 460) using a C18 column (Eurospher RP 18, particle size 5 µm, column size 250 × 4.0 mm). A pre-column (35 × 4.0) was used. The mobile phase was a degassed solution of 0.1 M citrate buffer, pH 2.4, with 16% methanol (v/v), 0.3 mM Na_2EDTA and 0.52 mM sodium 1-octansulfonate, and pumped at a flow rate of 1 ml/min. All chromatography was performed at 30°C, and the separations were achieved under isocratic conditions. The detector cell operated at +0.88 V. Standard solutions of 2-MDTIQ were injected at different concentrations, and the peak height increased linearly. The detection limit of 2-MDTIQ was approximately 10 pmol/ml.

The 2-MDTIQ peaks in each of the samples assessed by comparing the retention times of the biological compounds detected in the CSF to the retention times of the reference compound present in the standard. In order to confirm the *identity* of the two peaks, control CSF from non-parkinsonian patients is mixed with various concentrations of 2-MDTIQ standard. The chromatograms of these mixtures have to show sharp and isolated peaks with retention times identical to those of the original samples. Moreover, in those cases in which 2-MDTIQ is detected in lumbar CSF, the peaks have to be shifted, according to the two original relative concentrations after addition of the standard solution. In order to determine the *purity* of the putative peaks in the biological samples, voltammograms should be generated for known peaks in the standard and be compared with voltammograms from peaks thought to represent the same compounds in the biological samples. Figure 2 gives a typical voltammogram of standard solutions of dopamine and 2-MDTIQ, and Fig. 3 shows a typical chromatogram of CSF in which 2-MDTIQ could be detected.

2.2   Urine

No difference is made in the nutritional regime for both patients and control subjects. Forty-eight h prior to and during urine collection, the intake of cheese, chocolate, fresh and dried

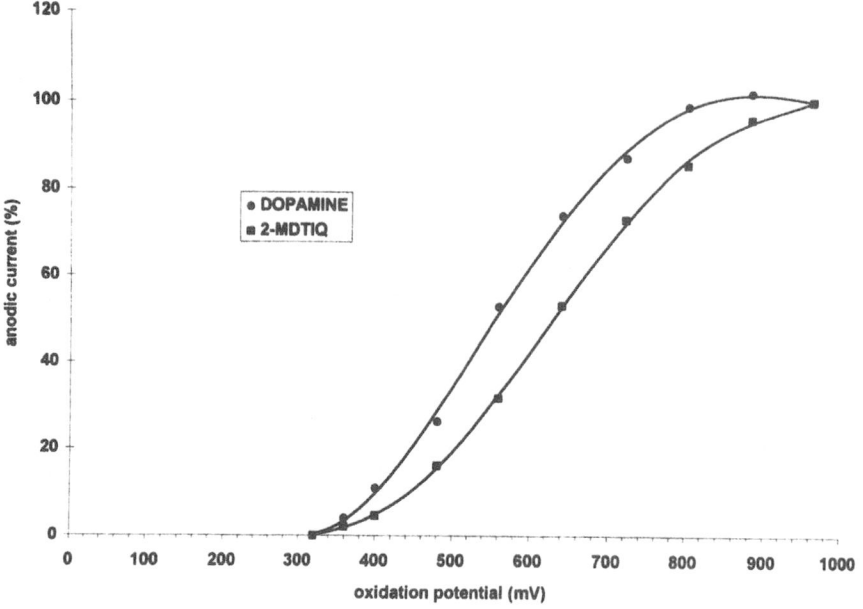

Fig. 2 Voltammogram of standard solutions of dopamine (1 μM) and 2-MDTIQ (1 μM). The anodic current is given at different voltages (mV) of the electrochemical detector.

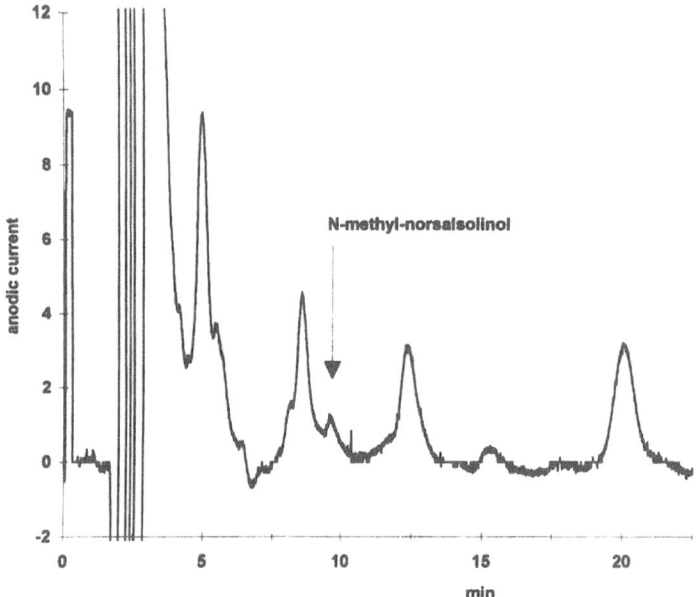

Fig. 3 Typical chromatogram of cerebrospinal fluid (CSF) of a parkinsonian patient in which N-methyl-norsalsolinol (2-MDTIQ) could be detected.

banana, soy sauce, all alcohol (especially beer), port and white wine should be forbidden (Strolin Benedetti et al. 1989).

2.2.1 Urine measurements of salsolinol: The 12 h urine samples are collected in the presence of 50 mg semicarbazide and Na_2EDTA. The following protocol gives the procedures of the analysis of total (free plus conjugated) salsolinol.

2.2.2 Affinity chromatography: Urine measurements can be performed according to Moser et al. (1995b, 1996a). After centrifugation (10 min, 200 g), the supernatant (500 µl) was added to acetate buffer, pH 5.0, arylsulfatase IV (EC 3.1.6.1) 5 U, and β-glucuronidase (EC 3.2.1.31) 350 U, and incubated 16 h at 30°C. After hydrolysis, 500 µl urine was brought to pH 8.6 (EPPS buffer with NaCl 0.15 M and MgCl2 0.01 M) and loaded into a freshly prepared m-amino-phenylboronic acid agarose cartridge (approximately 800–1000 µl). The cartridge was washed with H_2O and methanol, and salsolinol was eluted with 250 µl acetic acid 0.25 M. The recovery by affinity chromatography described above was approximately 60% (Fig. 4).

2.2.3 High performance liquid chromatography: Aliquots of 80 µl were injected into the HPLC system. A C18 column (Eurospher RP 18, 5 µm, column size 250 × 4.0 mm with pre-column 35 × 4.0 mm) was used. The mobile phase was a degassed solution of 0.1 M citrate buffer, pH 3.0, with 14.5% methanol (v/v), 0.3 mM Na_2EDTA and 0.52 mM sodium 1-octansulfonate and pumped at a flow rate of 1 ml/min. All chromatography was performed at 30°C. The detector cell operated at +0.8 V. The detection limit of salsolinol was approximately 5 pmol/ml.

Values should be corrected for urine volume of 1000 ml and expressed in nmol/ml.

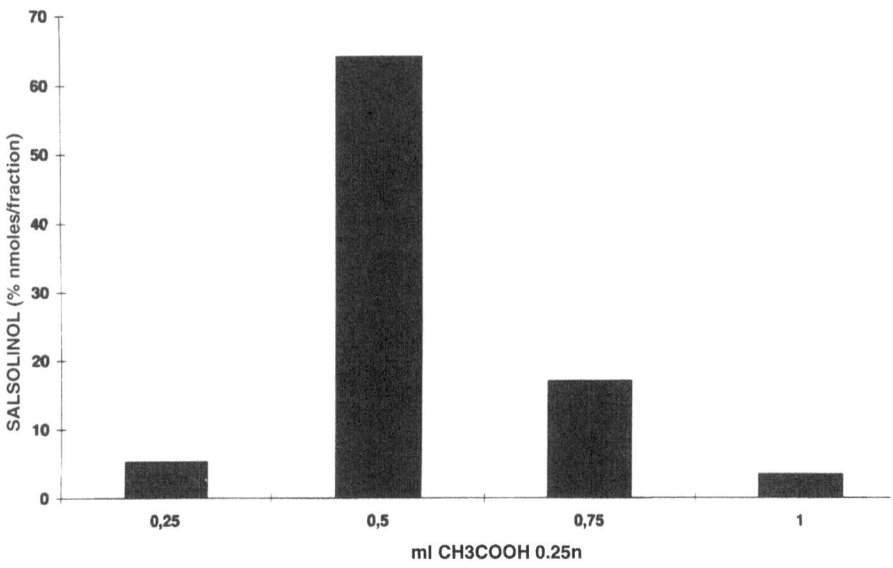

Fig. 4 Salsolinol was eluted with 250 µl acetic acid (0.25 M). The recovery of affinity chromatography was approximately 60% in fraction 2.

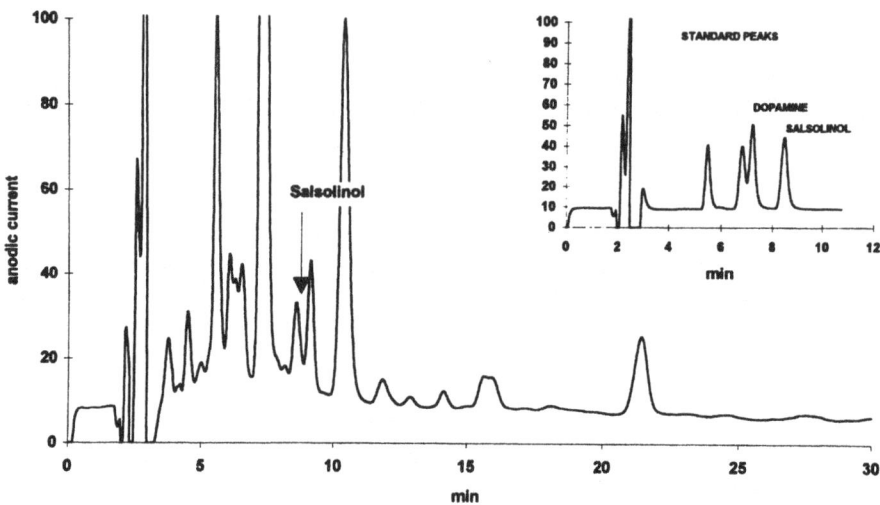

Fig. 5 Typical chromatogram of urine in which salsolinol could he detected. Standard peaks are also presented (small figure).

A resulting typical chromatogram of salsolinol is shown in Fig. 5 in which the standard peaks are also presented.

Validation of the peak for salsolinol is carried out by

(1)   comparison of peak retention times,
(2)   co-chromatography with a reference standard, and
(3)   comparison of voltammograms, as described in the CSF sections.

3. Frequency and TIQ Levels measured by HPLC-ECD

3.1   N-methyl-norsalsolinol (2-MDTIQ)

Niwa et al. (1991) identified 2-MDTIQ (N-methyl-norsalsolinol, 2-methyl-6,7-dihydroxy-1,2,3,4-tetrahydroisoquinoline) and 1,2-DDTIQ (2-methyl-salsolinol, 1,2-dimethyl-6,7-dihydroxy-1,2,3,4-tetrahydroisoquinoline) in *post mortem* human brain homogenates by means of gas chromatography combined with a double-focusing mass spectrometry. Brains were obtained from six patients with Parkinson's disease (from 68 to 80 years old) and from five patients with lung cancer, colon cancer, or chronic heart failure. Chemical ionization mass spectrometry was performed using isobutane as a reactant gas. Niwa et al. (1991) could detect 2-MDTIQ in frontal cortex homogenates of all 11 patients. The concentrations of 2-MDTIQ were estimated to be approximately 1 ng/g wet brain tissue.

Moser et al. (1995a) studied a large number of cerebrospinal fluids (CSFs) of 49 humans that included 34 patients with Parkinson's disease who all had symptoms of bradykinesia, resting tremor, and rigidity. The duration of illness ranged from 0.2 to 13 years. CSF of 15 normal subjects with a mean age of 55 ± 19 years who had symptoms requiring diagnostic lumbar puncture were also studied. 2-MDTIQ was found in nearly half of all patients with Parkinson's disease, but not in normal control subjects.

2-MDTIQ was present in CSF of patients *with l-dopa treatment*, but also in patients *without any treatment* for Parkinson's disease (Moser et al., 1995a). In the patient group presence of 2-MDTIQ in CSF was negatively correlated with duration of the disease, and most 2-MDTIQ positive CSFs were found during the first 2 years of the disease. After 8 years disease duration, 2-MDTIQ was present in only one out of four patients. Neither Webster rating scale scores, nor age seems to correlate with the presence of 2-MDTIQ.

3.2   Salsolinol

Dostert et al. (1993) measured salsolinol levels (1-methyl-6,7-dihydroxy-1,2,3,4-tetrahydroisoquinoline) by a gas chromatography/mass spectrometry with electron-capture negative-ion chemical ionization after derivatization with pentafluoropropionyl anhydride. They examined the urine of eight patients (mean age 70 ± 3.4 years) with Parkinson's disease, but without l-dopa treatment, and of eight control subjects (mean age 70 ± 3.6 years). In this study, daily urinary *excretion* of salsolinol level (*free*, glucuronide, sulfate, and *total*) was not different between the patient group and the control group. Dostert et al. (1993) also described that the variation of total salsolinol levels from *patient to patient* was repeatedly found to be high both in the patient group as well as in normal controls.

In a study of Moser et al. (1996a), salsolinol was examined in urine of 20 patients with Parkinson's disease and in 15 healthy volunteers with a mean age of 69 ± 10 years, without a history of drug or alcohol abuse, by means of reversed phase high performance liquid chromatography with electrochemical detection. All patients had symptoms of bradykinesia, resting tremor, and rigidity and were treated with l-dopa plus l-dopa decarboxylase inhibitor (mean l-dopa dose 327 ± 120 mg/d). The duration of illness ranged from 1.5 to 15 years with a mean age of 73 ± 11 years. In 75% of all the Parkinsonian patients salsolinol could be detected in urine, whereas very low levels of salsolinol were found in only 33% of controls. In Parkinsonian patients, urine levels of salsolinol were markedly enhanced, 10-fold in comparison to normal control subjects (0.028 ± 0.044 nmol/ml), and negatively correlated with the disease duration (Fig. 6). Additionally, the concentrations of urine salsolinol obtained from 20 patients with Parkinson's disease correlated with those found in CSF (R = 0.56; p = 0.045, Fig. 7, Moser et al, 1996a).

Combining the results of both authors, the discrepancy between urinary salsolinol levels implies that formation of salsolinol is associated with l-dopa treatment, and l-dopa treatment induces salsolinol formation. However, no correlation between daily l-dopa dose and urine salsolinol levels was observed (Moser et al., 1996a).

4. TIQ Derivatives and Dopamine Metabolites

Dopamine is mainly metabolized by monoamine oxidase (MAO, monoamine: oxygen oxidoreductase (deaminating), EC 1.4.3.4), which is one of the most important enzymes regulating the levels of catecholamines and serotonin in the mammalian brain (see also Chapter 11). 3,4-Dihydroxyphenylacetic acid (DOPAC) and homovanillic acid (HVA) are the main metabolites of dopamine (LeWitt et al., 1992). The DOPAC/dopamine ratio is often used to quantify dopamine turnover and monoamine oxidase activity since DOPAC is oxidized from dopamine by MAO. A more appropriate value is the homovanillic acid/3-O-methyl-dopa (HVA/MDOPA) ratio that reflects dopamine, as well as l-dopa, metabolism. MDOPA together with the HVA/MDOPA ratio is a very good long-term parameter of

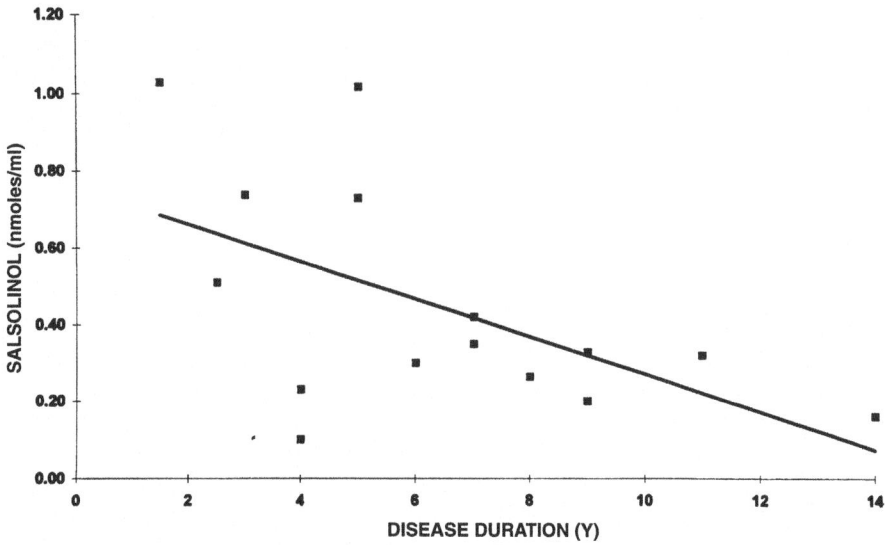

Fig. 6   In patients with Parkinson's disease, urine levels of salsolinol negatively correlated with disease duration.

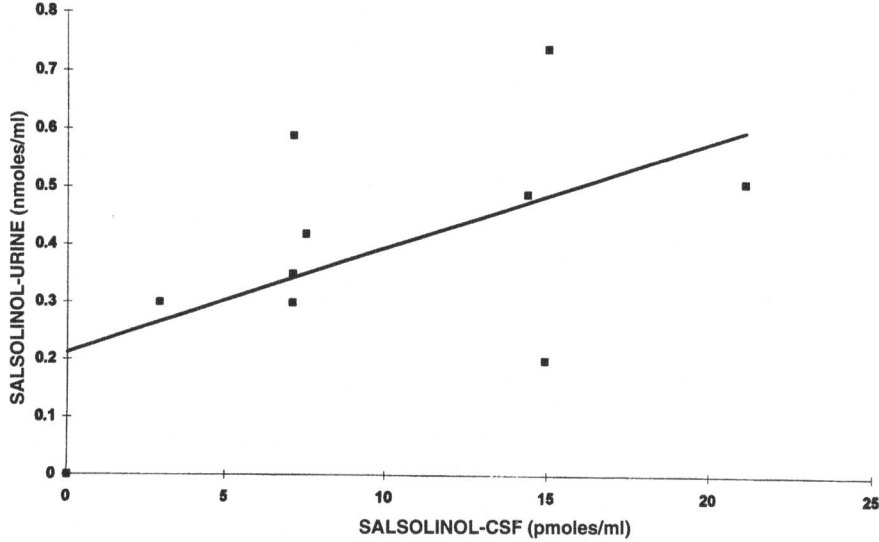

Fig. 7   In patients with Parkinson's disease, concentrations of urine salsolinol correlated with those found in cerebrospinal fluid (CSF).

L-dopa treatment and the corresponding dopamine metabolism (Melamed and Hefti, 1984; Gerlach et al., 1986).

HVA/MDOPA ratios were significantly higher in Parkinsonian patients with *N-methyl-norsalsolinol* (2-MDTIQ) present in the CSF, than in patients without the compound (Moser et al., 1995a). These findings are not related to different daily L-dopa doses since the mean daily L-dopa doses, the mean MDOPA levels, and the L-dopa/MDOPA ratio were nearly identical in comparison to patients without 2-MDTIQ in the CSF. In L-dopa treated patients with 2-MDTIQ, relative enhancement in levels of HVA (due to L-dopa treatment) was greater than the enhancement in MDOPA. This change in the HVA/MDOPA ratio was interpreted to signify an increased dopamine turnover in the remaining healthy striatal nerve endings (Moser et al., 1995a), which correlates with the increased firing rates of the dopaminergic nucleus A 9 neurons (Bernardini et al., 1990).

Thus, it is speculated that 2-MDTIQ is a result of the enhanced dopamine metabolism described above, and is endogenously synthesized. The hypothesis is also supported by the finding that 1-methyl-TIQ, another TIQ derivative, decreases in *substantia nigra* during progressive aging of the rat (Ayala et al., 1994): The reduction of 1-methyl-TIQ is definitely related to a decrease in dopamine content and a loss of dopamine neurons in different areas of the central nervous system during aging, while the dopamine neurons in the *substantia nigra* may be those with the highest loss during aging. According to Origitano et al. (1981) and Minami et al., (1992), salsolinol is also considered to be synthesized from dopamine *in situ* in dopaminergic neurons, since salsolinol and 2-MDTIQ cannot cross the blood-brain barrier. Thus, it is suggested that salsolinol also reflects L-dopa or dopamine metabolism of the mammals central nervous system, and salsolinol levels detected in urine may reflect the brain levels of free, not sulfo-conjugated dopamine, particularly since urine levels of this compound were found to be related to the HVA/MDOPA ratio in patients with Parkinson's disease (Dostert et al., 1990; Moser et al., 1996a).

5. Stereospecifity and Enantiomer Separation

The content of TIQ (1,2,3,4-tetrahydroisoquinoline) differs greatly in foods. High amounts of TIQ and 1-methyl-TIQ in cheese, white wine, and cacao are found by gas chromatography with mass spectrometry (Makino et al., 1988; Niwa et al., 1991). Salsolinol possesses an asymmetric center at C-1 position and exists as R- and S-enantiomers. The S-enantiomer of salsolinol is present in foods such as port wine and dried banana, while the endogenous salsolinol found in mammalian brains and urine of healthy subjects is apparently the R-enantiomer (Dostert et al., 1988; Strolin Benedetti et al., 1989). R-enantiomer of salsolinol is predominantly synthesized in the brain under physiological conditions by condensation with pyruric acid followed by decarboxylation (Minami et al., 1993). Additionally, salsolinol is formed by ring cyclation of dopamine with acetaldehyde (Pictet-Spengler condensation, non-enzymatic; Dostert et al., 1990). A first attempt to separate optical isomers of salsolinol was made by Dostert et al. (1989): After methylation of salsolinol with diazomethane, the resulting salsolidine was incubated with N-trifluoroacetyl-L-prolyl chloride as derivatizing agent and analyzed by gas chromatography. However, this method was not suitable for quantification of the derivative corresponding to the S-enantiomer.

A simple and rapid method is presented by Stammel and Thomas (1993) for direct separation of both enantiomers of salsolinol without derivatization by high performance liquid chromatography (HPLC) using β-cyclodextrin-bonded silica as chiral stationary phase. When this method is used, the time required for analysis and complete enantiomer separation is very short (less than 12 min). A separation of R- and S-enantiomers of salsolinol is also possible using reversed phase HPLC (Nucleosil 100, C18, 3 μM particle size) where β-cyclodextrin (0.03 M) is added to the mobile phase as a chiral selector. However, in experiments of Stammel and Thomas (1993), only a partial separation of the two enantiomers was achieved when β-cyclodextrin was employed in the mobile phase.

6. Cerebral Lesions Caused by TIQ Derivatives

6.1   TIQ, 1-Methyl-TIQ, 2-Methyl-TIQ

TIQ (1,2,3,4-tetrahydroisoquinoline, 20 mg/kg per day) induced L-dopa-sensitive parkinsonism in primates (squirrel monkeys) when injected subcutaneously (Nagatsu and
Yoshida, 1988; Yoshida et al., 1990). 2-methyl-TIQ, when administered intraperitoneally
and chronically to C57BL/6J mice (female), induced an atrophy of the central portion of
the substantia nigra pars compacta and pars lateralis with a reduction in tyrosine hydroxylase immunoreactivity (Fukuda, 1994). In a small study of Yoshida et al. (1993), 2-methyl-
TIQ was administered to two monkeys (20 mg/kg, s. c. per day, for 100 days). In this study,
behavioral scores of monkeys showed slight motor disturbances, but pathological examinations of the substantia nigra revealed no differences between the 2-methyl-TIQ treated
monkeys and controls. Tasaki et al. (1991) demonstrated that pretreatment of male C57BL
mice with 1-methyl-TIQ completely prevented MPTP- or TIQ-induced bradykinesia.

6.2   N-Methyl-R-salsolinol

Naoi et al. (1996) examined N-methyl-R-salsolinol (1R,2-dimethyl-6,7-dihydroxy-1,2,3,4-
tetrahydroisoquinoline) and salsolinol for their neurotoxicity for dopaminergic neurons by
stereotaxic injections into the left *corpus striatum* of male Wistar rats. 100 nmol of the compounds dissolved in Ringer solution were injected into the rat *striatum* at a flow rate of
1 µl/2 min (total volume 5 µl). Only N-methyl-R-salsolinol induced behavioral changes
very similar to those found in Parkinson's disease, including hypokinesia; stiff tail, limb
twitching, and postural abnormalities. In biochemical analysis, Naoi et al. (1996) could
show that after N-methyl-R-salsolinol application to the *striatum,* N-methyl-R-salsolinol
itself and its oxidation product accumulated in the *corpus striatum.* Dopamine and noradrenaline were reduced in the *corpus striatum* as well as in the *substantia nigra,* whereas
serotonin and its metabolites were unaffected. After a single injection of N-methyl-R-
salsolinol in the *striatum,* tyrosine hydroxylase activity markedly decreased in the *substantia nigra.* Also a mild necrosis was detected around the injected site with proliferation
of blood vessels and appearance of macrophages when N-methyl-R-salsolinol was administered, whereas the oxidation product of N-methyl-R-salsolinol caused massive necrosis
around the injected spot. Naoi et al. (1996) suggested that N-methyl-R-salsolinol may elicit
cytotoxicity by generating hydroxyl radicals during oxidation. The oxidation product was
found to accumulate in cells by binding to mitochondria and other subcellular compart-
ments. It is speculated that the potent cytotoxicity of the oxidation product of N-methyl-R-
salsolinol might be due to the inhibition of the mitochondrial respiratory chain in a similar
way as with MPTP (see also Chapter 3).

6.3   N-Methyl-norsalsolinol

N-methyl-norsalsolinol   (2-methyl-6,7-dihydroxy-1,2,3,4-tetrahydroisoquinoline)   (2-
MDTIQ, 8 µg/3 µl) was stereotactically injected into the left medial forebrain bundle, and
rotational behavior of animals as well as neurochemical changes in the brain were mea-

sured in female *Wistar rats* (Moser et al., 1996b). Three weeks after lesioning, rotational behavior was assessed following the administration of S-amphetamine (5 mg/kg) and apomorphine (0.1 mg/kg). The total number of rotations, induced by the drug, was counted during a 60-min period. Additionally, rotational behavior was assessed during 60 min by a rotation score (RS) which reflects well the uniformly-directed rotations performed by rats. The rotation score RS is given by $[(l - r)/(l + r)]^2$; 1, number of nose-to-tail rotations to the left (ipsiversive to the lesion) and r, number of nose-to-tail rotations to the right (contraversive to the lesion).

After 2-MDTIQ lesions, S-amphetamine caused animals to rotate, with *marked* preference, in the direction ipsiversive to the lesion (RS 0.94 ± 0.08). There was no response to apomorphine administration 3 weeks after lesioning (RS 0.04 ± 0.05), even if higher concentrations of apomorphine (0.1 mg/kg) were used. The reaction to S-amphetamine was not due to a reduction of dopamine metabolism of the ipsilateral caudate-putamen or mesencephalic structures, since dopamine and metabolite levels were not different when compared to control rats, and MAO activity was unchanged.

As expected from these neurochemical results, dopaminergic cell bodies of the *substantia nigra pars compacta* were also unaffected under the phase contrast (Fig. 8). It is suggested that the effect of 2-MDTIQ cannot be related to, for example, a partial nigrostriatal degeneration, but that it appears as a specific interaction between 2-MDTIQ and dopaminergic neurons activated by S-amphetamine (Moser et al., 1996b). One explanation is that the application of 2-MDTIQ leads to an insensitivity of the dopamine uptake/transporter system to S-amphetamine (Mintz et al., 1994; Moser et al., 1996b). This would result in a decline of ipsilateral dopamine release in the caudate-putamen with ipsiversive rotations to S-amphetamine. TIQ and salsolinol indeed meet the criteria for false neurotransmitter and can be accumulated and stored in rat brain synaptosomes (Heikkila et al., 1971; Stammel and Thomas, 1993). However, an effect of 2-MDTIQ on presynaptic membranes of dopaminergic synaptosomes has never been reported.

6.4   N-Methyl-4-hydroxy-norsalsolinol

In experiments of Liptrot et al. (1993), male *Wistar rats* received unilateral intrastriatal injections (10 or 100 nmol) or intraventricular infusion (100 or 200 nmol/µl/h for 3 h) of N-methyl-4-hydroxy-norsalsolinol (2-methyl-4,6,7-trihydroxy-1,2,3,4-tetrahydro-isoquinoline). After *intraventricular* infusion, N-methyl-4-hydroxy-norsalsolinol caused a reduction of dopamine levels in the *corpus striatum, substantia nigra,* dorsal raphe, hypothalamus, and a reduction in noradrenaline in the *locus coeruleus.* According to Liptrot et al. (1993), pretreatment of animals with a combination of monoamine oxidase A (clorgyline, 8 mg/kg, i. p.) and B (R-deprenyl, 10 mg/kg, i. p.) inhibitor completely prevented the N-methyl-4-hydroxy-norsalsolinol-induced dopamine reduction in the substantia nigra and hypothalamus. Unilateral *intrastriatal* injections of N-methyl-4-hydroxy-norsalsolinol produced marked ipsilateral reduction of dopamine concentrations compared to 57% concentration found in sham-operated controls. Most of the animals showed postural asymmetry and a tendency to circle towards the side of injection. No experiments with apomorphine or amphetamine application were performed by Liptrot et al. (1993). With these results, N-methyl-4-hydroxy-norsalsolinol should be evaluated further as a possible MPTP-like compound, which may derive from endogenous catecholamines.

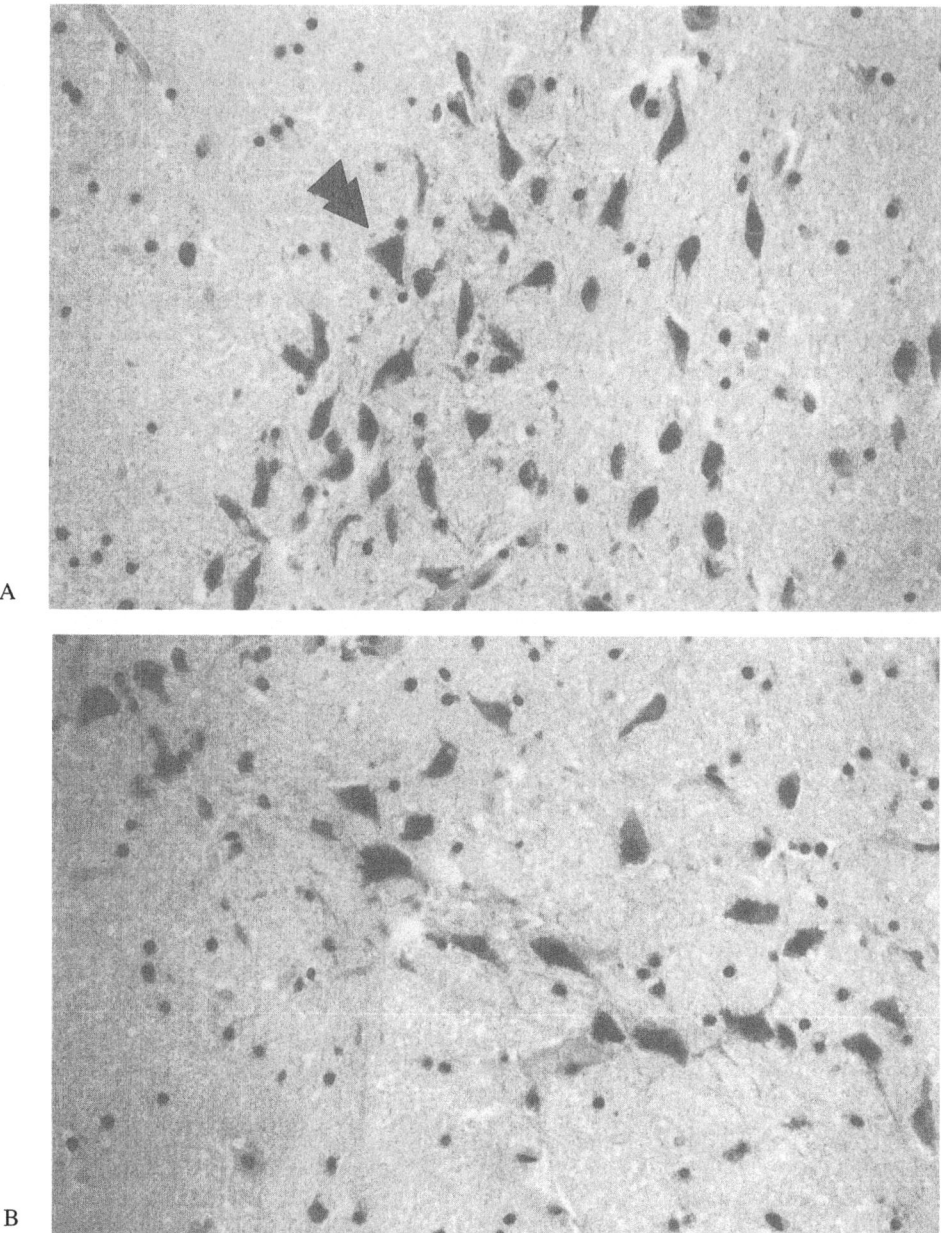

Fig. 8 Brain slices of the left substantia nigra photographed under phase contrast 3 weeks after stereotactically performed lesions by 2-MDTIQ (a) and controls (b). ➡ dopaminergic cell body.

7. Hallucinosis and TIQ Derivatives

At present, there is only one publication concerning hallucinations in patients with Parkinson's disease and TIQ derivatives (Moser et al., 1996a). In this study, 20 parkinsonian patients were divided into two groups according to the presence of visual hallucinations during the week before the CSF and urine collection. Group I consisted of 11 patients without any visual hallucinations; group II consisted of nine patients, with visual hallucinations, also treated with L-dopa plus L-dopa decarboxylase inhibitor (mean age 74 ± 7 years). One day before CSF and 12 h urine collection, the severity of Parkinson's disease was rated by the Webster rating scale (mean 16.2, range from 8 - 25; group I 15.8 ± 5.9; group II 16.6 ± 4.8). Mean Mini mental score was also not different between groups, 22.2 ± 6.3 vs 21.7 ± 5.7. No medication for treating visual hallucinations was given during the week prior to examination.

Salsolinol levels in urine of patients with hallucinations were significantly increased (almost three-fold of those found in patients without visual hallucinations). Since the mean daily L-dopa doses for both groups were nearly identical, this result is not related to different daily L-dopa doses, although Dostert et al. (1989) have found that daily urinary excretion of salsolinol was lower in untreated parkinsonian patients than in control subjects, and increased largely after L-dopa treatment.

Since either high values of the main serotonin metabolite 5-hydroxyindolacetic acid (HIAA, measured in CSF) or high L-dopa dose/MDOPA ratio, (which well reflects a degree of L-dopa inactivation by O-methylation) were found in parkinsonian patients with hallucinations, it is suggested that the serotonergic system as well as dopaminergic system, is involved in hallucinosis. The pathophysiology of visual hallucinations, which occur fairly frequently in the course of the pharmacological treatment of Parkinson's disease (Banerjee et al., 1989; Meco et al., 1990), has been ascribed either to dopamine receptor hypersensitivity (Cummings, 1992) or to overstimulation of serotonin receptors in the limbic areas (Zoldan et al., 1993; Lauterbach, 1993; Meco et al., 1994).

The precise mechanism causing hallucinosis in L-dopa treated patients with Parkinson's disease is not understood, but it seems to be associated with overstimulation of corticolimbic serotonergic receptors by serotonin flushed out of nerve terminals by dopamine that is probably formed there from exogenous L-dopa (Zoldan et al., 1993). The resulting imbalance between dopaminergic and serotonergic systems may be responsible for the hallucinations (Zoldan et al., 1993). In this respect, salsolinol probably reflects an overloaded dopaminergic system with a production of atypical dopamine metabolites. Alternatively, salsolinol itself might be capable of inducing hallucinations. As to its effect on receptors, salsolinol has been reported to bind to rat brain dopamine as well as to opiate receptors of the δ-type (Airaksinen et al., 1984; Stammel and Thomas, 1991). However, the induction of hallucinations by administration of TIQ derivatives has never been reported.

References

Airaksinen M.M., Saano V., Steidel E., Juvonen H., Huhtikangas A., and Gynther J. (1984) Binding of β-carbolines and tetrahydroisoquinolines by opiate receptors of the δ-type. Acta Pharmac. Toxicol. 55:380–385.

Allievi C., Dostert P., and Strolin Benedetti M. (1991) Determination of free salsolinol concentrations in human urine using gas chromatography-mass spectrometry. J. Chromatogr. Biomed. Appl. 568:271–279.

Ayala A., Parrado J., Cano J., and Machado A. (1994) Reduction of 1-methyl-1,2,3,4-tetrahydroisoquinoline level in substantia nigra of the aged rat. Brain Res. 638:334–336.

Banerjee A.K., Falkai P.G., and Savidge M. (1989) Visual hallucinations in the elderly associated with the use of levodopa. Postgrad. Med. J. 65:358–361.

Bernardini G.L., Specialte S.G., and German D.C. (1990) Increased midbrain dopaminergic cell activity following 2'CH$_3$-MPTP-induced dopaminergic cell loss: an *in vitro* electrophysiological study. Brain Res. 527:123–129.

Burns R.S., Chiueh C.C., Markey S.P., Ebert M.H., Jacobowitz D.M., and Kopin I.J. (1983) A primate model of Parkinsonsm: selective destruction of dopaminergic neurons in the pars compacta of the substantia nigra by N-methyl-4-phenyl-1,2,3,6-tetrahydropyridine. Proc. Natl. Acad. Sci. USA 80:4546–4550.

Coscia C.J., Burke W., Jamroz G., Lasala J.M., McFarlane J., Mitchell J., O'Toole M.M., and Wilson M.L. (1977). Occurrence of a new class of tetrahydroisoquinoline alkaloids in L-dopa-treated parkinsonian patients. Nature 269:617–619.

Cummings J.L. (1992) Psychosis in neurologic disease: neurobiology and pathogenesis. Neuropsychiatr. Neuropsychol. Behav. Neurol. 5:144–150.

Dostert P., Strolin Benedetti M., and Dordain G. (1988) Dopamine-derived alkaloids in alcoholism and in Parkinson's and Huntington's diseases. J. Neural Transm. 74:61–74.

Dostert P., Strolin Benedetti M., Dordain G, and Vernay D. (1989) Enantiomeric composition of urinary salsolinol in parkinsonian patients after Madopar. J. Neural Transm. 1:269–278.

Dostert P., Strolin Benedetti M., Bellotti V., Allievi C., and Dordain G. (1990) Biosynthesis of salsolinol, a tetrahydroisoquinoline alkaloid, in healthy subjects. J. Neural Transm. 81:215–223.

Dostert P., Strolin Benedetti M., Della Vedova F., Allievi C., La Croix R., Vernay D., and Durif F. (1993) Dopamine-derived tetrahydroisoquinolines and Parkinson's disease. Adv. Neurol. 60:218–223.

Fukuda T. (1994) 2-methyl-1,2,3,4-tetrahydroisoquinoline does dependently reduce the number of tyrosine hydroxylase-immunoreactive cells in the substantia nigra and the locus ceruleus of C57BL/6J mice. Brain Res. 639:325–328.

Gerlach M., Klaunzer N., and Pruntek H. (1986) Determination of L-dopa and 3-O-methyl dopa in human plasma by extraction using C$_{18}$ cartridges followed by high performance liquid chromatographic analysis with electrochemical detection. J. Chromatogr. 380:379–385.

Heikkila R., Cohen G., and Dembiec D. (1971) Tetrahydroisoquinoline alkaloids: uptake by rat brain homogenates and inhibition of catecholamine uptake. J. Pharmacol. Exp. Ther. 179:250–258.

Kaakkula S., and Wurtman R.J. (1993) Effects of catechol-O-methyltransferase inhibitors and L-3,4-dihydroxyphenylalanine with or without carbodopa on extracellular dopamine in the rat striatum. J. Neurochem. 60:137–144.

Langston J.W., Forno L.S., Rebert C.E., and Irwin I. (1984) Selective nigra toxicity after systemic administration of N-methyl-4-phenyl-1,2,3,6- tetrahydropyridine (MPTP) in the squirrel monkey. Brain Res. 292:390–394.

Lauterbach E.C. (1993) Dopaminergic hallucinosis with fluoxetine in Parkinson's disease. Am. J. Psychiatry 150:1750.

LeWitt P.A., Galloway M.P., Matson W., Milbury P., and McDermott M. (1992) Markers of dopamine metabolism in Parkinson's disease. Neurology 42:2111–2117.

Liptrot J., Holdup D., and Phillipson O. (1993) 1,2,3,4-Tetrahydro-2-methyl-4,6,7-isoquinolinetriol depletes catecholamines in rat brain. J. Neurochem. 61:2199–2206.

Makino Y., Ohta S., Tackikawa O., and Hirobe M. (1988) Presence of tetrahydroisoquinoline and 1-methyl-tetrahydroisoquinoline in foods, compounds related to Parkinson's disease. Life Sci. 43:373–378.

Meco G., Bonifati V., Cusimano G., Fabrizio E., and Vanacore N. (1990) Hallucinations in Parkinson's disease: neuropsychological study. Ital. J. Neurol. Sci. 11:373–379.

Meco G., Alessandria A., Bonivati V., and Giustini P. (1994) Risperidone for hallucinations in levdopa-treated Parkinson's disease patients. Lancet 343:1370–1371.

Melamed E., and Hefti F. (1984) Mechanism of action of short- and long-term L-dopa treatment in Parkinsonism: role of the surviving nigrostriatal dopaminergic neurons. Adv. Neurol. 40:149–170.

Minami M., Takahashi T., Maruyama W., Takahashi A., Dostert P., Nagatsu T., and Naoi M. (1992) Inhibition of tyrosine hydroxylase by R and S enantiomers of salsolinol, 1-methyl-6,7- dihydroxy-1,2,3,4-tetrahydroisoquinoline. J. Neurochem. 58:2097–2101.

Minami M., Maruyama W., Dostert P., Nagatsu T., and Naoi M. (1993) Inhibition of type A and B monoamine oxidase by 6,7-dihydroxy-l,2,3,4-tetrahydroisoquinolines and their N-methylated derivatives. J. Neural Transm. 92:125–135.

Mintz M., Gordon I., Roz N., and Rehavi M. (1994) The effect of repeated amphetamine treatment on striatal DA transporter and rotations in rats. Brain Res. 668:239–242.

Moser A., and Kömpf D. (1992) Presence of methyl-6,7-dihydroxy-1,2,3,4-tetrahydro-isoquinolines, derivatives of the neurotoxin isoquinoline, in parkinsonian lumbar CSF. Life Sci. 50:1885–1891.

Moser A., Scholz J., Nobbe F., Vieregge P., Böhme V., and Bamberg H. (1995a) Presence of N-methyl-norsalsolinol in the CSF: correlations with dopamine metabolites of patients with Parkinson's disease. J. Neurol. Sci. 131:183–189.

Moser A., Scholz J., and Siebecker F. (1995b) HPLC assay for quantitating salsolinol in the urine of patients with Parkinson's disease. Biol. Chem. Hoppe-Seyler 376:132.

Moser A., Siebecker F., Vieregge P., Jaskowski P., and Kömpf D. (1996a) Salsolinol, catecholamine metabolites, and visual hallucinations in L-dopa treated patients with Parkinson's disease. J. Neural Transm. 103:421–432.

Moser A., Siebecker F., Nobbe F., and Böhme V. (1996b) Rotational behaviour and neurochemical changes in unilateral N-methyl-norsalsolinol and 6-hydroxydopamine lesioned rats. Exp. Brain Res. 112:89–95.

Nagatsu T., and Yoshida M. (1988) An endogenous substance of the brain, tetrahydroisoquinoline, produces parkinsonism in primates with decreased dopamine, tyrosine hydroxilase and biopterin in the nigrostriatal regions. Neurosci. Lett. 87:178–182.

Naoi M., Maruyama W., Sasuga S., Deng Y., Dostert P., Ohta S., and Takahashi T (1994) Inhibition of type A monoamine oxidase by 2(N)-methyl-6,7-dihydroxyisoquinolinium ions Neurochem. Int. 25:475–481.

Naoi M., Maruyama W., Dostert P., Hashizume Y., Nakahara D., Takahashi T., and Ota M. (1996) Dopamine-derived endogenous 1[R],2(N)-dimethyl-6,7-dihydroxy-1,2,3,4-tetrahydro-isoquinoline, N-methyl-[R]-salsolinol, induced parkinsonism in rat: biochemical, pathological and behavioural studies. Brain Res. 709:285–295.

Niwa T., Takeda N., Yoshizumi H., Tatematsu A., Yoshida M., Dostert P., Naoi M., and Nagatsu T. (1991) Presence of 2-methyl-6,7-dihydroxy-l,2,3,4-tetrahydro-isoquinoline and 1,2-dimethyl- 6,7-dihydroxy-1,2,3,4-tetrahydroisoquinoline, novel endogenous amines, in parkinsonian and normal human brains. Biochem. Biophys. Res. Commun. 177:603–609.

Origitano T., Hannigan J., and Collins M.A. (1981) Rat brain salsolinol and blood-brain barrier. Brain Res. 224:446–451.

Sandler M., Bonham Carter S.W., Hunter K.R., and Stern G.M. (1973) Tetrahydroisoquinoline alkaloides: *in vivo* metabolite of L-dopa in man. Nature 241:439–443.

Stammel W., and Thomas H. (1991) Interaction of tetrahydroisoquinoline alkaloids with opiate receptors in the rat brain. Biol. Chem. Hoppe-Seyler 372:909–910.

Stammel W., and Thomas H. (1993) A simple and rapid method for the seperation of the [R]- and [S]-enantiomers of the tetrahydroisoquinoline alkaloid salsolinol by high performance liquid chromatography. Analyt. Lett. 26:2513–2524.

Strolin Benedetti M., Dostert P., and Carminati P. (1989) Influence of food intake on the enantiometric composition of urinary salsolinol in man. J. Neural Transm. 78:43–51.

Tasaki Y., Makino Y., Ohta S., and Hirobe M. (1991) 1-Methyl-1,2,3,4-tetrahydroisoquinoline, decreasing in 1-methyl-4-phenyl-1,2,3,6-tetrahydropyridine-treated mouse, prevents parkinsonism-like behaviour abnormalities. J. Neurochem. 57:1940–1943.

Yoshida M., Niwa T., and Nagatsu T. (1990) Parkinsonism in monkeys produced by chronic administration of an endogenous substance of the brain, tetrahydroisoquinoline: the behavioral and biochemical changes. Neurosci. Lett. 119:109–113.

Yoshida M., Ogawa M., Suzuki K., and Nagatsu T. (1993) Parkinsonism produced by tetrahydroisoquinoline or the analogues. Adv. Neurol. 60:207–211.

Zoldan J., Friedberg G., Goldberg-Stern H., and Melamed E. (1993) Ondansetron for hallucinosis in advanced Parkinson's disease. Lancet 341:562–563.

Chapter 3

An Animal Model of Parkinson's Disease Prepared by Endogenous N-Methyl(R)Salsolinol

Makoto Naoi, Wakako Maruyama and Philippe Dostert

Contents in Brief

1. Introduction

The discovery of 1-methyl-4-phenyl-1,2,3,6-tetrahydropyridine (MPTP) as a parkinsonism-inducing agent (Davis et al., 1979) suggests that there may be endogenous or xenobiotic neurotoxins to cause Parkinson's disease (PD) in humans. After transport into the brain through the blood-brain barrier, MPTP is oxidized into 1-methyl-4-phenyl-2,3-dihydropyridine by type B monoamine oxidase [monoamine: oxygen oxidoreductase (deaminating), EC 1.4.3.4, MAO], which is further auto-oxidized to 1-methyl-4-phenylpyridinium ion (MPP$^+$) (Chiba et al., 1984). MPP$^+$ is considered to be a true dopamine neurotoxin because of its selective uptake and accumulation in dopamine neurons and its potent cytotoxicity (see reviews, Singer et al., 1987; Tipton and Singer, 1993). The mechanism of the cell death is ascribed to either the inhibition of Complex I in the mitochondrial respiratory chain (Nicklas et al., 1985; Mizuno et al., 1987), the generation of reactive oxygen species, such as superoxide (Zang and Misra, 1992; Hasegawa et al., 1990) and hydroxyl radical (Chiueh et al., 1993), or to the DNA damage (Dipasquale et al., 1991).

The studies using MPTP suggest that dopaminergic neurotoxins may have common characteristics: oxidation into a cytotoxic cation, uptake and accumulation in dopaminergic cells by a dopamine transporter, inhibition of ATP synthesis, generation of reactive oxygen species and induction of apoptosis to cause selective cell death of dopamine neurons. In addition, endogenous neurotoxin should be produced and accumulated in the nigro-striatal system. Isoquinolines with a catechol structure (Naoi et al., 1995a and b, 1996c, 1997) and without one (Nagatsu and Yoshida, 1989), and also β-carbolines (Collins, 1994; Matsubara, 1996) have been proposed as candidates for naturally-occurring MPTP-like compounds.

As shown in Fig. 1, *N*-methylation of these toxin candidates produces compounds with structure similar to MPTP (Naoi et al., 1989a; Matsubara et al., 1992), and the oxidation produces those comparable to MPP⁺ (Naoi et al., 1989b). 1,2,3,4-Tetrahydroisoquinoline was detected in human brain (Niwa et al., 1987; Ohta et al., 1987) and reported to induce parkinsonism in monkey (Nagatsu and Yoshida, 1988). However, the depletion of dopamine neurons and the accumulation in the nigro-striatal system could not be confirmed for this isoquinoline.

We have examined the neurotoxicity of compounds with structures similar to dopamine and MPTP and found that the derivatives of a dopamine-derived catechol isoquinoline, 1-methyl-6,7-dihydroxy-1,2,3,4-tetrahydroisoquinoline (salsolinol, sal), are selective neuro-toxins for dopamine neurons (Naoi et al., 1995a and b, 1996a and c). Sal was detected in human urine after administration of L-dopa (Sandler et al., 1973) and also in human brain (Sjöquist et al 1982). Sal has been considered to be synthesized from dopamine and acetalde-hyde by a non-enzymatic Pictet-Spengler reaction as racemic (*R*)- and (*S*)-enantiomer. To support this non-enzymatic synthesis, racemic salsolinols were detected in bananas and wine (Strolin Benedetti et al., 1989). However, in urine of healthy subjects only (*R*)-enantiomer

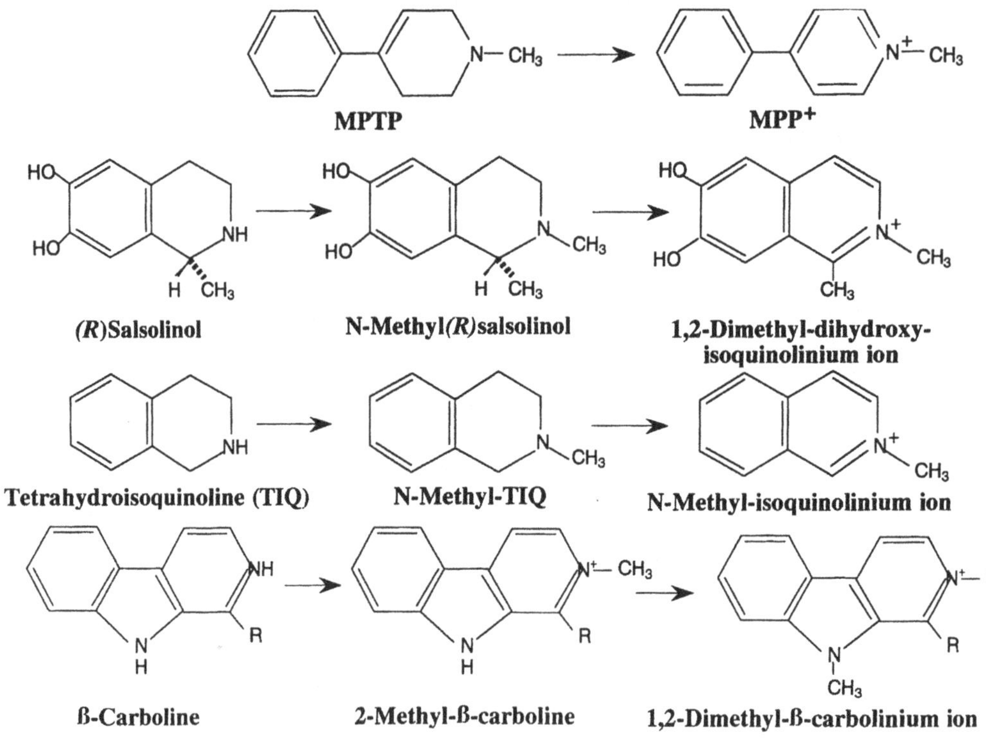

Fig. 1 Chemical structures of endogenous alkaloids, salsolinol and TIQ, and MPTP and MPP⁺. (*R*)Salsolinol and 1,2,3,4-tetrahydroisoquinoline (TIQ) are metabolized by a N-methyl-transferase into *N*-methyl(*R*)salsolinol and *N*-methyl-TIQ, and oxidized into 1,2-dimethyl-6,7-dihydroxyisoquinolinium ion and *N*-methylisoquinolinium ion, respectively.

of Sal was detected, suggesting that Sal may be produced by an enzyme (Dostert et al., 1987, 1990). In addition, Sal is not transported through the blood-brain barrier (Origitano et al., 1981), indicating that Sal in the brain should be synthesized *in situ.*

Recently, the enantiomeric structure and metabolism of salsolinol derivatives in the brain have been partially elucidated, as shown in Fig. 2. In human brain (Deng et al., 1995; Maruyama et al., 1997a), cerebrospinal fluid (Maruyama et al., 1996a) and intraventricular fluid (Maruyama et al., 1996b) only the (*R*)enantiomers of Sal and *N*-methylsalsolinol (*N*MSal) have been identified. We isolated a novel enzyme that can catalyze the stereo-specific synthesis of (*R*)Sal from dopamine and acetaldehyde (Naoi et al., 1996b). This (*R*) salsolinol synthase was purified from human brain cytosol with a molecular weight of 34.3 ± 8.3 KD. Dopamine was the only amine substrate, whereas acetaldehyde, formaldehyde and pyruvic acid were other substrates. *N*-Methylation of (*R*)Sal into *N*-methyl(*R*)salsolinol [*N*M(*R*)Sal] was proved by *in vivo* microdialysis (Maruyama et al., 1992). *N*M(*R*)Sal is further oxidized into 1,2-dimethyl-6,7-dihydroxyisoquinolinium ion (DMDHIQ$^+$) by non enzymatic (Maruyama et al., 1995a and b) and enzymatic oxidation (Naoi et al., 1995c).

For the study of neurodegenerative disorder pathogenesis, the preparation of animal models has several benefits to screen neurotoxins and to clarify the mechanism of the selective neurotoxicity. Using these catechol isoquinoline derivatives, we tried to set up an animal model of PD in rats. Out of Sal derivatives, only *N*M(*R*)Sal was found to induce parkinsonism in rats and to be a potent neurotoxin, specific to dopamine neurons (Naoi et al., 1996a). After injection of the catechol isoquinolines into the *striatum,* the behavioral, biochemical and histopathological changes were examined to assess neurotoxicity selective to dopaminergic cells. To confirm the cytotoxicity specific for dopamine system, the activity of the rate-limiting enzyme of catecholamine synthesis, tyrosine hydroxylase (tyrosine, tetrahydropteridine: oxygen oxidoreductase (3-hydroxylation); EC 1.4.16.2, TH), and the

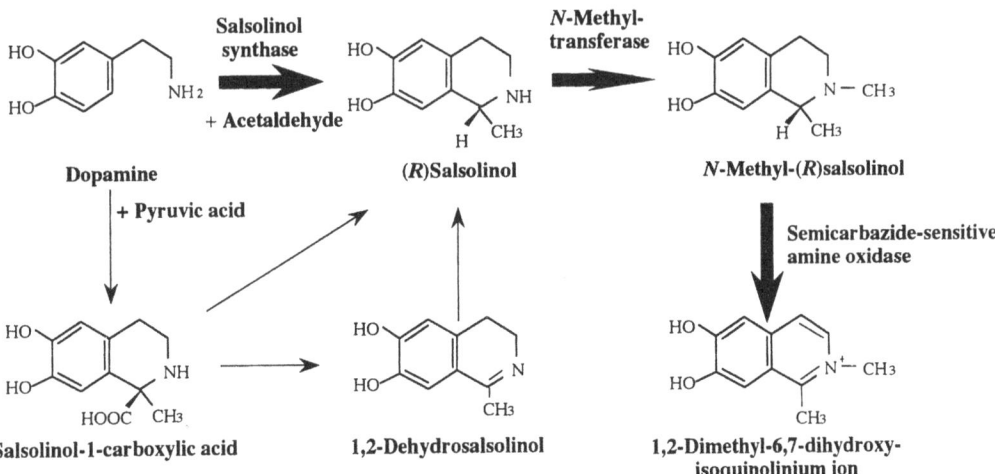

Fig. 2   Metabolic pathway of (*R*)-salsolinol in the brain. A (*R*)-salsolinol synthase enantio-selectively synthesizes (*R*)salsolinol and (*R*)salsolinol-1-carboxylic acid from dopamine and acetaldehyde or pyruvic acid, respectively. The decarboxylation of (*R*)salsolinol-1-carboxylic acid into 1,2-dehydrosalsolinol was found to be non-enzymatic, but enantio-selective synthesis of (*R*)Sal from (*R*)salsolinol-1-carboxylic acid has never been confirmed.

levels of biogenic monoamines and their metabolites were examined in the brain regions. In addition, by histopathological observation the density of TH-immuno-reactive cells was quantitatively examined in the *substantia nigra*. This review summarizes the preparation of an animal model of Parkinson's disease with *N*M(*R*)Sal and the methods to assess the behavioral, biochemical and pathological changes in dopaminergic neurons of the nigro-striatal system caused by the endogenous neurotoxin.

2. Preparation of a Rat Model of Parkinson's Disease

2.1 Materials

The (*R*)- and (*S*)-enantiomers of Sal and *N*MSal, and 2-methyl-6,7-dihydroxy-1,2,3,4-tetrahydroisoquinoline (*N*-methylnorsalsolinol) were synthesized according to a previously reported method (Teitel et al., 1972). DMDHIQ$^+$ was synthesized by the method of Bembenek et al. (1990). 6,7-Dihydroxy-1,2,3,4-tetrahydroisoquinoline (norsalsolinol) was purchased from Janssen (Beerse, Belgium), and sodium octanesulfonate was purchased from Aldrich (Milwaukee, Wis). The other chemicals were obtained from Nacalai Tesque (Kyoto, Japan).

2.2 Animal experiments

The experimental protocols of rat experiments were approved by the Ethics Committee of the Department of Biosciences, Nagoya Institute of Technology. The catechol isoquinolines were injected into the brains of male Wistar rats (body weight, about 250g). The microinjection probe was implanted in the left *striatum* according to the stereotaxic atlas of Paxinos and Watson (1986) (0.5 mm anterior to the bregma, + 3.0 mm lateral to the midline and 6.8 mm ventral to the dura). Twelve hours after the surgery, catechol isoquinolines (100 nmoles), dissolved in the Ringer solution, were injected into the rat *striatum* at a flow rate of 1 µl/2 min (a total volume of 5 µl). The behavioral changes were monitored by video and at regular intervals for 3 days. As control, rats were treated in a similar way and injected with the vehicle (the Ringer solution). For continuous infusion, *N*M(*R*)Sal was administered in the *striatum* for a week by attachment of a cannula to a mini-osmotic pump (Alzet, model 2002, 0.5 µl per hour, Palo Alto, CA) filled with *N*M(*R*)Sal solution (50 mmol/L in the Ringer solution) (Nitta et al., 1993). The site of the injection was confirmed by the histological study after the sacrifice.

3. Behavior Observation

3.1 Behavior changes due to perturbation in dopaminergic system

As shown in Figs. 3–5, after a single injection of *N*M(*R*)Sal into the left *striatum*, rats exhibited postural abnormality with the head and trunk deviating toward the lesioned side, lateral extension of the right hind limb and stiffness of the tail elevated above the ground (Fig.

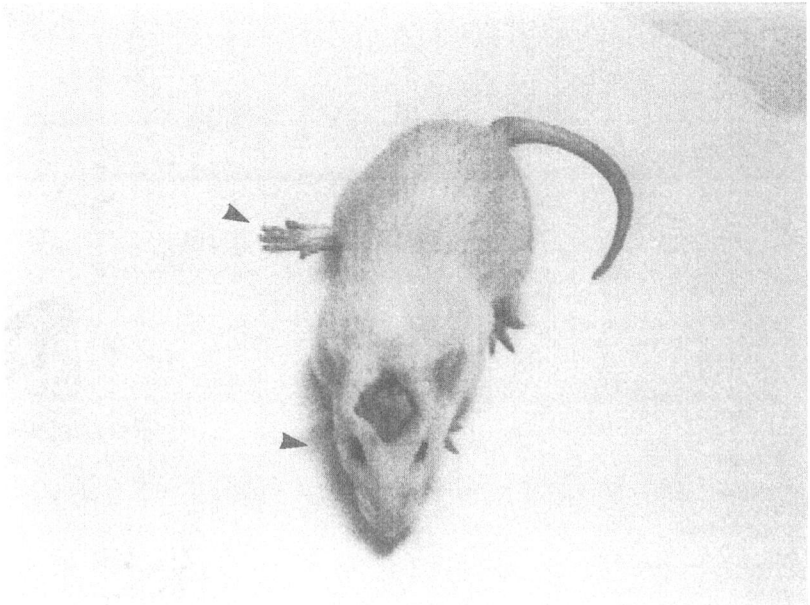

Fig. 3 Typical behavioral patterns induced in rats by *N*M(*R*)Sal injected in the left *striatum*. After a single injection of *N*M(*R*)Sal in the left *striatum*, the rat showed right hind limb extension (shown by an arrow) and reduced blinking of right eye (arrow).

3). The blinking of the right eye was markedly reduced. During spontaneous activity, the rats showed ipsilateral circulation toward the injection site (Fig. 4). Injection of *N*M(*R*)Sal into both sides of the *striatum* induced akinesia to rats, and they could not climb down from the edge of a bottle for several hours (Fig. 5). Some rats exhibited fine regular twitching of right limbs at rest, with a cycle of about 60/min. Twitching lasted for several hours, and the circulation was detected for 24 to 48 h after a single injection. A single injection of DMD-HIQ$^+$ in the left *striatum* induced hypokinesia in the right limbs, but no involuntary movement was detected. Other catechol isoquinolines, *N*-methyl(*S*)salsolinol, (*R*)- and (*S*)-salsolinol, norsalsolinol and *N*-methylnorsalsolinol, did not induce any behavioral changes to rats. By continuous infusion of *N*M(*R*)Sal with an osmotic mini pump, rats showed ipsilateral rotation for the first 48 h and, later, akinesia for 4 or 5 days.

We also injected salsolinol derivatives in the ventricles, and the behavioral changes induced in rats were not specific to dopamine depletion, but mixed with those due to other monoamines. Rats showed so-called "Serotonin Syndrome," a behavior response induced in rodents through stimulation of serotonin receptors (Glennon et al., 1991). The behaviors included so-called "wet-dog" behavior (Bedard and Pycock, 1977), namely shudder of the head, neck and trunk; sniffing or chewing, licking with typical mouth movements; and tremor in buccal muscles, associated with a chattering noise and tongue protraction (Spanos and Yamamoto, 1989; De Duffard et al., 1995). After the administration into the medial forebrain bundles, the behavioral changes were limited to postural abnormality and rotation, which may be due to the activation of the dopaminergic system (Robinson and Becker, 1986).

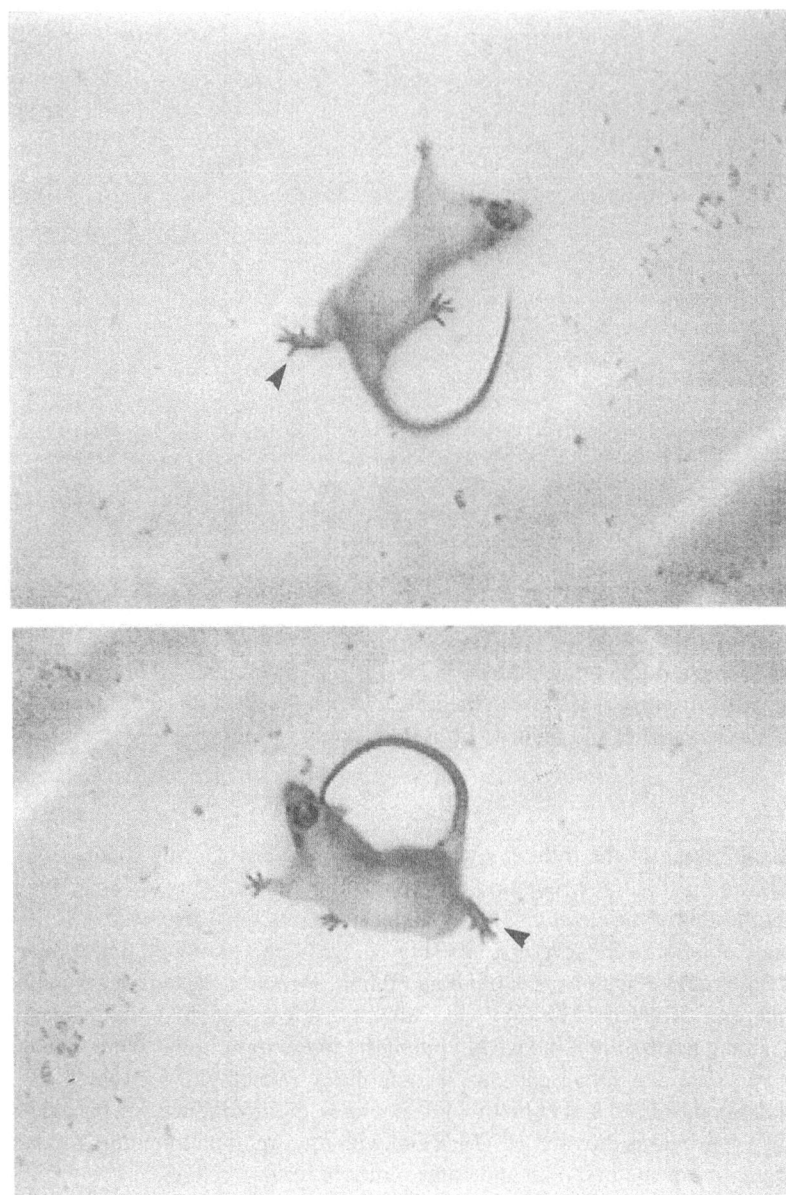

Fig. 4 Typical behavioral patterns induced in rats by *N*M(*R*)Sal injected in the right *striatum*. The circulation of the rat towards the lesioned side. The rat pivoted on the left hind limb (arrow) with the head and trunk deviated to the lesioned side.

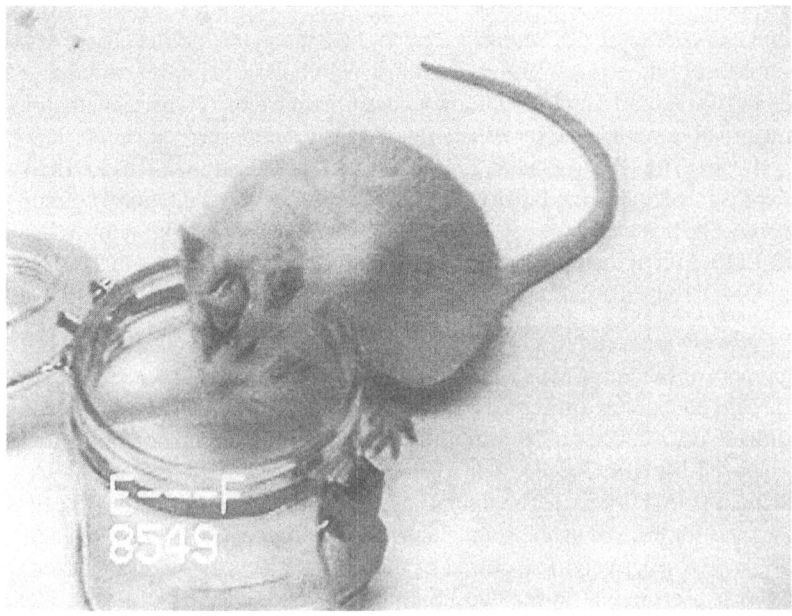

Fig. 5   Typical behavioral patterns induced in rats by *N*M(*R*)Sal injected in both sides of the *striatum*. The rat showed akinesia for several hours.

4. Biochemical Analysis in the Brain

4.1   Methods

4.1.1 Quantitative analysis of monoamines, their metabolites and isoquinolines: Three days after a single injection, the rat was sacrificed, and the brain was removed and cut in 2-mm-thick slices by coronal section with a Rodent Brain Matrix (Activational System, Pelco International, Redding, CA) and kept frozen at –80°C until analysis. The first and second (slice # 1 and # 2) and the seventh slice (slice # 7) from the rostral were confirmed to contain the *striatum* and the *substantia nigra,* respectively. The rat brain slices were weighed and homogenized in distilled water (1 ml/100 mg wet weight). The homogenate was mixed with 1/10 volume of 1 mol/L perchloric acid containing 1 mmol/L disodium EDTA and 1 mmol/L sodium metabisulfite, and centrifuged at 22,000 g for 10 min. The supernatant was filtered through a Millipore HV filter (pore size, 0.45 μm). Catecholamines, indoleamines and their metabolites and the reduced form of catechol isoquinolines were analyzed using high-performance liquid chromatography (HPLC) with a multi-electrochemical detection (ECD) system or with a Coulochem-II ECD (ESA, Chelmsford, MA) (Maruyama et al., 1992; Naoi et al., 1993). For the multi-ECD system the electrodes were set from 0 to 600 mV with a 60 mV increment. The parameters of a Coulochem-II ECD system connected to a Shimadzu LC-9A pump (Kyoto, Japan) were as follows: a model 5021 conditioning cell was set at +300 mV, and the first and second electrodes of a model 5011 analytical cell were set at +50 mV and –300 mV, respectively. The output of the second electrode was monitored.

For both HPLC-ECD systems, the column used was a reverse-phase Inertosil ODS-2 (4.6 mm i.d. × 250 mm, GL Sciences, Tokyo, Japan) and the mobile phase was composed of 90 mmol/L sodium acetate-35 mmol/L citric acid buffer, pH 4.35, containing 130 μmol/L disodium EDTA, 230 μmol/L sodium octanesulfonate and 120 ml/L methanol. DMDHIQ$^+$ was quantitatively analyzed by HPLC-fluorometric detection (Naoi et al., 1994; Maruyama et al., 1995b). The HPLC system consisted of a LC-9A pump, a RF-500LCA spectrofluorometer (Shimadzu, Kyoto, Japan) and a reverse-phase Inertosil ODS-3 column (4.6 mm i.d. × 150 mm, GL Sciences, Tokyo, Japan). The mobile phase was the same as the one used for HPLC-ECD, except that the methanol concentration was increased to 220 ml/L. For detection of DMDHIQ$^+$, the fluorescence at 500 nm was measured with excitation at 355 nm.

4.1.2 Enantiomeric analysis of salsolinol derivatives: For quantitation of (*R*)- and (*S*)-enantiomers of Sal and *N*MSal, the sample (225 μl) was mixed with 25 μl of 1 mol/L perchloric acid containing 1 mmol/L EDTA and sodium metabisulfite. After being mixed and centrifuged at 22 000 g for 10 min, the sample was filtered through a Millipore HV filter and analyzed by HPLC-ECD. The HPLC apparatus consisted of a LC-9A pump and a Coulochem-II ECD system. The oxidation voltage of a model 5020 guard cell was 350 mV, and the ones for the first and second electrodes of a model 5010 analytical cell were 50 mV and 300 mV, respectively. The output of the second electrode was monitored. The column used was a β-cyclodextrin-bonded column, Nucleodex β-OH (4.0 mm i.d. × 200 mm, Macherey-Nagel, Düren Germany) according to Sallström Baum and Rommelspacher (1994). Connected to it in series was a reverse-phase Inertosil ODS-3 column (4.6 mm i.d. × 150 mm). The mobile phase was 100 mmol/L sodium phosphate buffer, pH 3.6, containing 55 ml/L methanol. The flow rate was 0.4 ml/min.

4.1.3 Assay for TH activity: TH activity was measured by HPLC-ECD as reported previously (Naoi et al., 1988; Maruyama and Naoi, 1994). Tissue samples were incubated in L-tyrosine with (6*R*)-L-*erythro*-5,6,7,8-tetrahydrobiopterin in the presence of NSD-1015, an inhibitor of aromatic L-aminoacid decarboxylase, and L-dopa produced was measured by HPLC-ECD.

A comparison of biochemical data for rats treated with *N*M(*R*)Sal and DMDHIQ$^+$, with those for control rats was made using one-way analysis of variance (ANOVA) followed by Sheffe F-test.

4.2   Biochemical changes by infusion of NM(R)Sal and DMDHIQ$^+$

4.2.1 Changes of monoamines and their metabolites: Biochemical analyses of monoamines and their metabolites are summarized in Fig. 6. In the brain slices # 2 (Figure 6A), containing a portion of the *striatum,* and in # 7 (Fig. 6B), containing the *substantia nigra,* marked reduction in dopamine was observed after an injection of *N*M(*R*)Sal and DMDHIQ$^+$. The reduction was more pronounced with *N*M(*R*)Sal than with DMDHIQ$^+$ ($p <$ 0.05), and in the *substantia nigra* dopamine was lower than the detection limit, 0.025 pmol/injection. After *N*M(*R*)Sal injection, L-dopa was reduced in the *substantia nigra* ($p <$ 0.05), while the metabolites of dopamine, 3,4-dihydroxyphenylacetic acid (DOPAC) and 3-methoxy-4-hydroxyphenylacetic acid (homovanillic acid, HVA), did not change. Noradrenaline and its metabolite, 3-methoxy-4-hydroxyphenylethylene glycol (MHPG), were reduced in the *striatum* and *substantia nigra* after injection of *N*M(*R*)Sal ($p < 0.05$). By contrast, serotonin and its metabolite, 5-hydroxyindole acetic acid (5-HIAA), were not reduced

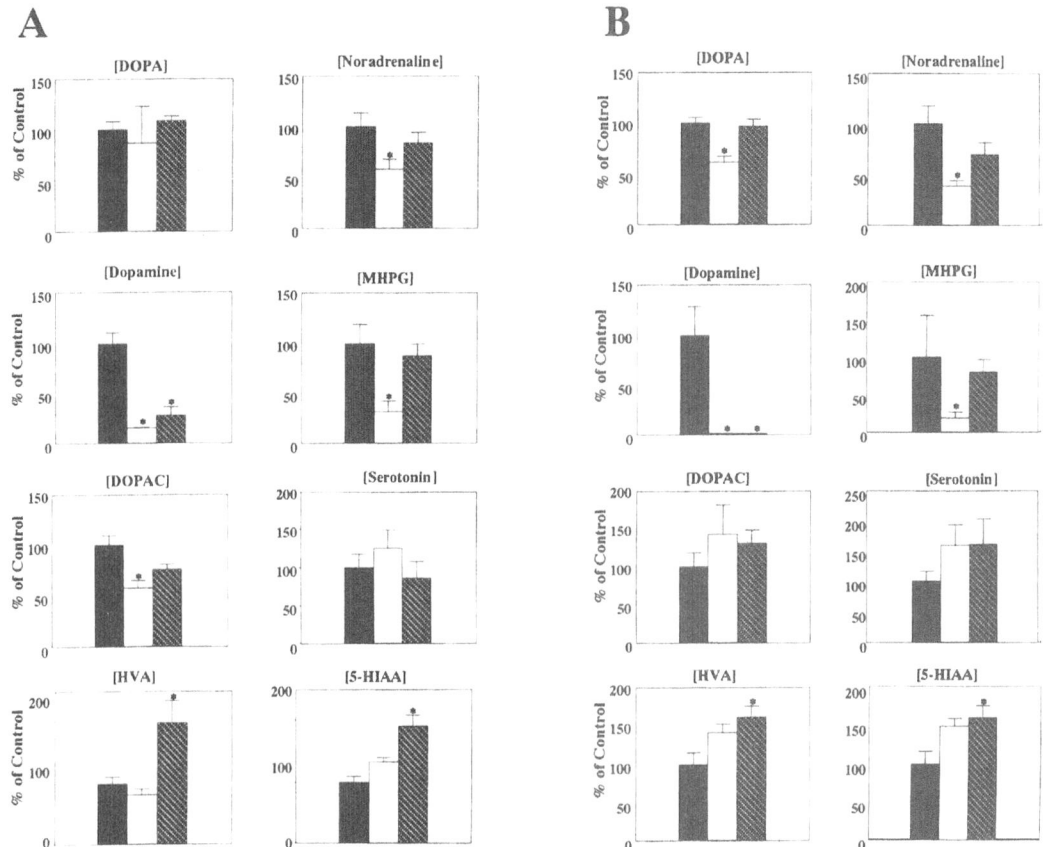

Fig. 6 Effects of the injection of *N*M(*R*)Sal and DMDHIQ⁺ on the levels of catecholamines and indoleamines in rat brain. A: in slice # 2 containing a potion of the striatum, B: in slice # 7 containing the substantia nigra. The column and bar represent the mean and SD of duplicate measurements of 6 rats for each compound. The difference from control is statistically significant (* p < 0.05). The filled column represents control, the hollow column after *N*M(*R*)Sal injection, and the hatched column after DMDHIQ⁺ injection. The rats were sacrificed 3 days after a single injection of 100 nmoles of each compound into the left striatum. The abbreviations used; DOPAC, 3,4-dihydroxyphenylacetic acid; HVA, 3-methoxy-4-hydroxyphenylacetic acid, homovanillic acid; MHPG, 3-methoxy-4-hydroxyphenylethylene glycol; 5-HIAA, 5-hydroxyindoleacetic acid.

In control rat the concentration of amines and their metabolites is as follows (pmol/mg wet weight brain tissue, mean ± SD). In slice # 2 (including the striatum) and slice # 7 (including the substantia nigra): DOPA; 12.24 ± 3.33, 14. 37 ± 2.47; DA; 20.48 ± 6.25, 0.34 ± 0.19; DOPAC; 12.24 ± 3.24, 0.51 ± 0.25; HVA; 1.49 ± 0.58, 0.48 ± 0.19; NE; 5.53 ± 2.67, 7.3 ± 4.41; MHPG; 3.60 ± 1.62, 2.98 ± 0.51; 5-HIAA; 1.61 ± 0.38, 2.09 ± 1.16; 5-HT; 0.42 ± 0.26, 0.33 ± 0.17.

Table 1.   Tyrosine hydroxylase activity in the *striatum* and *substantia nigra* of control rats and rats injected with $NM(R)$Sal and DMDHIQ$^+$

Brain slice containing	Tyrosine hydroxylase activity (pmol/min/mg wet weight) after injection of		
	Control	$NM(R)$Sal	DMDHIQ$^+$
Striatum	14.08 ± 0.62	6.46 ± 1.21***	17.89 ± 4.50
Substantia nigra	3.00 ± 1.42	0.003 ± 0.01***	2.92 ± 1.33

Rats were sacrificed 3 days after a single injection of $NM(R)$ Sal or DMDHIQ$^+$, or the vehicle for control.
The value represents the mean and SD of triplicate measurements of 6 rats.
Statistically significant ($p < 0.05$) by comparison with control (*) or from rats injected with DMDHIQ$^+$ (**).

after an injection of $NM(R)$Sal. After DMDHIQ$^+$ injection HVA and 5-HIAA were increased in the *striatum* and *substantia nigra,* which may be due to the inhibition of monoamine oxidase ($p < 0.05$). In other brain regions, the content of dopamine, noradrenaline, serotonin and their metabolites were not affected after an injection of $NM(R)$Sal or DMDHIQ$^+$.

4.2.2 Accumulation of NM(R)Sal and DMDHIQ$^+$: $NM(R)$Sal and DMDHIQ$^+$ were accumulated in rat brain 3 days after a single injection, as shown in Fig. 7. The amount of $NM(R)$Sal was 1.03 ± 0.17 and 1.71 ± 0.73 pmol/mg wet weight in slices # 1 and # 2 (the *striatum*), respectively. In the slices # 5 to # 7 no significant amounts of $NM(R)$Sal could be detected. However, large amounts of DMDHIQ$^+$, an oxidation product of injected $NM(R)$Sal, were identified in slices # 1 and # 2. In addition, substantial amounts of DMDHIQ$^+$ were found in slices # 6 and # 7 containing the substantia nigra; 0.45 ± 0.16 and 0.48 ± 0.09 pmol/mg wet weight, respectively. After an injection of DMDHIQ$^+$, remarkable amounts of DMDHIQ$^+$ were detected in slices # 1 - # 3, and the amount was the highest in slice # 1.

4.2.3 Reduction of TH activity: As summarized in Table 1, TH activity in the *striatum* and *substantia nigra* was significantly reduced after a single injection of $NM(R)$Sal in the striatum ($p < 0.05$), while DMDHIQ$^+$ did not affect TH activity. In other brain regions, no significant reduction of TH activity was detected after injection of $NM(R)$Sal or DMDHIQ$^+$.

5. Histological Study

5.1   Methods for histological analysis

Three days after a single injection of catechol isoquinolines or after 1 week of continuous infusion with a mini-osmotic pump in the left side of the *striatum,* the rat was anesthesized with sodium pentobarbital (50 mg/kg) and was perfused transcardially with a solution of physiological saline followed by fixation with a 200 ml/L solution of formaldehyde. The brain was removed from the skull and postfixed with the formaldehyde solution overnight at 4°C. The brain was cut into sections of 8 μm thickness using a microtome, and the sections were stained by the hematoxylin-eosin (H-E) and Klüver-Barrera (K-B) method. Immunohistochemical examination of paraffin-embedded material was performed by the streptavidin-biotin complex method with rabbit anti-TH antibody (Chemicon International,

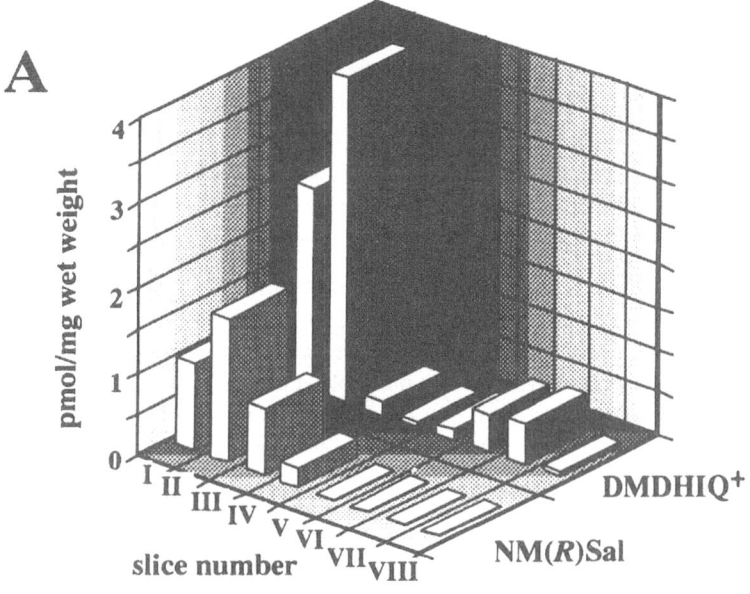

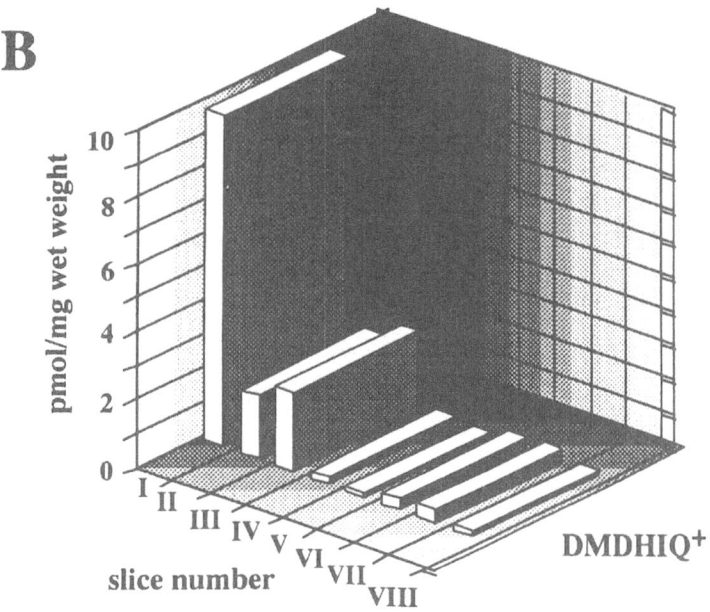

Fig. 7 Concentration of *N*M(*R*)Sal and DMDHIQ⁺ in the rat brain. Three days after a single injection of *N*M(*R*)Sal (A) and DMDHIQ⁺ (B) in the striatum (slice # 1 and # 2), the rats were sacrificed and brain slices of 2 mm thickness were prepared. Slice # 7 was identified to contain the substantia nigra. *N*M(*R*)Sal was quantitatively measured by HPLC-ECD and DMD-HIQ⁺ by HPLC-fluorometric detection. The column represents the mean of duplicate measurements of six rats, expressed as pmol/mg wet weight.

Temecula, CA). Cells were counted as neurons on the following basis: the presence of Nissl body stained by K-B staining and a visible nucleolus (Whitehouse et al., 1992). The number of dopamine neurons stained with anti-TH antibody was counted in a 15 μm × 15 μm area in the brain region, containing the *substantia nigra* according to the atlas of Paxinos and Watson (1986).

5.2   Cytotoxicity in the striatum

The *striatum* of the rats after a single injection of *N*M(*R*)Sal and DMDHIQ$^+$ is shown in Fig. 8. In the *striatum* of control rats administered with the vehicle, necrosis was not observed (Fig. 8A), whereas after *N*M(*R*)Sal administration, mild necrosis was detected around the injected site (shown by an arrow) with a proliferation of blood vessels and the appearance of macrophages (Fig. 8B). DMDHIQ$^+$ administration caused massive necrosis around the injected spot, and numerous macrophages were observed (Fig. 8C). K-B staining also showed massive destruction of myelin structure after injection of DMDHIQ$^+$, whereas *N*M(*R*)Sal did not cause significant changes in the structure as compared with control.

5.3   Depletion of dopamine neurons in the substantia nigra

After 1 week of continuous injections of *N*M(*R*)Sal into the left *striatum,* the density of neurons stained with anti-TH antibody was reduced markedly in the *substantia nigra* of the treated side (Fig. 9B), as compared with the control side (Fig. 9A). Table 2 shows that the number of TH-positive neurons was significantly reduced in the *substantia nigra* of the injected side, as compared with that of the opposite side ($p < 0.05$). By staining with K-B method, the number of neurons containing Nissl body was reduced slightly in the injected side of the *substantia nigra,* although a statistically significant difference was not reached. TH-positive neurons in the ventral tegmental area were not affected by the injection of *N*M(*R*)Sal. The reduction of TH-positive neurons in the *substantia nigra* was not found 3 days after a single injection or after 3 daily injections of *N*M(*R*)Sal or DMDHIQ$^+$.

6. Discussion

The principal neurological signs of PD are akinesia, muscle rigidity and tremor. Many animal models of PD have been prepared and used to examine the effects of various compounds as anti-parkinsonian drugs. However, a valid and reliable model has not been created yet. Even the potent dopaminergic neurotoxin MPTP could not induce permanent behavioral changes in rodents. The rotation model was prepared by unilateral lesion of the *substantia nigra* with 6-hydroxydopamine (6-OHDA) in rat (Ungerstedt et al., 1973). However, unilateral nigral lesions in rat induced sporadic bursts of head and neck tremor, but did not elicit akinesia or muscular rigidity (Buonamici et al., 1986). The treatment of rats with reserpine induced all three neurological signs of PD (Colpaert, 1987), but it depleted almost all biogenic monoamines, both in the brain and periphery.

The bilateral injection of 6-OHDA into the medial forebrain bundle at the level of the anterolateral hypothalamus induced a marked hypokinesia in rats (Ervin et al., 1977), and such injection into posterolateral hypothalamus itself caused tremor and muscular rigidity in addition to hypokinesia (Jolicoeur et al., 1991). In these papers, the semi-quantitative

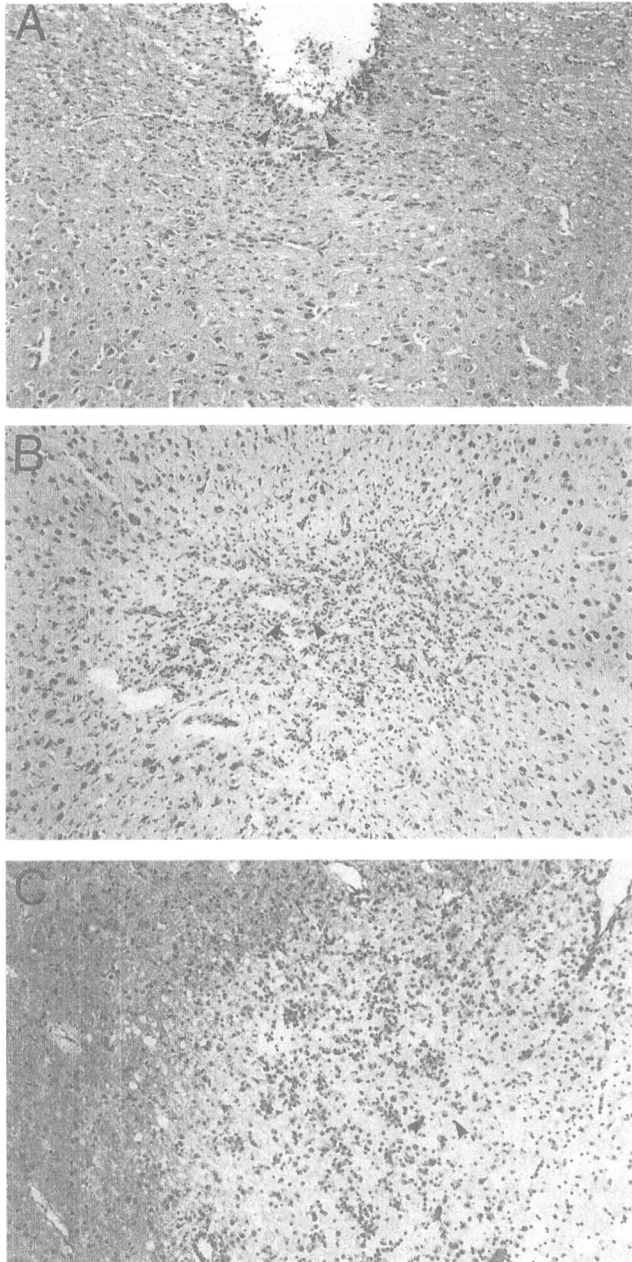

Fig. 8 Morphological change in the *striatum* of rats after injection of *N*M(*R*)Sal and DMDHIQ$^+$. Three days after a single injection of the compound in the left *striatum,* the rats were sacrificed and the striatum was stained by H-E staining. (A) control, no necrosis; (B) after *N*M(*R*)Sal injection, the necrosis was limited around the injected site; and C, DMDHIQ$^+$ injection, massive necrosis with activated macrophages. The injected site was shown by an arrow. Magnification × 25.

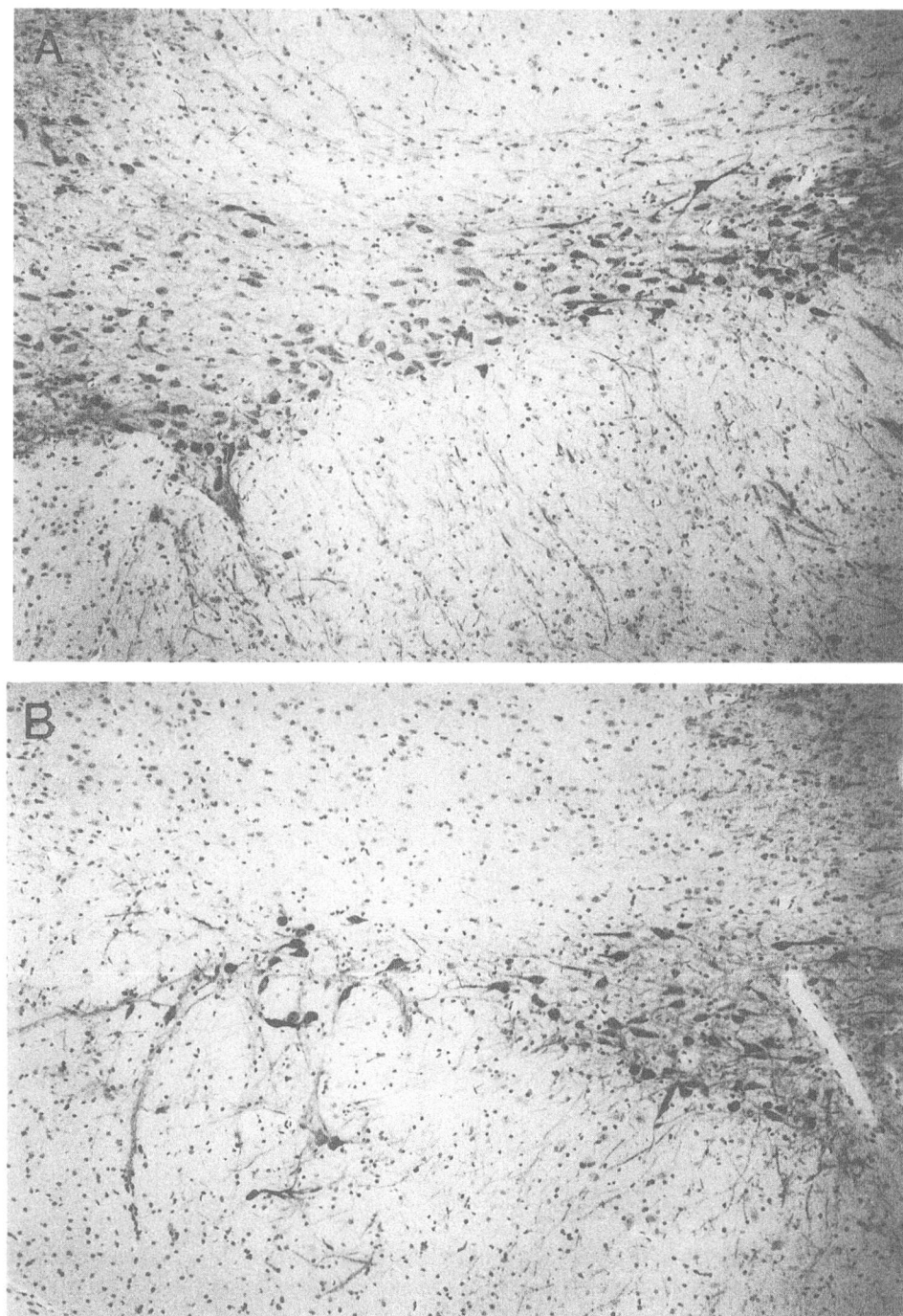

Fig. 9   The substantia nigra of rats injected with *N*M(*R*)Sal. Immuno-staining for tyrosine hydroxylase. The rats were sacrificed after 1 week of continuous infusion of *N*M(*R*)Sal in the left
striatum. (A) The right control side and (B) the left injected side of the substantia nigra. The
number of TH positive neurons was decreased in the substantia nigra of the injected side
compared with control. Magnification × 25.

Table 2. The density of neurons stained with anti-TH antibody and K-B method in the *substantia nigra* after 1 week of continuous infusion of *N*M(*R*)Sal in the left side of the *striatum.*

	Density of neurons (number/225μm^2)	
	Injected side	Control side
Stained with anti-TH antibody	3.090 ± 0.315*	6.687 ± 0.618
Stained with K-B staining	5.943 ± 0.335	6.890 ± 0.191

The value represents the mean and SD and the number of rats were 8.
*p < 0.05, calculated by paired *t*-test.
The left side of the striatum was continuously infused by *N*M(*R*)Sal using a mini pump, and the control side was not treated.

methods of studying the behavioral abnormalities due to dopamine depletion, such as catalepsy, muscular rigidity by prolonged grasping, rigidity and tremor were described. The evaluation of 6-OHDA-induced parkinsonism as an animal model of PD is reviewed by Reading and Dunnett (1994).

Our work reports the setting up of an animal model of PD using *N*M(*R*)Sal, an endogenous catechol isoquinoline present in the human brain. The effects of this isoquinoline on the nigro-striatal dopaminergic system were studied systematically via behavioral, biochemical and histopathological observations. As shown by behavioral assessment, only *N*M(*R*)Sal induced hypokinesia, postural abnormality, involuntary movement and stiffness of the tail. These behavioral changes may be appropriate for a rat model of PD. Previously, salsolinol derivatives were examined for behavioral changes after injection in the brain. Costal et al. (1976) reported that Sal and *N*MSal induced minor behavioral changes after bilateral injection into the nucleus accumbens of rats.

Another dopamine-derived isoquinoline, 1,2,3,4-tetrahydro-6,7-dihydroxy-1-(3,4-dihydroxybenzyl)-isoquinoline (tetrahydropapaveroline) was reported to induce behavioral changes in rats after an injection in lateral ventricle (Myers and Oblinger, 1977). However, no biochemical and pathological data for the brain were presented. An adrenaline-derived isoquinoline, 2-methyl-4,6,7-trihydroxy-1,2,3,4-tetrahydroisoquinoline, was reported to deplete catecholamines in rat brain after ventricular injection (Liptrot et al., 1993). However, this isoquinoline was synthesized by the Pictet-Spengler reaction and has never been identified in the human brain. Our newly purified (*R*)-salsolinol synthase does not catalyze the condensation of adrenaline with formaldehyde (Naoi et al., 1996b). Most of these previous studies were aimed to examine the effects of isoquinolines in alcoholism (Cohen, 1976), and the biochemical and pathological data have never been presented to demonstrate the selective neurotoxicity to dopamine neurons in the nigro-striatal system.

A possible mechanism of the selective neurotoxicity of *N*M(*R*)Sal to dopamine neurons in the *substantia nigra* is summarized in Fig. 10. Using human dopaminergic neuroblastoma SH-SY5Y cells, only *N*M(*R*)Sal was found to be accumulated in the cells by the dopamine transport system, but the (*S*)-enantiomer of *N*MSal and other catechol isoquinolines were not (Takahashi et al., 1994). In a rat model of PD, *N*M(*R*)Sal injected in the *striatum* may be taken up into dopaminergic terminals by a dopamine transport system. *N*M(*R*)Sal is transported by retrograde axonal flow to cell body in the *substantia nigra,* oxidized into DMD-HIQ$^+$ and accumulated, as shown by analysis of the rat brain regions. Recently, *N*M(*R*)Sal

Dopamine neuron

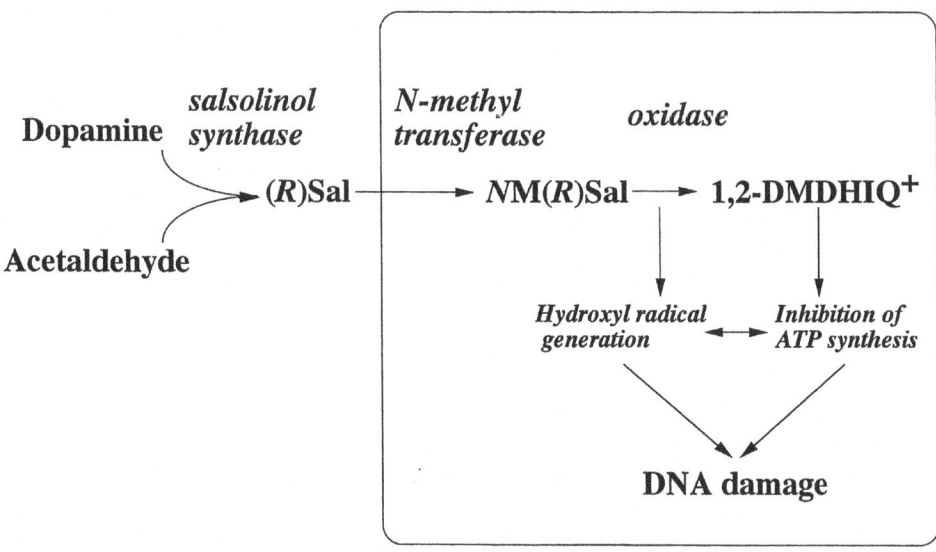

Fig. 10 The mechanism of cytotoxicity of *N*M(*R*)Sal to dopamine neurons. (*R*)Sal is biosynthesized from dopamine and acetaldehyde by a (*R*)salsolinol synthase. *N*-Methylation of
(*R*)Sal into *N*M(*R*)Sal increases the selectivity to dopamine neurons and oxidation of this
catechol isoquinoline generates hydroxyl radical and a potent neurotoxin, 1,2-DMDHIQ⁺.
Hydroxyl radical itself is cytotoxic, and also induces DNA damage.

and DMDHIQ⁺ were found to accumulate in the nigro-striatal system in the human brain
(Maruyama et al., 1997a). This catechol isoquinolinium ion is more cytotoxic than the
reduced isoquinoline (Naoi et al., 1996c). Oxidation of *N*M(*R*)Sal simultaneously produces
hydroxyl radicals, as shown by *in vivo* (Maruyama et al., 1995b) and *in vitro* studies
(Maruyama et al., 1995a). The selective depletion of dopamine neurons was confirmed in
the *substantia nigra,* where, however, no remarkable necrotic tissue reaction was observed.
These results suggest that the cell death of dopamine neurons caused by *N*M(*R*)Sal may be
not necrotic, but apoptotic, whereas an injection of DMDHIQ⁺ induced necrosis. Indeed,
recently we found that apoptotic DNA damage is induced by *N*M(*R*)Sal, but not by DMD-
HIQ⁺ or by other catechol isoquinolines (Naoi et al., 1997; Maruyama et al., 1997b).

    In relation to pathogenesis of PD, we analyzed the cerebrospinal fluid of untreated
patients with PD, and the *N*M(*R*)Sal level was found to increase significantly by comparison with control or with a disease control, the multiple system atrophy (Maruyama et al.,
1996a). The level of *N*M(*R*)Sal in cerebrospinal fluid was 8.32 ± 2.89 nM (mean $\pm$ SD) for
parkinsonian patients, whereas 4.55 ± 2.08 and 3.59 ± 1.52 nM for control and for patients
with multiple system atrophy, respectively. We should emphasize that, in the human brain,
*N*M(*R*)Sal is synthesized by a series of enzymatic reactions; (*R*)-salsolinol synthase enan-
tio-specifically synthesizes (*R*)-salsolinol and a *N*-methyltransferase *N*M(*R*)Sal. The activity of these enzymes and a *N*M(*R*)Sal oxidase may be the endogenous factors involved in

the pathogenesis of PD. The quantitative analysis of these catechol isoquinolines and of the enzymes related to the metabolism are now underway in human brain and in clinical samples.

Acknowledgment

This work was supported by a Grant-In-Aid for Scientific Research on Priority Area and P.D. from the Ministry of Education, Science and Culture, Japan.

References

Bedard P., and Pycock C.J. (1977) "Wet-dog" shake behaviour in the rat: A possible quantitative model of central 5-hydroxytryptamine activity. Neuropharmacology 16:663–670.

Bembenek M.E., Abell C.W., Chrisey L.A., Rowadowska M.D., Gessner W., and Brossi A. (1990) Inhibition of monoamine oxidase A and B by simple isoquinoline alkaloids: racemic and optically active 1,2,3,4-tetrahydro-, 3,4-dihydro-, and fully aromatic isoquinolines. J. Med. Chem. 33:147–152.

Buonamici M., Maj R., Pagani F., Rossi A.C., and Khazan, N. (1986) Tremor at rest episodes in unilaterally 6-OHDA-induced substantia nigra lesioned rat; EEG-EMG and behaviour. Neuropharmacology 25:323–325.

Chiba K., Trevor A.J., and Castagnoli Jr. N. (1984) Metabolism of the neurotoxic amine, MPTP by brain monoamine oxidase. Biochem. Biophys. Res. Commun. 120:574–578.

Chiueh C.C., Miyake H., and Peng M.-T. (1993) Role of dopamine autoxidation, hydroxyl radical generation, and calcium overload in underlying mechanisms involved in MPTP-induced parkinsonism. Adv. Neurol. 60:251–258.

Cohen G. (1976) Alkaloid products in the metabolism of alcohol and biogenic amines. Biochem. Pharmacol. 25:1123–1128.

Collins, M.A. (1994) Potential parkinsonian protoxicants within and without. Neurobiol. Aging 15:277–278.

Colpaert F.C. (1987) Pharmacological characteristics of tremor, rigidity and hypokinesia induced by reserpine in rat. Neuropharmacology 9:1431–1440.

Costal B., Naylor R.J., and Pinder R.M. (1976) Hyperactivity induced by tetrahydroisoquinoline derivatives injected into the nucleus accumbens. Eur. J. Pharmacol. 39:153–160.

Davis G.C., Williams A.C., Markey S.P., Ebert M.H., Caine E.D., Reichert C.W., and Kopin I.J. (1979) Chronic parkinsonism secondary to intravenous injection of meperidine analogous. Psychiatry Res. 1:249–254.

De Duffard A.M.E., Bortolozzi A., and Duffard R.O. (1995) Altered behavioral responses in 2,4-dichlorophenyoxyacetic acid treated and amphetamine challenged rats. Neuro. Toxicology 16:479–488.

Deng Y., Maruyama W., Dostert P., Takahashi T., Kawai M., and Naoi M. (1995) Determination of the (R)- and (S)-enantiomers of salsolinol and N-methylsalsolinol by use of a chiral HPLC column. J. Chromatogr. B. 670:47–54.

Dipasquale B., Marini A.M., and Youle R.J. (1991) Apoptosis and DNA degradation by

1-methyl-4-phenylpyridinium ion in neurons. Biochem. Biophys. Res. Commun. 181:1442–1448.

Dostert P., Strolin Benedetti M., and Dedieu M. (1987) Ratio of enantiomers of salsolinol in human urine. Pharmacol. Toxicol. (Supplement 1) 60:13.

Dostert P., Strolin Benedetti M., Belotti V., Allievi C., and Dordain G. (1990) Biosynthesis of salsolinol, a tetrahydroisoquinoline alkaloid, in healthy subjects. J. Neural Transm. (GenSect) 81:215–223.

Ervin G.N., Fink J.S., Young R.C., and Smith G.P. (1977) Different behavioral responses to L-dopa after anterolateral hypothalamic injections of 6-hydroxydopamine. Brain Res. 132:507–520.

Glennon R., Darmani N., and Martin B. (1991) Multiple population of serotonin receptors may modulate the behavioral effects of serotonergic agents. Life Sci. 48:2493–2498.

Hasegawa E., Takeshige K., Ohishi T., Murai Y., and Murakami S. (1990) 1-Methyl-4-phenylpyridinium ion (MPP$^+$) induces NADH-dependent superoxide formation and enhances NADH-dependent lipid peroxidation in bovine heart submitochondrial particles. Biochem. Biophys. Res. Commun. 170:1049–1055.

Jolicoeuer F.B., Rivest R., and Drumheller A. (1991) Hypokinesia, rigidity, and tremor induced by hypothalamic 6-OHDA lesions in the rat. Brain Res. Bull. 26:317–320.

Liptrop J., Holdup D., and Phillipson O. (1993) 1,2,3,4-Tetrahydro-2-methyl-4,6,7-isoquinolinetriol depletes catecholamines in rat brain. J. Neurochem. 61:2199–2206.

Maruyama W., Nakahara D., Ota M., Takahashi T., Takahashi A., Nagatsu T., and Naoi M. (1992) N-Methylation of dopamine-derived 6,7-dihydroxy-1,2,3,4-tetrahydroisoquinoline, (R)-salsolinol, in rat brains: *In vivo* microdialysis study. J. Neurochem. 59: 395–400.

Maruyama W., and Naoi M. (1994) Inhibition of tyrosine hydroxylase by a dopamine neurotoxin, 1-methyl-4-phenylpyridinium ion: Depletion of allostery to the biopterin cofactor. Life Sci. 55:207–212.

Maruyama W., Dostert P., Matsubara K., and Naoi M. (1995a) N-Methyl(R)salsolinol produces hydroxyl radicals: Involvement to neurotoxicity. Free Rad. Biol. Med. 19:67–75.

Maruyama W., Dostert P., and Naoi M. (1995b) Dopamine-derived 1-methyl-6,7-dihydroxyisoquinolines as hydroxyl radical promoters and scavengers in the rat brain: *In vivo* and *in vitro* studies. J. Neurochem. 64:2635–2643.

Maruyama W., Abe T., Tohgi H., Dostert P., and Naoi M. (1996a) A dopaminergic neurotoxin, (R)-N-methylsalsolinol increases in parkinsonian CSF. Ann. Neurol. 40:199–122.

Maruyama W., Narabayashi H., Dostert P., and Naoi M. (1996b) Stereospecific occurrence of a parkinsonism-inducing catechol isoquinoline, N-methyl(R)salsolinol, in the human intraventricular fluid. J. Neural Transm. 103:1069–1076.

Maruyama W., Sobue G., Matsubara K., Hashizume Y., Dostert P., and Naoi M. (1997a) A dopaminergic neurotoxin, 1(R),2(N)-dimethyl-6,7-dihydroxy-1,2,3,4-tetrahydroisoquinoline, N-methyl(R)salsolinol, and its oxidation product, 1,2(N)-dimethyl-6,7-dihydroxyisoquinolinium ion, accumulate in the nigrostriatal system of the human brain. Neurosci. Lett. 223:61–64.

Maruyama W., Naoi M., Kasamatsu T., Hashizume Y., Takahashi T., Kohda K., and Dostert P. (1997b) An endogenous dopaminergic neurotoxin, N-methyl-(R)-salsolinol, induces DNA damage in human dopaminergic neuroblastoma SH-SY5Y cells. J. Neurochem. 69:322–329.

Matsubara K., Neafsey E.J., and Collins M.A. (1992) Novel S-adenosylmethionine-dependent indole-N-methylation of β-carboline in brain particulate fractions. J. Neurochem. 59:511–518.

Matsubara K. (1996) Occurrence of neurotoxin β-carbolinium cations in mammalian central nervous system. Biogenic Amines 12:161–169.

Mizuno Y., Saitoh T., and Sone N. (1987) Inhibition of mitochondrial NADH-ubiquinone oxidoreductase activity by 1-methyl-4-phenylpyridinium ion. Biochem. Biophys. Res. Commun. 143:294–299.

Myers R.D., and Oblinger M.M. (1997) Alcohol drinking in the rat induced by acute intracerebral infusion of two tetrahydroisoquinolines and a β-carboline. Drug Alcohol Depend. 2:469–483.

Nagatsu T., and Yoshida M. (1988) An endogenous substance of the brain, tetrahydroisoquinoline, produces parkinsonism in primates with decreased dopamine, tyrosine hydroxylase and biopterin in the nigrostriatal regions. Neurosci. Lett. 87:178–182.

Naoi M., Takahashi T., and Nagatsu T. (1988) Simple assay procedure for tyrosine hydroxylase activity by high-performance liquid chromatography employing coulometric detection with minimal sample preparation. J. Chromatogr. 427:229–238.

Naoi M., Matsuura S., Takahashi T., and Nagatsu T. (1989a) A N-methyltransferase in human brain catalyzes N-methylation of 1,2,3,4-tetrahydroisoquinoline in N-methyl-1,2,3,4-tetrahydroisoquinoline, a precursor of a dopaminergic neurotoxin, N-methylisoquinolinium ion. Biochem. Biophys. Res. Commun. 161:1213–1219.

Naoi M., Matsuura S., Parvez H., Takahashi T., Hirata Y., and Nagatsu T. (1989b) Oxidation of N-methyl-1,2,3,4-tetrahydroisoquinoline into N-methylisoquinolinium ion by monoamine oxidase. J. Neurochem. 52:653–655.

Naoi M., Maruyama W., Acworth I.N., Nakahara D., and Parvez H. (1993) Multi-electrode detection system for determination of neurotransmitters. In: Methods in Neurotransmitter and Neuropeptide Research (Parvez H., Naoi M., Nagatsu T., and Parvez S. eds.), Vol. 1. pp. 1–39, Elsevier, Amsterdam.

Naoi M., Maruyama W., and Dostert P. (1994) Binding of 1,2(N)-dimethyl-6,7-dihydroxyisoquinolinium ion to melanin: effects of ferrous and ferric ion on the binding. Neurosci. Lett. 171:9–12.

Naoi M., Maruyama W., Dostert P., Nakahara D., Takahashi T., and Nagatsu T. (1995a) Metabolic bioactivation of endogenous isoquinolines as dopaminergic neurotoxins to elicit Parkinson's disease. In: Alzheimer's and Parkinson's diseases; Recent Development (Hanin I. S., Yoshida M., and Fisher A., eds.), pp. 553–559, Plenum, New York.

Naoi M., Maruyama W., and Dostert P. (1995b) Dopamine-derived 6,7-dihydroxy-1,2,3,4-tetrahydroisoquinolines; Oxidation and neurotoxicity. Prog. Brain Res. 106:227–239.

Naoi M., Maruyama W., Zhang J.H., Takahashi T., Deng Y., and Dostert P. (1995c) Enzymatic oxidation of the dopaminergic neurotoxin, 1(R),2(N)-dimethyl-6,7-dihydroxy-1,2,3,4-tetrahydroisoquinoline, into 1,2(N)-dimethyl-6,7-dihydroxyisoquinolinium ion. Life Sci. 57:1061–1066.

Naoi M., Maruyama W., Dostert P., Hashizume Y., Nakahara D., Takahashi T., and Ota M. (1996a) Dopamine-derived endogenous 1(R),2(N)-dimethyl-6,7-dihydroxy-1,2,3,4-tetrahydroisoquinoline, N-methyl-(R)-salsolinol, induced parkinsonism in rat: Biochemical pathological and behavioral studies. Brain Res. 709:285–295.

Naoi M., Maruyama W., Dostert P., Kohda K., and Kaiya T. (1996b) A novel enzyme enantio-selectively synthesizes (R)salsolinol, a precursor of a dopaminergic neurotoxin, N-methyl(R)salsolinol. Neurosci. Lett. 212:183–186.

Naoi M., Maruyama W., Dostert P., and Hashizume Y. (1996c) Animal model of Parkinson's disease induced by naturely-occurring 1(R), 2(N)-dimethyl-6,7-dihydroxy-1,2,3,4-tetrahydroisoquinoline. Biogenic Amines 12:135–147.

Naoi M., Maruyama W., Dostert P., and Hashizume Y. (1997) N-Methyl-(R)salsolinol as a dopaminergic neurotoxin: From an animal model to an early marker of Parkinson's disease. J. Neural Transm. (Suppl) 50:89–105.

Nicklas W.J., Vyas I., and Heikkila R.E. (1985) Inhibition of NADH-linked oxidation in brain mitochondria by 1-methyl-4-phenylpyridine, a metabolite of the neurotoxin, 1-methyl-4-phenyl-1,2,3,6-tetrahydropyridine. Life Sci. 36:2503–2508.

Nitta A., Murase Y., Furukawa Y., Hayashi K., Hasegawa T., and Nabeshima T. (1993) Memory impairment and neural dysfunction after continuous infusion of anti-nerve growth factor antibody into the septum in adult rats. Neuroscience 57:495–499.

Niwa T., Takeda N., Kaneda N., Hashizume Y., and Nagatsu T. (1987) Presence of tetrahydroisoquinoline and 2-methyltetrahydroquinoline in parkinsonian and control brains. Biochem. Biophys. Res. Commun. 144:1084–1089.

Ohta S., Kohno M., Makino Y., Tachikawa O., and Hirobe M. (1987) Tetrahydroisoquinoline and 1-methyl-tetrahydroisoquinoline are present in the human brain; Relation to Parkinson's disease. Biomed. Res. 8:453–456.

Origitano T., Hamingen J., and Collins M.A. (1961) Rat brain salsolinol and blood-brain-barrier. Brain Res. 274:446–451.

Paxinos G. and Watson C. (1986) The rat brain in stereotaxic coordinates, 2nd Ed. Academic Press, Sidney.

Reading P.J., and Dunnett S.B. (1996) 6-Hydroxydopamine lesions of nigrostriatal neurons as an animal model of Parkinson's disease. In: Toxin-induced models of neurological disorders (Woodruff M.L. and Nonneman A.J. eds.), pp. 89–119, Plenum Press, New York, London.

Robinson T.E., and Becker J.B. (1986) Enduring change in brain and behavior produced by chronic amphetamine administration: A review and evaluation of animal models of amphetamine psychosis. Brain Res. Rev. 11:157–198.

Sallström Baum S., and Rommelspacher H. (1994) Determination of total dopamine, R- and S-salsolinol in human plasma by cyclodextrin bonded-phase liquid chromatography with electrochemical detection. J. Chromatogr. B. 600:235–241.

Sandler M., Carter S.B., Hunter K.R., and Stern G.M. (1973) Tetrahydroisoquinoline alkaloids, *in vivo* metabolism of L-dopa in man. Nature 241:439–443.

Singer T.P., Castagnoli Jr. N., Ramsay R.R., and Trevor A.J. (1987) Biochemical events in the development of parkinsonism induced by 1-methyl-4-phenyl-1,2,3,6-tetrahydropyridine. J. Neurochem. 49:1–8.

Sjöquist B., Eriksson A., and Winblad B. (1982) Salsolinol and catecholamines in human brain and their relation to alcoholism. Prog. Clin. Biol. Res. 90:57–67.

Spanos L.J., and Yamamoto B.K. (1989) Acute and subchronic effects of methylenedioxymethamphetamine [(±)MDMA] on locomotion and serotonin syndrome behavior in the rat. Pharmacol. Biochem. Behavior 32:835–840.

Strolin Benedetti M., Belloti V., Pianezola E., Carminati P., and Dostert P. (1989) Ratio of the R and S enantiomers of salsolinol in food and human urine. J. Neural Transm. 77:47–53.

Takahashi T., Deng Y., Maruyama W., Dostert P., Kawai M., and Naoi M. (1994) Uptake of a neurotoxin-candidate, (R)-1,2-dimethyl-6,7-dihydroxy-1,2,3,4-tetrahydroisoquinoline into human dopaminergic neuroblastoma SH-SY5Y cells by dopamine transport system. J. Neural Transm. (GenSect) 98:107–118.

Teitel S., O'Brien J., and Brossi A. (1972) Alkaloids in mammalian tissues, synthesis of (+) and (-) substituted 6,7-dihydroxy-1,2,3,4-tetrahydroisoquinolines. J. Med. Chem. 15:845–846.

Tipton K.F., and Singer T.P. (1993) Advances in our understanding of the mechanisms of the neurotoxicity of MPTP and related compounds. J. Neurochem. 61:1191–1206.

Ungerstedt U., Avemo A., Avemo E., Ljungberg T., and Ranje C. (1973) Animal models of parkinsonism. In: Advances in Neurology, Vol. 3 (Calne D. B., ed.), pp. 257–271, Raven Press, New York.

Whitehouse P.J., Price D.L., Struble R.G., Clark A.W., Coyle J.T., and DeLong M.R. (1982) Alzheimer's disease and senile dementia: Loss of neurons in the basal formation. Science 215:1237–1239.

Zang L.-Y., and Misra H.P. (1992) EPR kinetic studies of superoxide radicals generated during the autoxidation of 1-methyl-4-phenyl-2,3-dihydroxypyridine, a bioactivated intermediate of Parkinsonism-inducing neurotoxin, 1-methyl-4-phenyl-1,2,3,6-tetra-hydropyridine. J. Biol. Chem. 267:23601–23608.

Putative Endogenous Neurotoxins Derived from the Biogenic Amine Neurotransmitters

Glenn Dryhurst

Contents in Brief

1. Introduction

5-Hydroxytryptamine (5-HT; serotonin) and the catecholamines dopamine (DA), norepinephrine (NE), and epinephrine (EPI) together are known as the biogenic amine neurotransmitters in the central and peripheral nervous systems. Only a minute fraction of the many billions of neurons in the brain employ biogenic amines as neurotransmitters. However, probably owing to their remarkable axonal divergence and wide distribution throughout the brain, serotonergic, dopaminergic and noradrenergic neurons appear to play disproportionately important roles in many physiological processes. Furthermore, a remarkable number of psychoactive drugs that include neuroleptics, antidepressants and stimulants in addition to many hallucinogens mediate their effects in large part as a consequence of their interactions with one or more biogenic amine neuronal pathways in the brain. Such observations have led to a number of hypotheses implicating disturbances of serotonergic, dopaminergic, and noradrenergic systems in the brain with mental illnesses such as schizophrenia and affective psychoses.

It is also of interest that the two major neurodegenerative disorders of the brain, Alzheimer's disease (AD) and Parkinson's disease (PD), both result in the progressive and severe degeneration of a subset of neurons that include selected biogenic amine pathways. Similarly, transient cerebral ischemia (ischemia-reperfusion or stroke) and drugs of abuse such as methamphetamine (MA) and related amphetamines also evoke profound degeneration of certain biogenic amine pathways in the brain. Such observations raise an important question concerning reasons why only selected biogenic amine pathways are vulnerable to degeneration in these brain disorders while others are spared. Furthermore, the possibility arises that the biogenic amine neurotransmitters or unusual metabolites derived from them might play roles in the neurodegenerative processes.

Of potential relevance to this suggestion are growing lines of evidence implicating oxidative stress in neuronal death in anatomically selective regions of the brain in AD, PD, ischemia-reperfusion and as a consequence of neurotoxic doses of MA and other amphetamine drugs. Oxidative stress refers to a condition when the production of partially reduced or reactive oxygen species (ROS) such as superoxide radical anion ($O_2-\cdot$), hydrogen peroxide (H_2O_2), and hydroxyl radical (HO·) exceeds the protective capacities of endogenous defense mechanisms of the cell (Simonian and Coyle, 1996). It is widely assumed that cellular damage caused by ROS in the brain is sustained by lipids, proteins, and nucleic acids (Halliwell and Gutteridge, 1987; Floyd, 1990; Halliwell, 1992a,b).

However, the biogenic amines share one chemical property that distinguishes them in a very important way from all other known or putative neurotransmitters: ease of oxidation. Thus, under pathological conditions when oxidative stress develops in regions of the brain innervated by biogenic aminergic neurons it is extremely unlikely, from a chemical perspective, that these neurotransmitters could escape oxidation while lipids, proteins, and nucleic acids undergo oxidative modifications. This statement applies most particularly to biogenic amines that are present in the neuronal cytoplasm or synaptic cleft. This also raises the possibility that the resulting oxidative metabolites of 5-HT, DA, and NE might play roles in neurodegenerative processes in the brain and, indeed, in chemical reactions responsible for the initial generation or potentiation of oxygen radical formation.

Such a possibility provides one plausible rationalization for the selective degeneration of certain biogenic amine pathways in neurodegenerative disorders such as AD and PD. This idea also draws some support from the fact that very minor oxidative modification to 5-HT and DA, for example, results in the formation of powerful (and widely used) neurotoxins. For example, 5,6-dihydroxytryptamine (5,6-DHT) and 5,7-dihydroxytryptamine (5,7-DHT) are serotonergic neurotoxins (Baumgarten et al., 1975; Baumgarten and Björklund, 1976; Jacoby and Lytle, 1978; Tabatabaie and Dryhurst, 1997) and 6-hydroxydopamine (6-OHDA) is a catecholaminergic neurotoxin (Kostrzewa and Jacobowicz, 1974).

In this chapter evidence will be reviewed that demonstrates the vulnerability of particular biogenic amine neurotransmitter pathways to degeneration in AD, as a consequence of ischemia-reperfusion, and neurotoxic doses of MA. These apparently disparate brain disorders and drug regimen have been selected for consideration for a number of reasons. Thus, ischemia-reperfusion and MA both evoke the degeneration of certain biogenic amine terminals and it is likely that the initial stages of AD affects nerve terminals rather than cell bodies. Furthermore, oxidative stress is an important factor in the degeneration that occurs in the brain in AD and as a result of ischemia-reperfusion and MA administration. Experiments with laboratory animals increasingly point to the conclusion that the neurodegeneration of biogenic amine terminals resulting from ischemia-reperfusion and MA might be mediated either by their neurotransmitters or aberrant oxidative metabolites. Furthermore, several lines of evidence suggest that one biogenic amine neurotransmitter or an aberrant metabolite might also contribute to the degeneration of a second biogenic aminergic neuronal system and, indeed, other neuronal systems. Evidence that oxygen radical-mediated or some other form of aberrant oxidative metabolism of biogenic amines actually occurs in the brain in AD or as a result of ischemia-reperfusion or MA administration and that such processes or resulting metabolites play roles in selective neurodegeneration is scientifically weak.

However, very recent experiments begin to provide some support for this hypothesis. Key questions, therefore, relate to the identities of putative aberrant oxidative metabolites of the biogenic amines and their neurobiological properties. The possibility of trapping, isolating, and unequivocally identifying such metabolites formed in the brain, which are likely to be evanescent species, is remote. Nevertheless, studies of the *in vitro* oxidation chemistry of 5-HT, DA and NE under conditions that approximate their physiological environment permits the isolation and identification of their putative oxidative metabolites, and subsequent evaluation of their neurochemical, neurobehavioral, and neurobiological properties. Accordingly, the present status of the *in vitro* oxidation chemistry of the biogenic amines will be reviewed along with relevant *in vitro* and *in vivo* properties of the resulting reaction products.

2. Alzheimer's Disease

Alzheimer's disease (AD) is a progressive neurodegenerative disorder that affects multiple neurotransmitter systems, but in rather remarkably selective anatomic regions of the brain. To illustrate, AD is characterized by degeneration of pyramidal neurons in the frontal and temporal cortex, hippocampus and amygdala (Ball, 1977; Pearson et al., 1985; Hubbard and Anderson, 1985; Hyman et al., 1987; Proctor et al., 1988; Palmer, 1991). Substantial losses of glutamatergic neurons occur in these regions (Hyman et al., 1987; Proctor et al., 1988) of the brain along with decreased levels of somatostatin (Beal et al., 1986) and perhaps vasoactive intestinal peptide (Arai et al., 1984). In addition, long cholinergic (Davies and Maloney, 1976; Perry et al., 1977; Bowen et al., 1983; Palmer and Bowen, 1990), noradrenergic (Mann et al., 1982; Tomlinson et al., 1982; Palmer et al., 1987a), and serotonergic (Bowen et al., 1983; Yamamoto and Hirano, 1985; Palmer et al., 1987b; D'Amato et al., 1987; Tejani-Butt et al., 1995) neurons that project from subcortical cell bodies in the nucleus basalis of Meynert (NBM), locus ceruleus (LC), and raphe nuclei (RN), respectively, to the cortex and hippocampus also degenerate in AD. Thus, neurons that undergo the most profound degeneration in AD are either located entirely within certain regions of the cortex or hippocampus/amygdala complex or project from subcortical cell bodies and connect to the latter structures.

The apparent importance of the connectivity of subcortical neurons with the cortex draws support, for example, from the observation that noradrenergic neurons that project from rostral regions of the LC to the cortex undergo severe degeneration in AD, whereas more caudal LC cell bodies that project to the cerebellum and spinal cord are spared (Marcyniuk et al., 1986; German et al., 1987). Such a selective pattern of neuronal degeneration suggests it is the anatomic location of neurons that is important to their vulnerability to degeneration in AD. Indeed, it has been argued that such an anatomically-selective pattern of neuronal damage in AD does not support a random appearance of brain lesions, but rather points to a progression of the disease from defined starting points along specific connecting neuronal pathways (Saper et al., 1987). Such a *system neurodegeneration* might therefore point to the transfer of one or more pathogens between connected neurons.

A number of lines of evidence suggest that the primary lesions in AD occur in nerve terminals located in the association areas of the cortex and hippocampus, sites of intense senile plaque (SP) formation (Perry et al., 1982; Mann, 1988). SPs are extraneuronal markers of degenerating nerve terminals and are one of the characteristic neuropathological hallmarks of AD. Hardy et al. (1985) have suggested that AD might be initiated by some form of chronic attack on the axon terminals of long serotonergic, noradrenergic and, perhaps, cholinergic neurons that project from subcortical cell bodies where they innervate blood capillaries in certain regions of the cortex and hippocampus (Edvinsson et al., 1983; Kaleria et al., 1989). These investigators further hypothesized that an environmental toxicant, virus or other pathogen might enter these nerve terminals from microvessels and evoke retrograde degeneration of these and connected neurons by transneuronal transfer of the toxin. This concept provides an elegant rationale for the anatomic selectivity of the neurodegeneration that occurs in AD, i.e., why certain neuronal pathways are vulnerable, whereas others utilizing identical neurotransmitters but in other regions of the brain are spared. However, there is little evidence for the involvement of a specific environmental toxicants or other exogenous pathogens in initiating and propagating the neurodegeneration that occurs in AD.

There are, however, many lines of evidence that oxidative stress plays an important role in the pathogenesis of AD. To illustrate, increased levels of protein oxidation (Smith et al., 1991) increased activities of superoxide dismutase (SOD) (Zemlan et al., 1989; Pappolla et al., 1992), glucose-6-phosphate dehydrogenase (Martins et al., 1986) and glutathione peroxidase (Annarén et al., 1986) and increased lipid peroxidation (Hajimohammadadreza and Brammer, 1990; Subbarao et al., 1990; Palmer and Burns, 1994) all occur in regions of the brain that degenerate in AD. Indeed, recent evidence suggests that low molecular weight products of lipid peroxidation crosslink apolipoprotein E (Montine et al., 1996). Apolipoprotein E genotype is a major determinant of vulnerability to late onset AD. Furthermore, there is evidence that oxygen radicals play a role in the transformation of soluble β-amyloid peptide (βAP) into the aggregated form found at the core of SPs (Dyrks et al., 1992). βAP appears to be toxic towards cultured neurons, particularly in its aggregated form (Koh et al., 1990; Yanker et al., 1990; Pike et al., 1993), leading to the hypothesis that AD is caused by this peptide. Indeed, introduction of suspensions of SP cores from postmortem AD brains into the rat hippocampus evokes localized neurodegeneration (Frautshy et al., 1991). Furthermore, *in vitro* studies reveal that βAP fragments into free radical peptides that potentiate oxygen radical formation which, in turn, might contribute to lipid peroxidation and damage to proteins (Hensley et al., 1994). Polymerization of tau protein, the major component of neurofibrillary tangles (NFTs), has also been associated with oxidative stress (Troncoso et al., 1993).

NFTs are intraneuronal markers for degenerating cell bodies and are another neuropathological hallmark of AD. Elevated levels of heme oxygenase-1, induced by oxidative stress, have been found in SPs, neurons containing NFTs, and glial cells in AD brains (Smith et al., 1994; Schipper et al., 1995). Furthermore, a major increase of mitochondrial 8-hydroxydeoxyguanosine, a marker for oxygen radical-mediated oxidation of DNA, has been measured in the AD brain (Mecocci et al., 1994). Key questions that emerge from the preceding information concern the source(s) of abnormally elevated levels of oxygen radical species and, particularly, the issue of the anatomic selectivity of the neurodegeneration that occurs in AD. In other words, whether the neurodegenerative mechanisms are directly caused by oxidative stress and/or βAP neurotoxicity or other mechanisms, it seems to be of paramount importance to address the reasons why neurons utilizing diverse neurotransmitters are damaged/destroyed in certain regions of the AD brain but spared in others.

Both $O_2-\cdot$ and H_2O_2 are byproducts of many normal metabolic processes. Furthermore, mitochondria are a major source of intracellular oxygen radicals (Freeman and Crapo, 1982). Normally, $O_2-\cdot$ is rapidly transformed into H_2O_2 and molecular oxygen by SOD, and then H_2O_2 is converted to water and molecular oxygen by glutathione peroxidase or catalase. However, under abnormal conditions these protective mechanisms may be inadequate with the result that $HO\cdot$ is formed from H_2O_2 by the Fenton reaction (Eq. 1) or from $O_2-\cdot$ and H_2O_2 in the Haber-Weiss

$$Fe^{2+} + H_2O_2 \rightarrow Fe^{3+} + HO^- + HO\cdot \tag{1}$$

$$Fe^{3+} + O_2-\cdot \rightarrow Fe^{2+} + O_2^{2-}$$

$$HO^- + HO\cdot \qquad\qquad H_2O_2 \tag{2}$$

reaction (Eq. 2). Both of these reactions require the presence of catalytic amounts of low molecular weight iron or certain other transition metal ion species (Pryor, 1986; Halliwell and Gutteridge, 1987). Formation of $O_2-\cdot$ also occurs by reaction between low molecular weight Fe^{2+} and molecular oxygen (Eq. 3). Hydroxyl radical ($HO\cdot$) is an extraordinarily reactive species and one of the most powerful oxidants known (Slivka and Cohen, 1985). Superoxide ($O_2-\cdot$) is generally considered to be a less aggressive oxidant, although it is capable of oxidizing catecholamines (Cohen, 1994) and 5-HT (Wrona and Dryhurst, unpublished results). Clearly, therefore, low molecular weight iron species have the potential to mediate oxygen radical formation.

$$Fe^{2+} + O_2 \rightarrow Fe^{3+} + O_2-\cdot \tag{3}$$

Thus, it may be of some significance to note that AD patients have increased cerebrospinal fluid (CSF)/serum ratios for immunoglobin and albumin and greatly elevated CSF albumin levels (Alafuzoff et al., 1983) that, together with localization of immunoglobins and other serum proteins within brain parenchyma (Wisniewski and Kozlowski, 1982; Mann, 1988), are consistent with an increased blood-brain barrier (BBB) permeability (Mann, 1988). Furthermore, SPs in the AD brain are always geographically close to or present in blood capillaries (Miyakawa et al., 1982) which also points to a hematogeneous role in the disease (Mann, 1988). Indeed, increased levels of iron have been detected in NFTs (Good et al., 1992). In addition, head trauma is a risk factor for AD (French et al., 1985; Mortimer et al., 1985; Shalat et al., 1986) and liberates low molecular weight iron, increases oxygen radical formation (Wei and Kontos, 1987; Aust, 1988; Hall and Braughler, 1988; Halliwell, 1992a,b; Hall et al., 1994), and leads to βAP formation (Roberts et al., 1991) and neuropathological features in the brain similar to those in AD (Rudelli et al, 1982). Thus, an early event in the pathogenesis of AD might be traced to the permeability of the BBB caused, *inter alia,* by head trauma, exposure to certain environmental toxicants, and/or genetic factors. Bleeding releases hemoglobin (Halliwell, 1992a) and low molecular weight iron species (Gutteridge, 1986) from erythrocytes that can mediate oxygen radical formation (Eqs. 1–3) (Puppo and Halliwell, 1988). Oxygen radicals and iron within or in close proximity to serotonergic or noradrenergic nerve terminals that innervate blood capillaries could therefore contribute not only to lipid peroxidation, protein, and DNA oxidation, but also to oxidation of 5-HT and NE. Should such oxidations of 5-HT and NE lead to products and byproducts (e.g., oxygen radicals) that are toxic towards not only serotonergic and noradrenergic neurons, respectively, but also to connected neurons as a consequence of transneuronal transfer, then a plausible rationalization for the anatomically-selective system neurodegeneration in AD emerges.

Many hypotheses have been advanced to explain the neurodegeneration that occurs in AD. These include genetic defects (Brumbach and Leech, 1994), the βAP hypothesis discussed earlier, excitotoxic mechanisms mediated by excitatory amino acid neurotransmitters (e.g., glutamate) acting on N-methyl-D-aspartate (NMDA) receptors (Greenamyre et al., 1985; Greenamyre and Young, 1989), altered intraneuronal Ca^{2+} homeostasis (Colvin et al., 1991; Mattson, 1992; Ito et al., 1994), mitochondrial abnormalities (Sims et al., 1987; Blass et al., 1990), and others. Interestingly, oxidative glutamate neurotoxicity (Murphy et al., 1989; Choi, 1992) appears to be dependent on uptake of biogenic amines into target neurons and intraneuronal oxidation by an unknown enzyme in reactions that generate cytotoxic levels of oxygen radicals (Maher and Davis, 1996).

However, these hypotheses fail to adequately address reasons for the anatomic selectivity of the neurodegeneration that occurs in AD. By contrast, in the event that 5-HT and NE or aberrant oxidative metabolites of these neurotransmitters formed in the terminals of serotonergic and noradrenergic axon terminals in the cortex and hippocampus mediate the retrograde degeneration of these and connected neurons as a result of axonal and transneuronal transport, then a plausible and experimentally testable hypothesis for the system degeneration in AD emerges. Evidence for such biogenic amine/aberrant metabolite - mediated system degeneration mechanisms can be drawn from animal studies of ischemia-reperfusion and MA administration.

3. Ischemia-Reperfusion

Experimentally-induced ischemia in laboratory animals evokes a massive release of 5-HT (Pulsinelli et al., 1982), NE (Globus et al., 1989), and DA (Brannan et al., 1987; Phebus and Clemens, 1989) with a smaller, more transient release of glutamate and aspartate (Benveniste et al., 1984). Upon reperfusion (reoxygenation), following transient forebrain ischemia, serotonergic, noradrenergic, and dopaminergic terminals (Weinberger et al., 1983), CA1 cells of the hippocampus, and cells in layers 3, 5 and 6 of the cortex (Pulsinelli and Brierley, 1979; Volpe et al., 1984; Sapolsky and Pulsinelli, 1985) degenerate in rat brain. Accumulating evidence suggests that tissue injury occurs almost exclusively during the reperfusion phase and is mediated directly or indirectly by oxygen radicals (Floyd, 1990; Oliver et al., 1990). For example, the generation of $O_2-\cdot$ (Kontos and Wei, 1986) and H_2O_2 (Hyslop et al., 1995) has been demonstrated during reperfusion of ischemic brain, and increased lipid peroxidation occurs (Yoshida et al., 1984; Oliver et al., 1990; Sakamoto et al., 1991). Furthermore, transgenic mice that overexpress Cu-Zn SOD are provided with significant protection against reperfusion injury following an ischemic insult (Kinouchi et al., 1991; Yang et al., 1994). Similarly, antioxidants reduce brain damage resulting from ischemia-reperfusion (Hall et al., 1988; Clemens et al., 1993). Because depletion of striatal DA levels protects medium-sized striatal neurons against ischemia-reperfusion-induced damage (Clemens and Phebus, 1988), it has been suggested that the MAO-mediated metabolism and autoxidation of this neurotransmitter generates cytotoxic levels of H_2O_2, and $O_2-\cdot$, respectively (Hyslop et al., 1995).

During the ischemic period intraneuronal levels of ATP fall, xanthine accumulates

(Onodera et al., 1986), and Ca^{2+} influx triggers proteolytic cleavage of xanthine dehydrogenase to form xanthine oxidase (XOD) (Kinuta et al., 1989). Thus, when oxygen is restored upon reperfusion, XOD catalyzes oxidation of xanthine to uric acid with concomitant formation of $O_2-\cdot$ and H_2O_2. Blood capillaries in the brain are probably the prime site of $O_2-\cdot$ and H_2O_2 formation by this mechanism (Betz, 1985). The resulting endothelial injury could thus cause an increase in capillary permeability (Del Maestro et al., 1981) and a breakdown of the BBB (Chan et al., 1984) with release of hemoglobin and low molecular weight iron. Furthermore, $O_2-\cdot$ is also capable of releasing iron from storage proteins such as ferritin (Yoshida et al., 1995). Thus, ischemia-reperfusion not only leads to the release of the biogenic amine neurotransmitters, but also a number of mechanisms exist by which ROS could potentially be generated that in turn could oxidize these compounds. That the biogenic amines and/or aberrant oxidative metabolites play roles in the neurodegeneration is supported by many lines of evidence. To illustrate, surgical or pharmacologic manipulations that deplete NE or DA in certain brain regions protect against neuronal damage caused by ischemia-reperfusion (Busto et al., 1985; Weinberger et al., 1985; Globus et al., 1987; Siesjö, 1988). It is of particular interest that α-methyl-*p*-tyrosine (AMT), a DA and NE synthesis inhibitor, attenuates not only damage to dopaminergic and noradrenergic terminals but also protects glutamatergic neurons against ischemia-reperfusion-induced damage (Weinberger and Cohen, 1983; Weinberger et al., 1985; Clemens and Phebus, 1988).

Ischemia-reperfusion also results in the depletion of glutathione (GSH) in the cortex, but without any corresponding increase in glutathione disulfide (GSSG) (Rehncrona et al., 1980; Cooper et al., 1980). This apparently irreversible loss of GSH becomes more pronounced with time after reperfusion of the brain. Protection against neuronal damage is also provided by NMDA receptor antagonists (Gill et al., 1987), other Ca^{2+} channel blockers (Nakayama et al., 1988), ω-conotoxin (N-type calcium channel) receptor antagonists (Ooboshi et al., 1992), and pharmacologic agents that elevate extracellular levels of gamma aminobutyric acid (GABA) (Sternau et al., 1989). Taken together, the preceding observations might point to a very complex but interconnected sequence of events that mediate the neurodegeneration that occurs following ischemia-reperfusion. Thus, not only do dopaminergic, noradrenergic, and serotonergic terminals degenerate, but one or more of the neurotransmitters employed by these neurons or unusual metabolites derived from them appear to be involved both in their degeneration and of glutamatergic and possibly other neurons by mechanisms that involve oxygen radicals, glutamate and NMDA receptors, ω-conotoxin receptors, GABA receptors, altered Ca^{2+} homeostasis, and mitochondrial abnormalities (Pulsinelli et al., 1982; Pulsinelli and Duffy, 1983; Choi, 1988; Siesjö, 1992; Meldrum, 1993; Coyle and Puttfarcken, 1993), and the irreversible consumption of GSH (Cooper et al., 1980; Rehncrona et al., 1980).

4. Methamphetamine (MA)

Administration of MA to the rat evokes release of large quantities of 5-HT, DA and NE (O'Dell et al., 1991; Bowyer et al., 1993; Bowyer and Holson, 1995), a rapid and profound decrease of tryptophan hydroxylase (TPH) activity and, using a multiple dose regimen, decreased tyrosine hydroxylase (TH) activity (Bakhit and Gibb, 1981; Peat et al., 1985). Repeated low doses or a single large dose of MA to the rat results in the degeneration of serotonergic and dopaminergic nerve terminals in certain regions of the brain (Gibb et al., 1994; Bowyer and Holson, 1995; Seiden and Sabol, 1995) and a subpopulation of unidentified cell bodies in the somatosensory cortex (Commins and Seiden, 1986), although nora-drenergic terminals are apparently spared (Wagner et al., 1980; Ricaurte et al., 1984). The neurodegeneration evoked by MA does not appear to be mediated directly by either the drug or any of its known metabolites (Gibb et al., 1994; Seiden and Sabol, 1995). However, many lines of evidence implicate oxygen radicals in the neurodegenerative and other neu-robiological changes induced by MA. To illustrate, antioxidants attenuate MA-induced depletions of 5-HT and DA in rat brain (DeVito and Wagner, 1989). Similarly, Cu-Zn SOD transgenic mice are protected against MA-induced depletions of DA (Cadet et al., 1994; Hirata et al., 1995, 1996), whereas SOD inhibition exacerbates decrements of DA and 5-HT (DeVito and Wagner, 1989). Decreased THP activity that occurs rapidly following MA administration also appears to result from oxidation of sulfhydryl residues within the enzyme molecule presumably by oxygen radicals (Stone et al., 1989). Indeed, evidence has been presented that MA induces HO· formation in the brains of mice (Kondo et al., 1992, 1993). That DA, NE or aberrant metabolites of these neurotransmitters play important roles in the neurodegenerative effects of MA can be inferred from the observations that AMT attenuates the MA-induced degeneration of striatal dopaminergic terminals, serotonergic terminals in cortex and hippocampus, and unknown cell bodies in the somatosensory cor-tex (Commins and Seiden, 1986; Axt et al., 1990). The cortex and particularly the hip-pocampus and somatosensory cortex have little or, in the latter structure, negligible dopaminergic input. Thus, such results strongly point to NE or an abnormal metabolite of this neurotransmitter in mediating MA-induced degeneration of serotonergic terminals in the hippocampus and cortex and unknown cell bodies in the somatosensory cortex. Along the same lines, selective DA uptake inhibitors protect striatal dopaminergic terminals, and perhaps might attenuate damage to serotonergic terminals in the cortex and hippocampus, against MA-induced damage (Schmidt and Gibb, 1985; Schmidt et al., 1985). Similarly, selective 5-HT uptake inhibitors protect serotonergic terminals, but exacerbate MA-induced damage to dopaminergic terminals (Ricaurte et al., 1983). Although several lines of evidence suggest an intact DA system is necessary for MA-induced neurotoxicity towards both dopaminergic and serotonergic terminals in certain brain regions (Wagner et al., 1983; Schmidt et al., 1985; Axt et al., 1990), perhaps mediated by DA or an aberrant metabolite (Wagner et al., 1983; Sonsalla et al., 1986), it is worth again stressing the point that studies leading to this conclusion almost always neglect the fact that pharmacologic agents that interfere with dopaminergic neurons also often affect noradrenergic neurons.

Furthermore, as Seiden and Sabol (1995) have noted, the MA-induced damage to sero-tonergic terminals often occurs in brain regions having little or no dopaminergic innerva-tion. The somatosensory cortex, for example, has virtually undetectable levels of DA yet MA evokes degeneration of unidentified cell bodies in this structure. However, this degen-eration is attenuated by AMT. Because AMT inhibits not only DA but also NE synthesis, it becomes possible that the latter neurotransmitter and/or 5-HT or aberrant metabolites might also be involved in MA-induced neurodegeneration.

In parallel with their ability to attenuate neuronal damage caused by ischemia-reper-fusion, NMDA receptor antagonists protect against MA-induced damage to dopaminergic (Sonsalla et al., 1991) and serotonergic terminals (Farfel et al., 1992), although this may be related to a temperature effect (Bowyer and Holson, 1995), as do pharmacologic agents that elevate extracellular GABA levels in the brain (Hotchkiss and Gibb, 1980a). MA-induced dopaminergic neurotoxicity can also be prevented by DA_1 or DA_2 receptor antagonists (Buening and Gibb, 1974; Hotchkiss and Gibb, 1980b, Sonsalla et al., 1986). The turnover of DA in mice treated with such receptor antagonists and MA is much greater than with MA alone, indicating that it is not only the amount of DA released into the synapse but also its subsequent postsynaptic actions that are important in generating neurotoxicity (Sonsalla et al., 1991).

The results of studies into the neurodegenerative consequences of ischemia-reperfusion and MA strongly implicate DA or an unknown metabolite in the processes that mediate degeneration of dopaminergic terminals. However, these studies also point to a role for DA and NE or unknown metabolites of these neurotransmitters in the degeneration of serotonergic terminals and other non-biogenic aminergic neurons. Experiments designed to investigate 5-HT depletion on the degeneration of serotonergic terminals or other neurons remain to be carried out. Nevertheless, the fact that 5-HT uptake inhibitors protect serotonergic terminals but exacerbate MA-induced damage to dopaminergic terminals implicate 5-HT or an unknown metabolite in the neurodegeneration of both serotonergic and dopaminergic terminals. In other words, as has been suggested in AD, it appears that both ischemia-reperfusion and MA evoke a system neurodegeneration in which 5-HT, DA and NE or aberrant metabolites in some way contribute not only the degeneration of their parent terminals but also, perhaps by transneuronal transfer of toxins, the degeneration of connected neurons. While there is some evidence that DA and NE might themselves be neurotoxins under certain conditions (see later discussion) the clear involvement of oxidative stress in AD, ischemia-reperfusion, and MA-induced neurodegeneration suggests that all of the easily oxidized biogenic amines might be oxidized to aberrant metabolites that might be neurotoxic. The following section, therefore, summarizes the *in vitro* oxidation chemistry of 5-HT, DA, and NE.

5. *In Vitro* Oxidation Chemistry of the Biogenic Amine Neurotransmitters

Rather than present a detailed mechanistic review of the very complex oxidation chemistry of 5-HT, DA and NE, an effort has been made to focus only on key intermediates and major identified products of the reactions. In almost all instances, oxidation reactions of the biogenic amines generate highly electrophilic intermediates and/or products. It is extremely unlikely that such species would escape reactions with nucleophiles that are present *in vivo,* particularly GSH, L-cysteine (CySH) and cysteinyl residues of proteins. Thus, considerable discussion will be devoted to the influence of GSH and CySH on the oxidation chemistry of the biogenic amine neurotransmitters.

5.1 *In vitro* oxidation chemistry of 5-hydroxytryptamine

Although the MAO-mediated oxidative deamination of 5-HT to 5-hydroxyindole-3-acetic acid (5-HIAA) is very well known (Udenfriend et al., 1956), many other enzyme systems also mediate oxidation of this neurotransmitter. These include ceruloplasmin (Porter et al., 1957; Eriksen et al., 1960; Martin et al., 1960; Walaas and Walaas 1961; Barrass et al., 1973; Richards, 1983), mitochondrial MAO (Blashko and Hellman, 1953; van Woert et al., 1967), horseradish and mammalian peroxidases (Nelson and Huggins, 1975), and microsomes (Uemura et al., 1980) to form initially colored solutions and ultimately dark melanin-like pigments. Molecular oxygen, Ag^+ and many other chemical oxidants oxidize 5-HT (Eriksen et al., 1960; Alivisatos and Williams-Ashman, 1964; Borg, 1965; Perez-Reyes and Mason, 1981).

Until recently, however, little was understood about the chemistry and products formed in these various enzyme-mediated and chemical oxidations of 5-HT. The first investigations to successfully isolate and identify major products of oxidation of 5-HT employed electro-chemical methods in acidic aqueous solution (Wrona and Dryhurst, 1987, 1988, 1989, 1990a). Under these conditions a radical intermediate is formed that, at millimolar concentrations, serves as a precursor of a number of dimers of 5-HT. However, a major product formed when very low (micromolar) concentrations of 5-HT are electro-oxidized at high potentials and low pH is tryptamine-4,5-dione (T-4,5-D) (Wrona and Dryhurst, 1987). At physiological pH, the electrochemically-driven oxidation ($2e$, $1H^+$) of 5-HT generates a cationic intermediate represented by resonance structures 1 and 2 in Scheme 1 (Wrona and Dryhurst, 1990b). This very electrophilic intermediate undergoes a number of follow-up reactions. Nucleophilic addition of water to the C(4)-centered carbocation 2 yields 4,5-dihydroxytryptamine (4,5-DHT) that is immediately oxidized ($2e$, $2H^+$) to T-4,5-D (Scheme 1).

Alternatively, 5-HT can attack carbocation 2 to give the carbon-carbon linked dimer 5,5'-dihydroxy-4,4'-bitryptamine (3) or the ether linked dimer 5-[[3-(2-aminoethyl)-1H-indol-4-yl]oxy]-3-(2-aminoethyl)-1H-indole (4). Carbocation 2 can also attack dimers 3 and 4 to give trimers and more complex oligomers, although these are only minor products. Oxidation ($2e$, $1H^+$) of dimer 3 gives the putative carbocation 5 that can undergo intramolecular cyclization to spiro compound 6 or, following nucleophilic attack by water, T-4,5-D and 5-HT. Dimer 4 is also readily oxidized to T-4,5-D and 5-HT by a similar pathway as conceptualized in Scheme 1. Oxidations of 5-HT by peroxidase/H_2O_2, ceruloplasmin/O_2, or tyrosinase/O_2 at physiological pH generate similar products to those observed in the electrochemically-driven reaction (Wrona and Dryhurst, 1991). In the presence of GSH the electrochemically-driven and various enzyme-mediated oxidations of 5-HT (Scheme 1) are partially diverted because of the facile nucleophilic addition of the tripeptide to carbocation 2 to give 4-S-glutathionyl-5-hydroxytryptamine (4-S-Glu-5-HT, Scheme 2) (Wrona et al., 1995a). GSH also reacts with T-4,5-D to give initially 7-S-glutathionyl-4,5-dihydroxy-tryptamine (7-S-Glu-4,5-DHT) that is immediately oxidized to 7-S-glutathionyl-trypta-mine-4,5-dione (7-S-Glu-T-4,5-D). CySH also intervenes in the electrochemically-driven oxidation of 5-HT at pH 7.4 by scavenging carbocation 2 to give 4-S-cysteinyl-5-hydroxy-tryptamine (4-S-CyS-5-HT) (Scheme 3) (Wrona et al., 1994). However, unlike 4-S-Glu-5-HT, 4-S-CyS-5-HT is much more easily oxidized than 5-HT to p-quinone imine 11 that cyclizes to 12. In the presence of free CySH 12 undergoes a complex sequence of reactions leading ultimately to 8-(2-aminoethyl)-1,2,3,4,6,9-hexahydro-5,9-dioxo-pyrrolo[3,2g][1,4]benzothiazine-2-carboxylic acid (13, Scheme 3). CySH also attacks T-4,5-D in a reaction sequence that leads to N-[7-[-(2-amino-2-carboxyethyl)thio]-3(2-aminoethyl)-1,4-dihydro-4-oxo-5H-indol-5-ylidene]-L-cysteine (10), a rather unstable compound that decomposes to 5-amino-tryptamine-4,7-dione (14). Much remains to be learned, however, about the reactions of CySH with T-4,5-D.

When incubated with an HO·−generating system (ascorbic acid/Fe^{2+}-EDTA/O_2/H_2O_2) at pH 7.4, 5-HT is very rapidly oxidized initially to a mixture of 2,5-, 4,5-, and 5,6-dihy-droxytryptamine (DHT) *via* intermediate radicals 15, 16 and 17, respectively (Scheme 4) (Wrona et al., 1995b). Under the experimental conditions employed in this investigation, 2,5-DHT was the major reaction product which, at pH 7.4, exists as its keto tautomer 5-hydroxy-3-ethylamino-2-oxindole (5-HEO). Rapid autoxidation of 4,5-DHT gives T-4,5-D that reacts with the C(3)-centered carbanion of 5-HEO (19) to give dimer 20 that is rapidly autoxidized to 3,3'-bis(2-aminoethyl)-5-hydroxy-[3,7'-bi-1H-indole]-2,4',5'-3H-trione (21). The latter dimer then slowly cyclizes to 22 that is autoxidized to 3'-(2-aminoethyl)-1',6',7',8'-tetrahydro-5-hydroxy-spiro[3H-indole-3,9'-[9H]pyrrolo[2,3-f]quinoline]-2,4',5'

Scheme 1

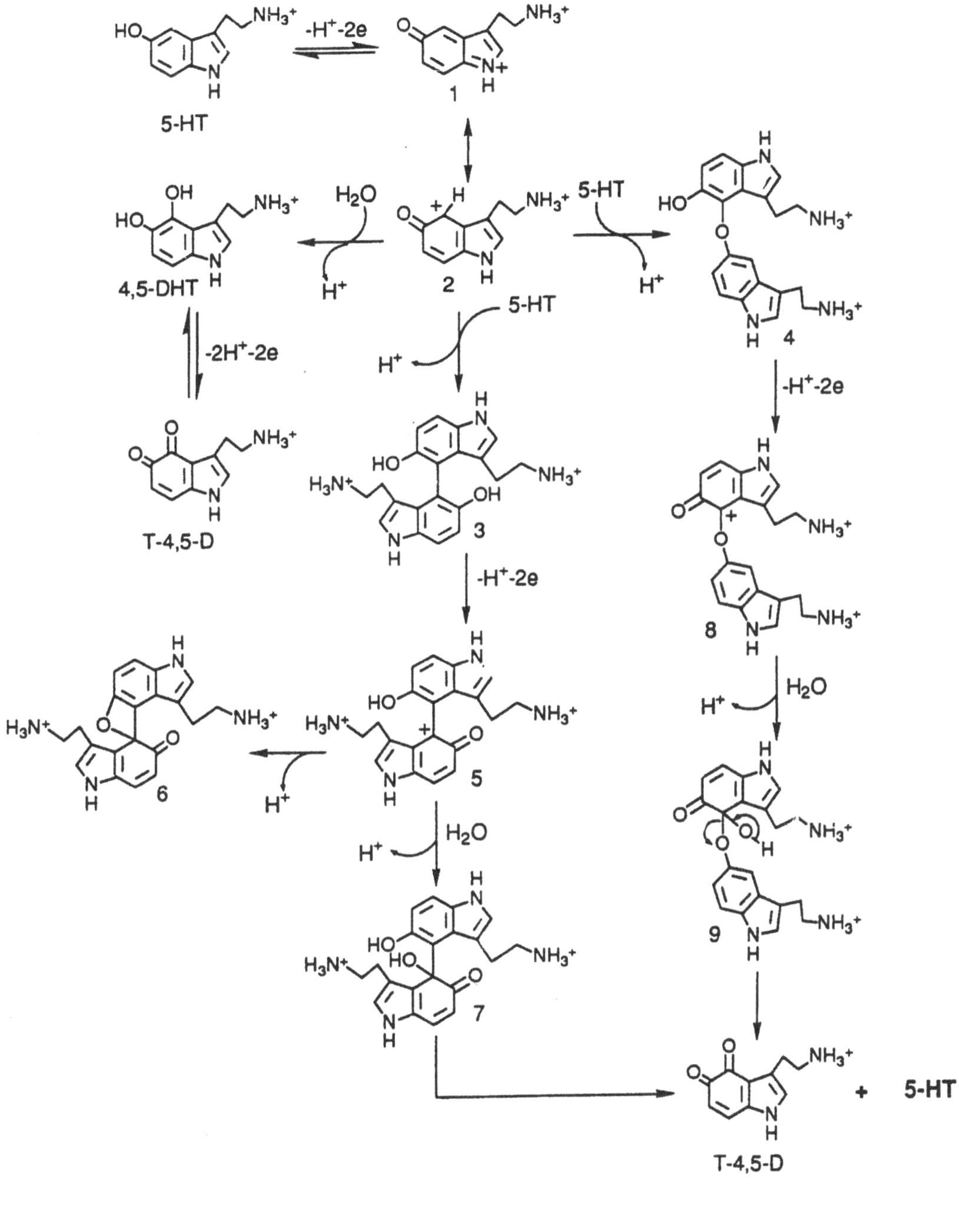

Scheme 2

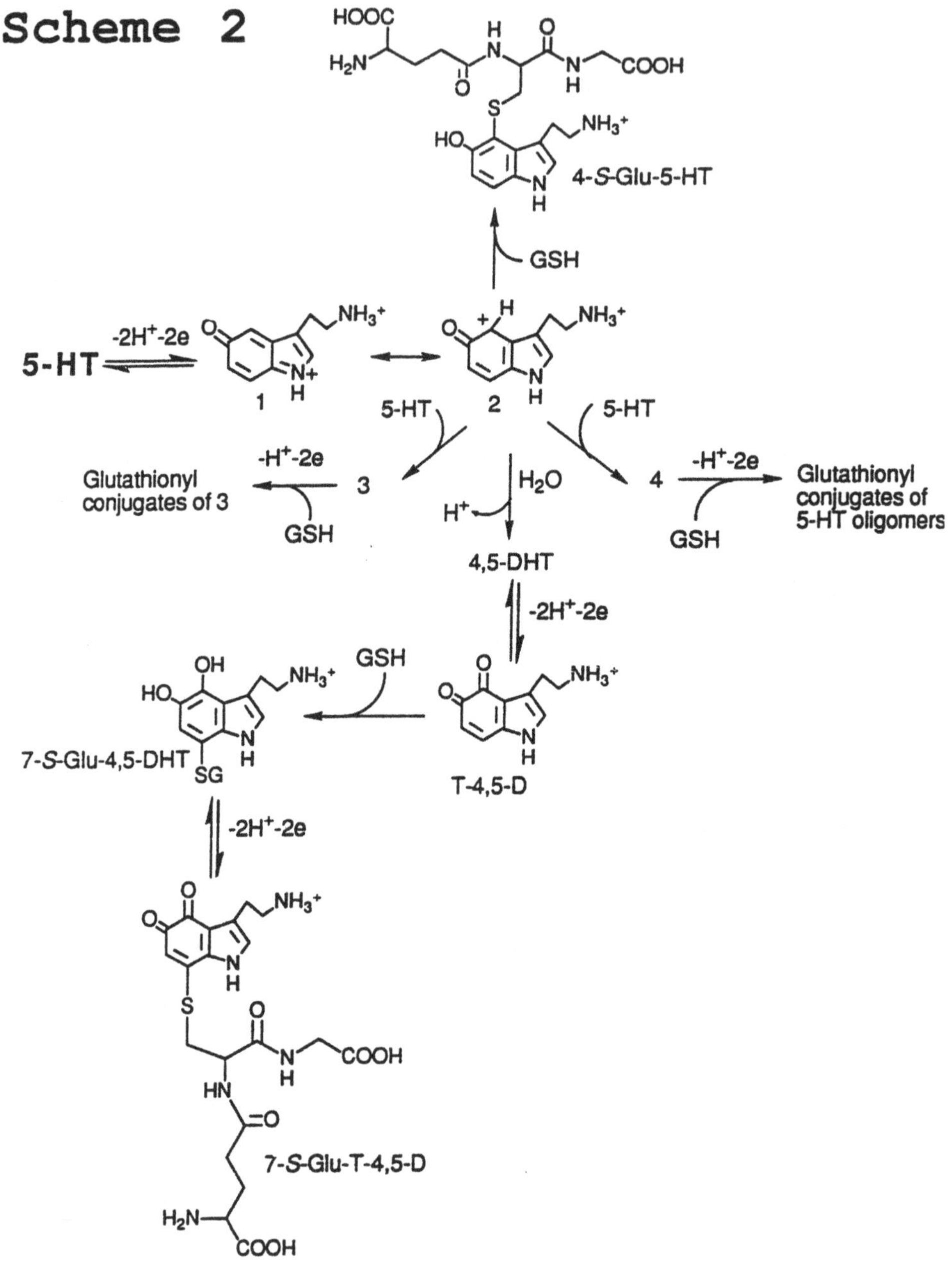

(1*H*)-trione (23) (Scheme 4). GSH interferes with the reaction between T-4,5-D and 5-HEO by preferentially reacting with the former dione to give 7-*S*-Glu-T-4,5-D. Thus, in the presence of GSH the yields of 5-HEO increase in the HO·—mediated oxidation of 5-HT. Because T-4,5-D reacts so readily with 5-HEO (to give 21) or GSH (to give 7-*S*-Glu-T-4,5-D), it is not observed in the free form (Wrona et al., 1995b). 5,6-DHT is a relatively minor product of the HO·—mediated oxidation of 5,6-DHT (Wrona et al., 1995b). In part this is

Scheme 3

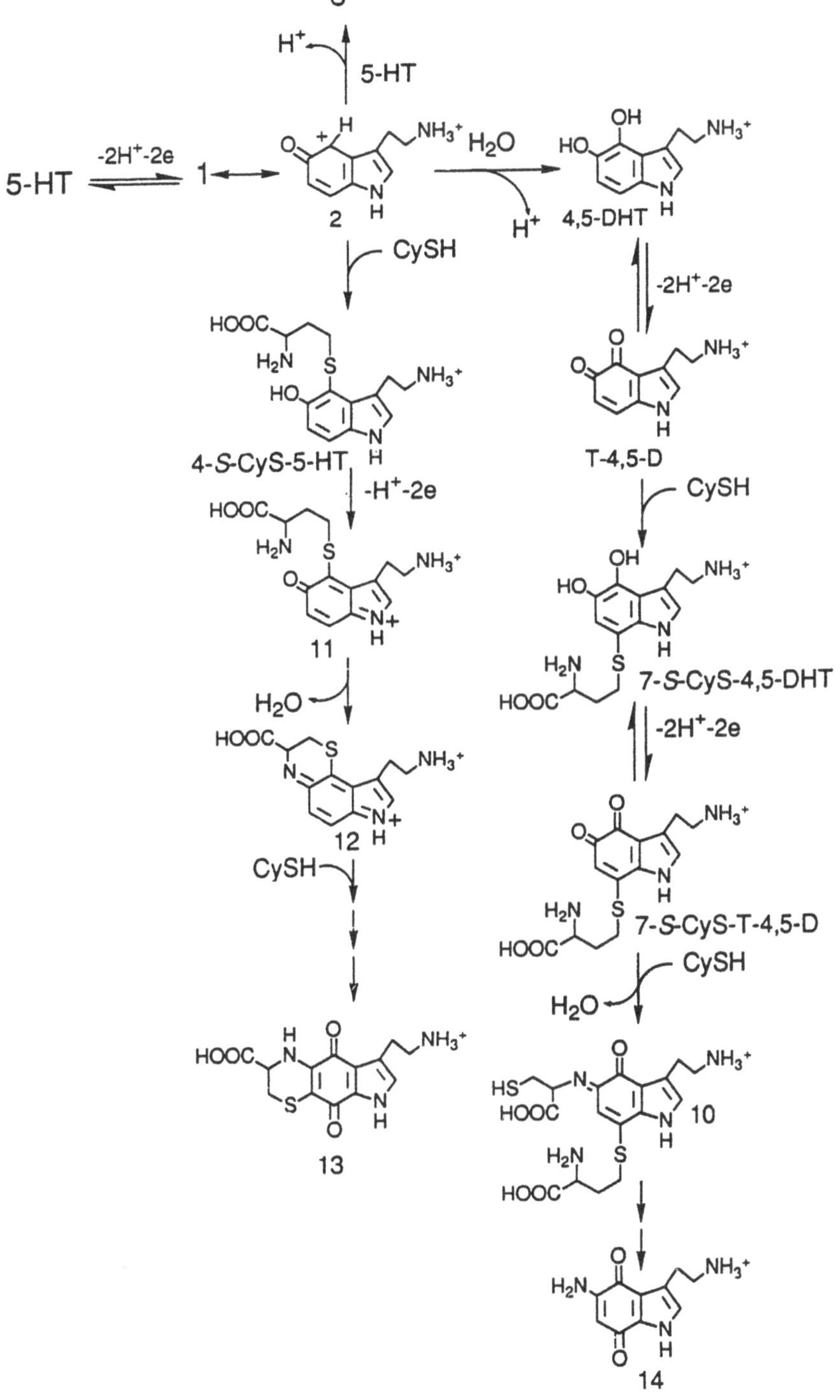

Scheme 4

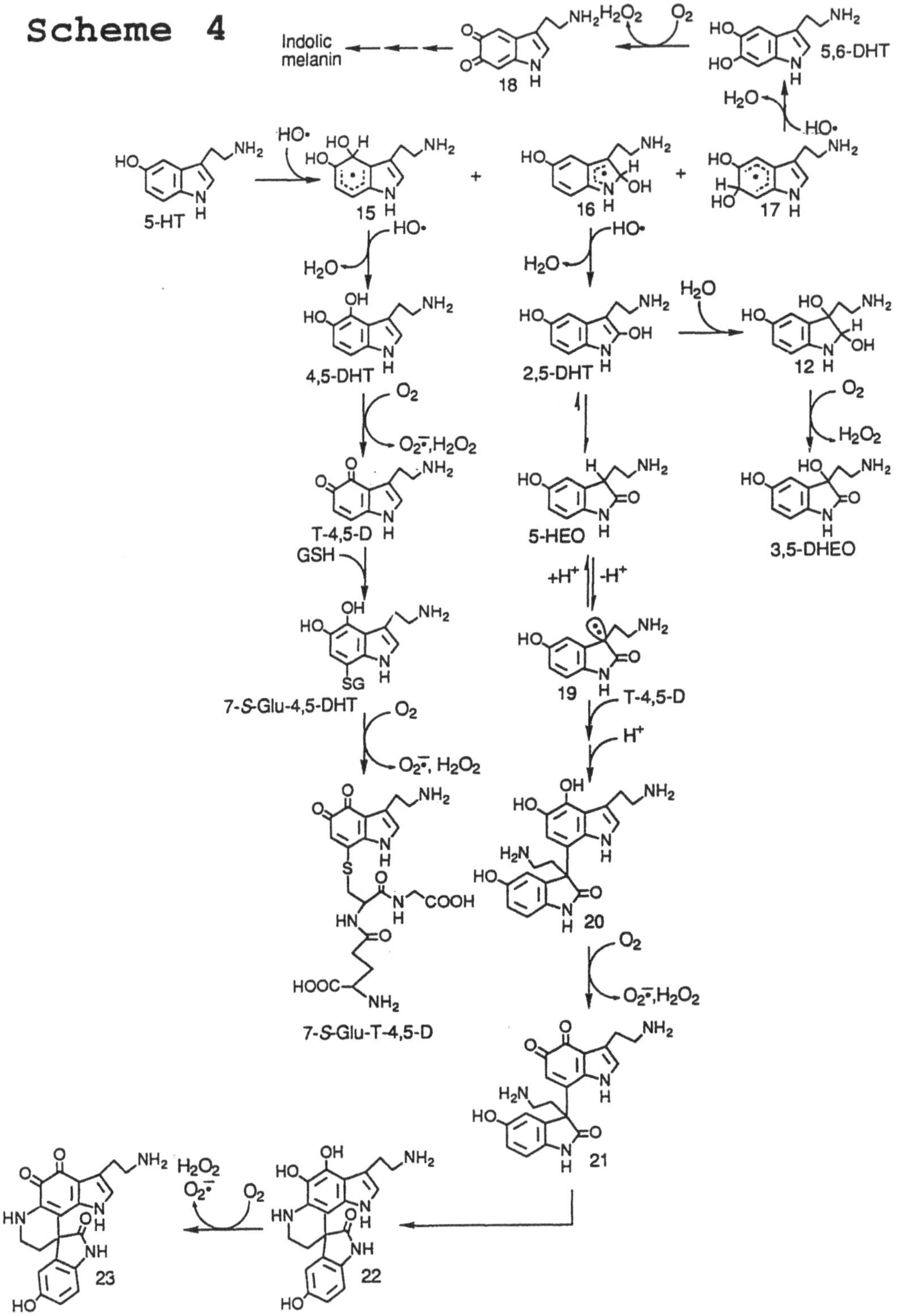

due to the facile autoxidation of 5,6-DHT to *p*-quinone imine 18 that subsequently oligomerizes and polymerizes to dark-colored indolic melanin (Singh et al., 1990; Singh and Dryhurst, 1990). However, recent studies (work in progress) indicate that the relative yields of 5,6-DHT and 5-HEO are dependent on the experimental conditions employed to generate HO ·. For example, in the presence of large molar excesses of H_2O_2 over Fe^{2+}, 5,6-DHT becomes a major reaction product compared to 5-HEO.

The O_2^{-}–mediated oxidation of 5-HT at pH 7.4 (O_2^{-}· being generated by the xanthine/XOD system) generates T-4,5-D as the major reaction product (Wrona and Dryhurst, unpublished results). 5-HEO is not a detectable product of this reaction.

By monitoring the autoxidation of 5-HT in buffered aqueous solution at pH 7.4 using HPLC with electrochemical detection in the oxidative mode (HPLC-EC$_{ox}$), it is evident that the neurotransmitter is rather rapidly oxidized. To illustrate, within 10 min in air-saturated pH 7.4 phosphate buffer at 37°C, 5-HT (200 µM) is oxidized to 5-HEO (major identified product), dimer 3 and a third compound tentatively identified as a trihydroxytryptamine (Wrona et al., 1996). However, only approximately 0.1 percent of the 5-HT is oxidized after this short time. The autoxidation reactions appears to be catalyzed by trace levels of transition metal ion contaminants in the buffer system because desferrioxamine and other strong transition metal ion complexing agents inhibit the reaction, whereas added Fe^{2+}, Cu^{2+} and (to a lesser extent) Fe^{3+} potentiate the reaction. Interestingly, at low concentrations, the intracellular antioxidant ascorbic acid (200 µM) dramatically increases the rate of autoxidation of 5-HT (200 µM) with resultant increases in the yields of 5-HEO and trihydroxytryptamine and the appearance of 5,6-DHT. However, ascorbic acid inhibits formation of dimer 3. Using HPLC-EC$_{ox}$ it is not possible to detect low levels of T-4,5-D. However, dimers 21 and 23, formed by reaction between 5-HEO and T-4,5-D (Scheme 4), can be detected as products when 5-HT is incubated at pH 7.4 with ascorbic acid and molecular oxygen. The mechanisms that underlie the transition metal ion-catalyzed oxidation of 5-HT by molecular oxygen remain to be elucidated. However, in the presence of ascorbic acid it appears that the autoxidation of the latter species serves as a source of H_2O_2 and hence, by transition metal ion-catalyzed Fenton chemistry, HO· that oxidizes 5-HT. GSH also fails to protect 5-HT against autoxidation in a reaction that generates 5-HEO and 3 although other products remain to be identified.

Because it appears to be formed as an intermediate or product of all known oxidations of 5-HT, T-4,5-D has been targeted as a potential aberrant oxidative metabolite of this neurotransmitter in AD (see later discussion). However, many of the biological studies on this compound have failed to recognize its great reactivity with the result that properties attributed to T-4,5-D are probably those of different compounds. A pure (≥95 percent) *solution* of T-4,5-D can be prepared by controlled potential electro-oxidation of a very dilute solution of 5-HT (≤35 µM) dissolved in 10 mM HCl using a strongly oxidizing applied potential (Wrona et al., 1987; Wong and Dryhurst, 1990). Oxidations of higher 5-HT concentrations result in formation of dimer 3. After complete oxidation of a 35 µM solution of 5-HT in 10 mM HCl, additional 5-HT (≤35 µM) can be added to the very dilute solution of T-4,5-D and the electro-oxidation continued until complete. By repeating this procedure numerous times it is possible to obtain relatively pure solutions of T-4,5-D at concentrations as high as approximately 1 mM (Wrona et al., 1996). However, such solutions exhibit significant secondary reactions of T-4,5-D after a few hours. At higher concentrations (e.g., 20 mM) T-4,5-D rapidly dimerizes in an acid-catalyzed reaction to 7,7'-bi-(5-hydroxytryptamine-4-one) (7,7'-D, Scheme 5) (Singh et al., 1992; unpublished results). Adjustment of the pH to 7.4 results in the autoxidation of 7,7'-D to 7,7'-bi-(tryptamine-4,5-dione)

Scheme 5

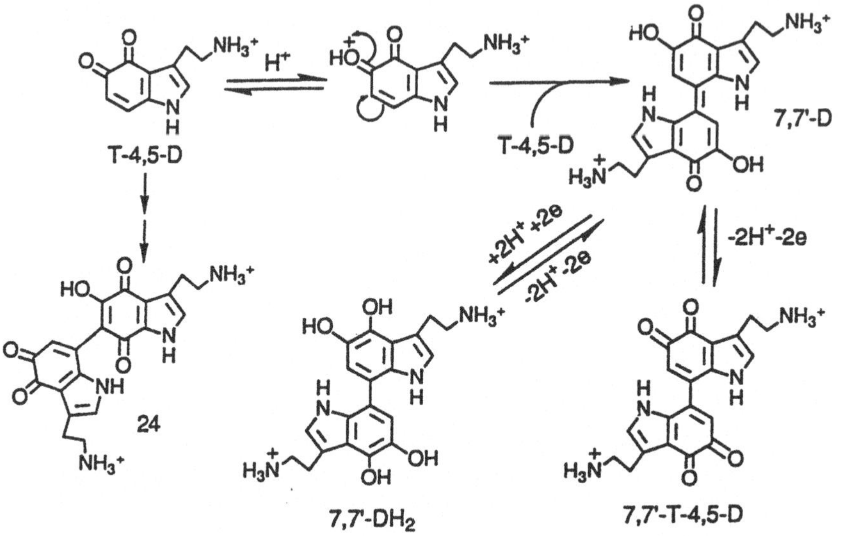

(7,7'-T-4,5-D) (Wrona and Dryhurst, 1988). In dilute aqueous solution at pH 7.4, T-4, 5-D (≤200 μM) slowly transforms into 3-(2-aminoethyl)-6-[3'-(2-aminoethyl)indol-4', 5'-dione-7-yl]-5-hydroxyindole-4,7-dione (24, Scheme 5) (Singh et al., 1992) and 7,7'-T-4,5-D.

When incubated with physiological reductants/antioxidants such as ascorbic acid (AA), NADPH, or GSH and molecular oxygen at pH 7.4, 7-*S*-Glu-T-4,5-D redox cycles in a reaction that generates H_2O_2, probably via intermediary formation of O_2^-· (Scheme 6) (Wong et al., 1993). However, in the presence of GSH nucleophilic addition reactions also occur to give glutathionyl conjugates such as 25 and 27 that are readily autoxidized to 26 and 28, respectively (Scheme 6). Trace levels of transition metal ions (e.g., Fe^{2+}) catalyze the decomposition of H_2O_2 to HO· that then attacks 7-*S*-Glu-T-4,5-D to give radical 29 that is further oxidized to 30 (Scheme 6). There is evidence that 30 can condense with free GSH to give the Schiff base 31 that exists in equilibrium with 30 as long as the tripeptide is available (Wong et al., 1993).

The electrochemically driven and various enzyme-mediated oxidation reactions of 5-hydroxytryptophan (5-HTPP) have also been studied. The key intermediate in these oxidation reactions that appear to proceed by very similar chemical pathways is the formation of the C(4)-centered carbocation (33b, Scheme 7) that reacts with available nucleophiles (Humphries et al., 1993). Reaction of 33b with water yields 4,5-dihydroxytryptophan (34) that is rapidly further oxidized to tryptophan-4,5-dione (35). Reaction of 33b with 5-HTPP gives diastereomers of 5,5'-dihydroxy-4,4'-bi-tryptophan (36) or the ether-linked dimer 37. Additional, more complex oligomers are formed as a result of attack of 33b on dimers 36 and 37 (not shown in Scheme 7). In the presence of GSH, carbocation 33b reacts to give 4-*S*-glutathionyl-5-hydroxytryptophan (38) that can be further oxidized to carbocation 39b (Scheme 7) (Wu and Dryhurst, 1996). Nucleophilic addition of water to 39b yields 40 that eliminates GSH giving dione 35. Reaction of 35 with the eliminated GSH then gives the 7-*S*-glutathionyl conjugate of the dione 42 (Scheme 7). In the absence of free GSH, conjugate

Scheme 6

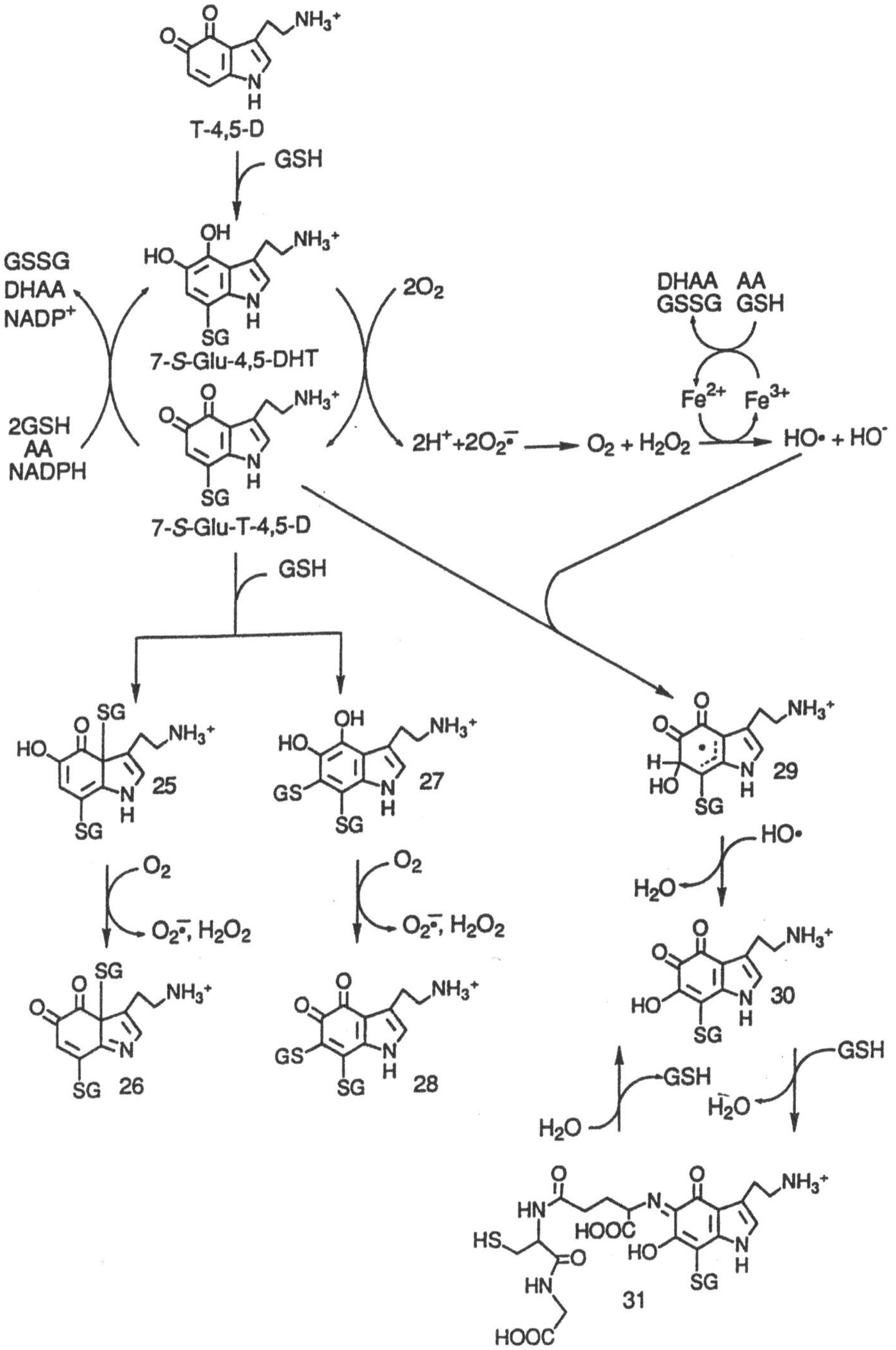

T-4,5-D

GSH

GSSG
DHAA
NADP+

7-*S*-Glu-4,5-DHT

2GSH
AA
NADPH

2O₂

7-*S*-Glu-T-4,5-D

GSH

DHAA AA
GSSG GSH

Fe²⁺ Fe³⁺

$2H^+ + 2O_2^{\overline{\cdot}} \longrightarrow O_2 + H_2O_2 \longrightarrow HO\cdot + HO^-$

25   27   29

O_2 O_2 HO•

$O_2^{\overline{\cdot}}, H_2O_2$ $O_2^{\overline{\cdot}}, H_2O_2$ H_2O

26   28   30

H_2O GSH $\overline{H}_2O$ GSH

31

Scheme 7

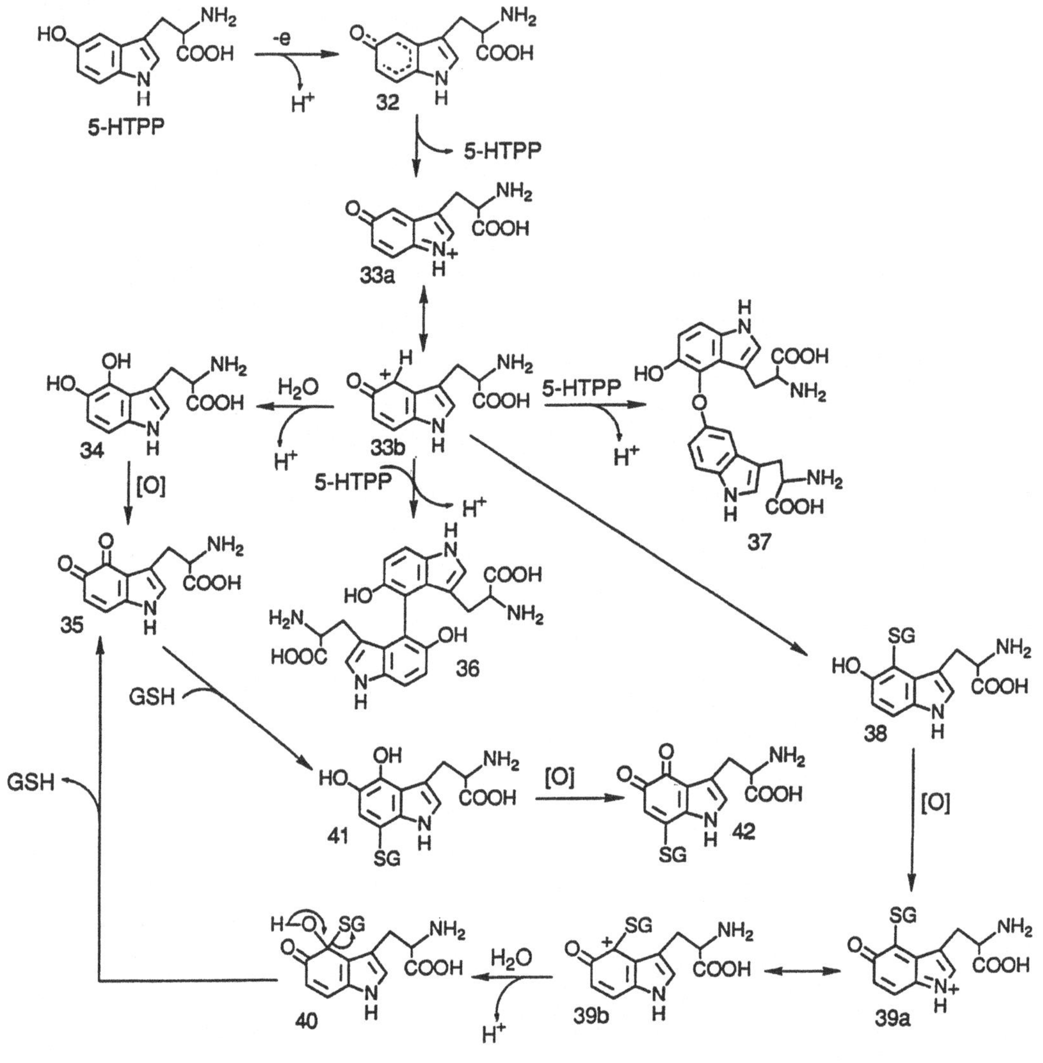

42 slowly dimerizes to 48 and 49 (Scheme 8). In the presence of GSH additional products include the bi-*S*-glutathionyl conjugates 43 and 44 and pyrroloquinolines 45–47 (Wu and Dryhurst, 1996).

Dimer 37 is formed as a result of the electrochemically-driven and various enzyme-mediated oxidations of 5-HTPP at pH 7.4 (Scheme 7) (Humphries et al., 1993). However, this dimer is appreciably more easily oxidized than 5-HTPP. Under weakly oxidizing conditions, i.e., where 5-HTPP is not significantly oxidized, 37 is oxidized (2*e*, 1H$^+$) to a cationic intermediate represented by the C(4)-centered carbocation (50a)/quinone iminium (50b) resonance structures (Scheme 9) (Wu et al., 1995). Nucleophilic addition of water to the C(4)-position of 50a then yields 51 that fragments into an equimolar mixture of 5-HTPP

Scheme 8

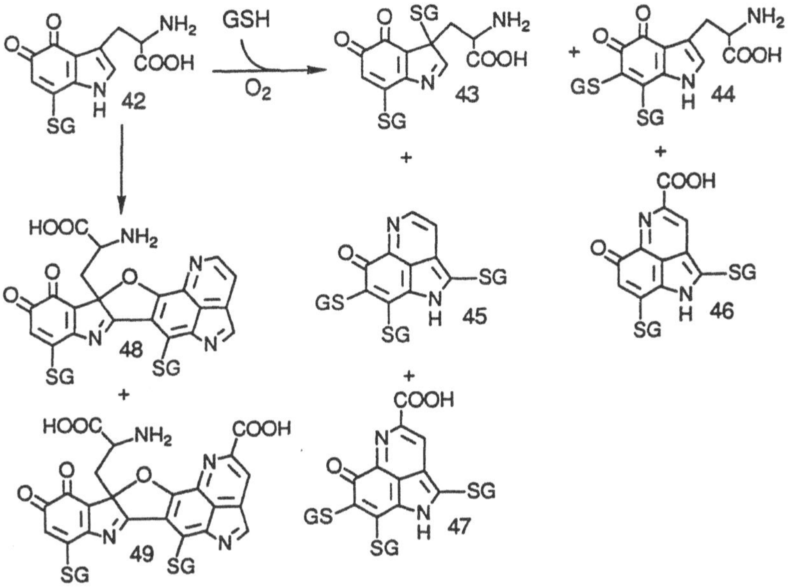

and dione 35. Under more strongly oxidizing conditions, however, oxidation of 5-HTPP formed in this reaction also occurs to give carbocation 33b that reacts with the free hydroxyl residue of 37 to form trimer 52 and, by similar pathways, tetramer 53 and larger oligomers (Scheme 9). However, all of these oligomers are ultimately oxidized to dione 35.

5.2   *In vitro* oxidation chemistry of dopamine (DA)

The HO−· mediated oxidation of DA at pH 7 leads to the formation of 2-, 5-, and 6-OHDA, the yields of the latter neurotoxin being lowest (Slivka and Cohen, 1985). Based upon studies of both the autoxidation (Scheulen et al., 1975; Graham, 1978) and electrochemically-driven (Tse et al., 1976; Young and Babbitt, 1983; Zhang and Dryhurst, 1993) oxidation of DA, it can be concluded that the initial step in the reaction with molecular oxygen involves formation of DA-*o*-quinone (54, Scheme 10), presumably via an intermediary phenoxyl radical, along with two mols of $O_2-\cdot$. The deprotonated form of *54,* i.e., *55,* then undergoes intramolecular cyclization to 5,6-dihydroxyindoline (56). Because 56 is much more easily oxidized than DA, it is chemically oxidized by 54 to dopaminochrome 57 that rearranges to 5,6-dihydroxyindole (5,6-DHI). Further oxidation of 5,6-DHI gives *p*-quinone imine 58 that reacts with other precursor molecules to give, ultimately, a dark, insoluble melanin polymer. The last known intermediate in the melanin pathway is 5,6-DHI (Zhang and Dryhurst, 1993). GSH can efficiently divert this melanin-forming pathway by scavenging *o*-quinone 54 to give, initially, 5-*S*-glutathionyldopamine (5-*S*-Glu-DA, Scheme 11) (Zhang and Dryhurst, 1995). The latter conjugate is more easily oxidized than DA to *o*-quinone 59 that reacts with free GSH to give 2,5-bi-*S*-glutathionyldopamine (2,5-bi-*S*-Glu-DA), an even more easily oxidized compound. The proximate oxidation product of 2,5-bi-

Scheme 9

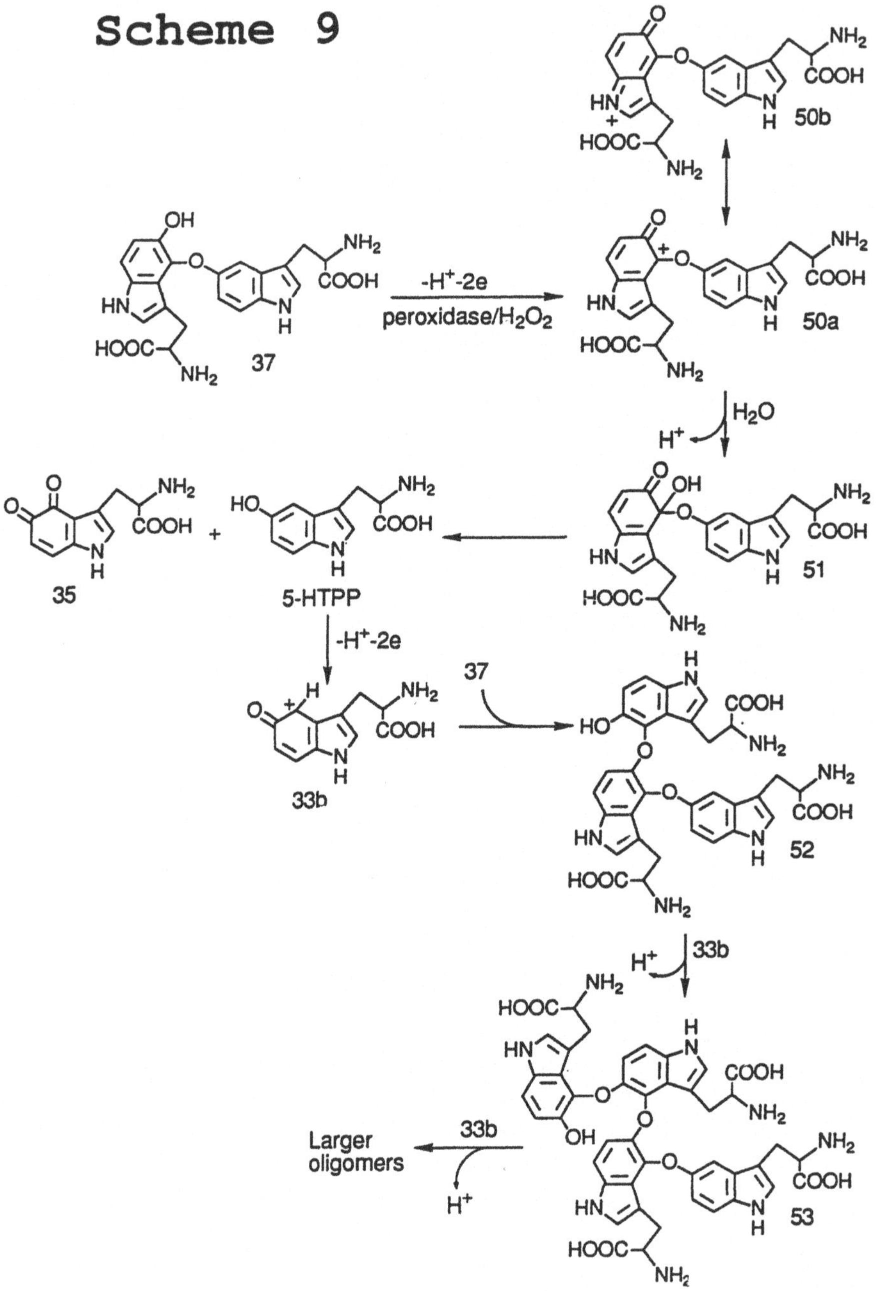

S-Glu-DA is o-quinone 60 (Scheme 11) that reacts by several pathways. Nucleophilic addition of GSH to 60 gives 2,5,6-tri-S-Glu-DA. Deprotonation of 60 to 61 followed by intramolecular cyclization yields 2,5-bi-S-glutathionyl-5,6-dihydroxyindoline (62) that is very readily oxidized to p-quinone imine 63. Rearrangement of 63 yields 4,7-bi-S-glutathionyl-5,6-dihydroxyindole (4,7-bi-S-Glu-5,6-DHI, Scheme 11). Ortho-quinone 60 also tautomerizes to p-quinone methide 64 that is the precursor of glutathionyl conjugates 65

Scheme 10

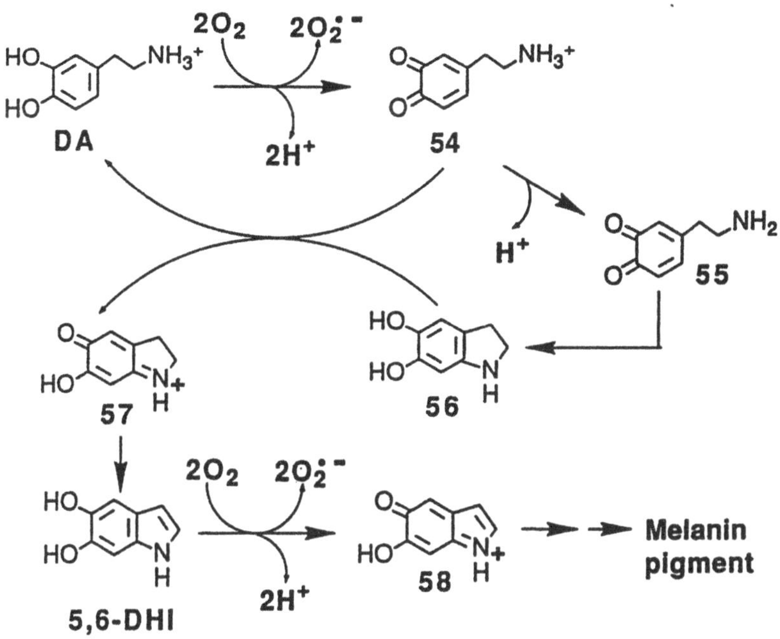

and 67 containing glutathionyl residues substituted at the β-position of the ethylamino side chain of DA.

CySH also diverts the normal oxidation of DA to melanin polymer, by scavenging *o*-quinone 54 to give 5-*S*-cysteinyldopamine (5-*S*-CyS-DA; major product) and 2-*S*-cysteinyldopamine (2-*S*-CyS-DA; minor product) (Scheme 12) (Zhang and Dryhurst, 1994; Shen and Dryhurst, 1996a). These cysteinyl conjugates, however, are more easily oxidized than DA. The resulting products are dependent on the relative concentration of free CySH. In the presence of large molar excesses of CySH, more highly substituted cysteinyl conjugates of DA, particularly 2,5,6-tri-*S*-CyS-DA, are the major products. These are formed as a consequence of the facile oxidations of 5-*S*-CyS-DA and 2-*S*-CyS-DA to *o*-quinones 68 and 69, respectively (Scheme 12). Nucleophilic addition of free CySH to 68 and 69 yields 2,5-bi-*S*-CyS-DA that is even more easily oxidized to *o*-quinone 70. Addition of CySH to 70 yields 2,5,6-tri-*S*-CyS-DA. Addition of CySH to *o*-quinone 68 gives 5,6-bi-*S*-CyS-DA (a very minor pathway) that is oxidized to *o*-quinone 71 and attacked by CySH providing an alternative pathway to 2,5,6-tri-*S*-CyS-DA. At a point in these reactions when CySH is depleted, or when DA is oxidized in the presence of low relative molar excesses of free CySH, alternative reaction pathways predominate that result in the formation of a number of dihydrobenzothiazines (DHBTs) and benzothiazines (BTs). This can be illustrated by the oxidation of 5-*S*-CyS-DA to 7-(2-aminoethyl)-3,4-dihydro-5-hydroxy-2*H*-1,4-benzothiazine-3-carboxylic acid (DHBT-1) in Scheme 13 (Zhang and Dryhurst, 1994; 1995; Shen and Dryhurst, 1996a). Thus, the proximate oxidation product of 5-*S*-CyS-DA, *o*-quinone 68, undergoes intramolecular cyclization (condensation) to the bicyclic *o*-quinone imine 72.

Compound 72 is unusual in that it can oxidize 5-*S*-CyS-DA, from which it is derived, to *o*-quinone 68 forming radical 73 that disproportionates to DHBT-1 and 72. The reaction

Scheme 11

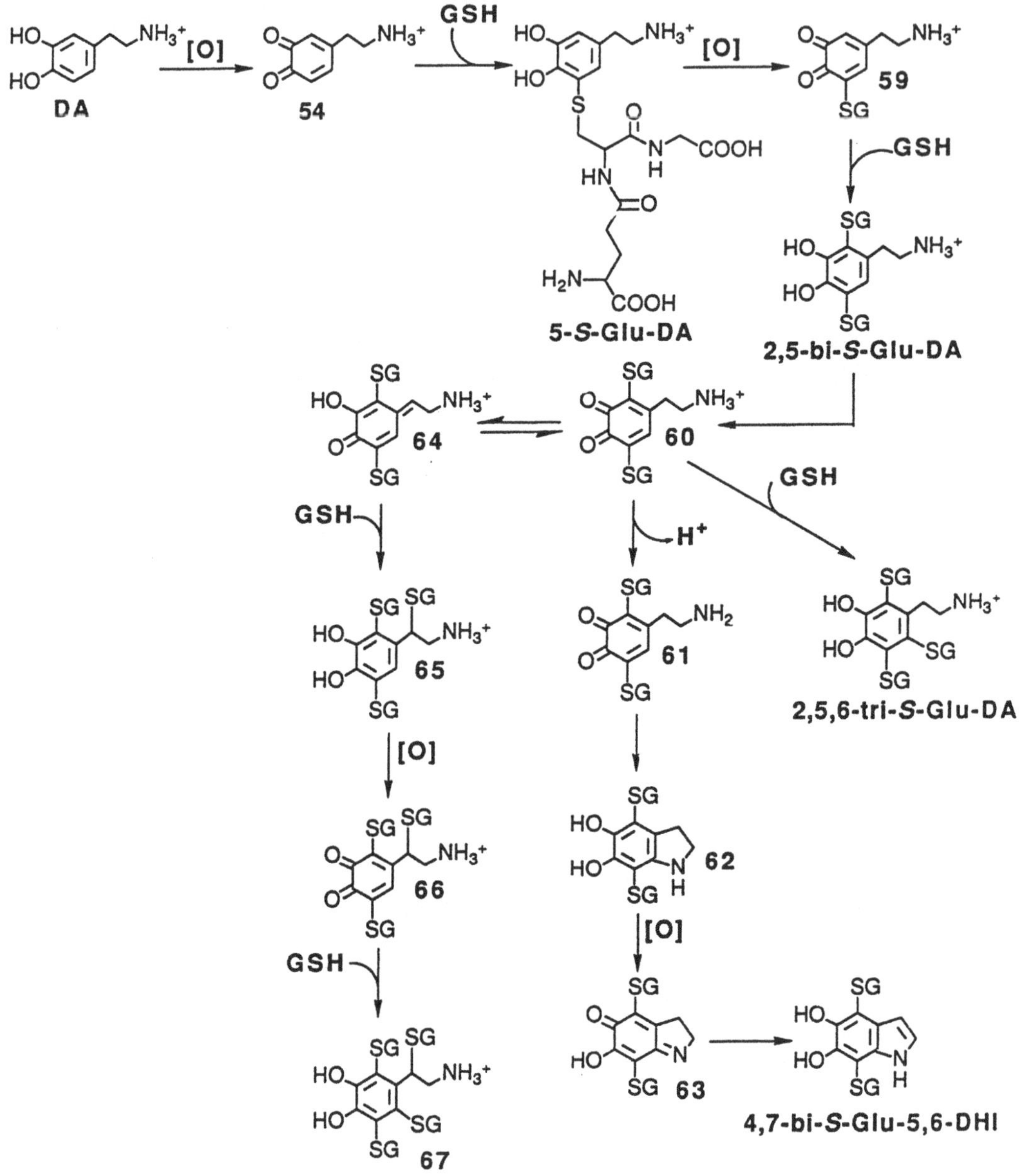

pathway shown in Scheme 13 occurs when 5-S-CyS-DA is oxidized electrochemically (Zhang and Dryhurst, 1995) or by $O_2^-\cdot$, $HO\cdot$ or molecular oxygen at pH 7.4, particularly in the presence of Fe^{2+} or Fe^{3+} (unpublished results). However, at pH 7.4, o-quinone imine 72 partially rearranges to benzothiazine BT-1. At higher pH values (e.g., 10–11) autoxidation of 5-S-CyS-DA to DHBT-1 is extremely rapid giving, initially, DHBT-1 in almost quantitative yield. A summary of the known products formed when DA is oxidized in the

Scheme 12

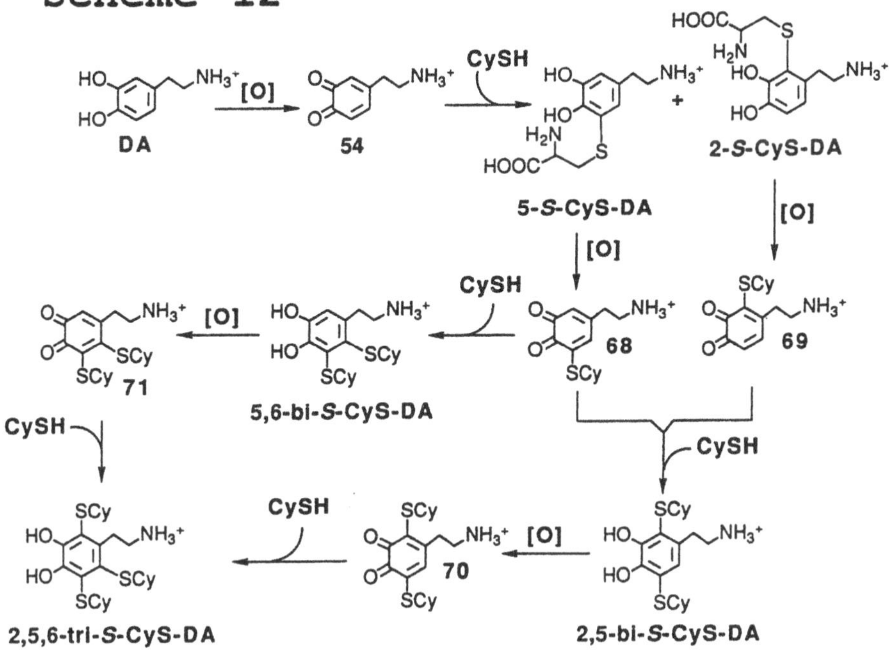

Scheme 13

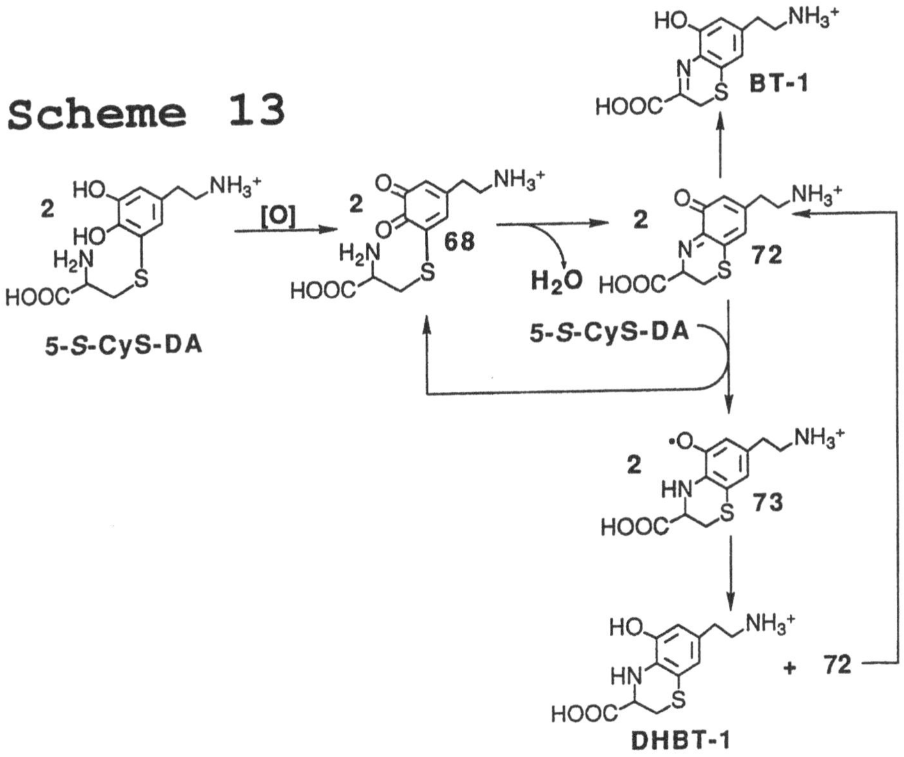

Scheme 14

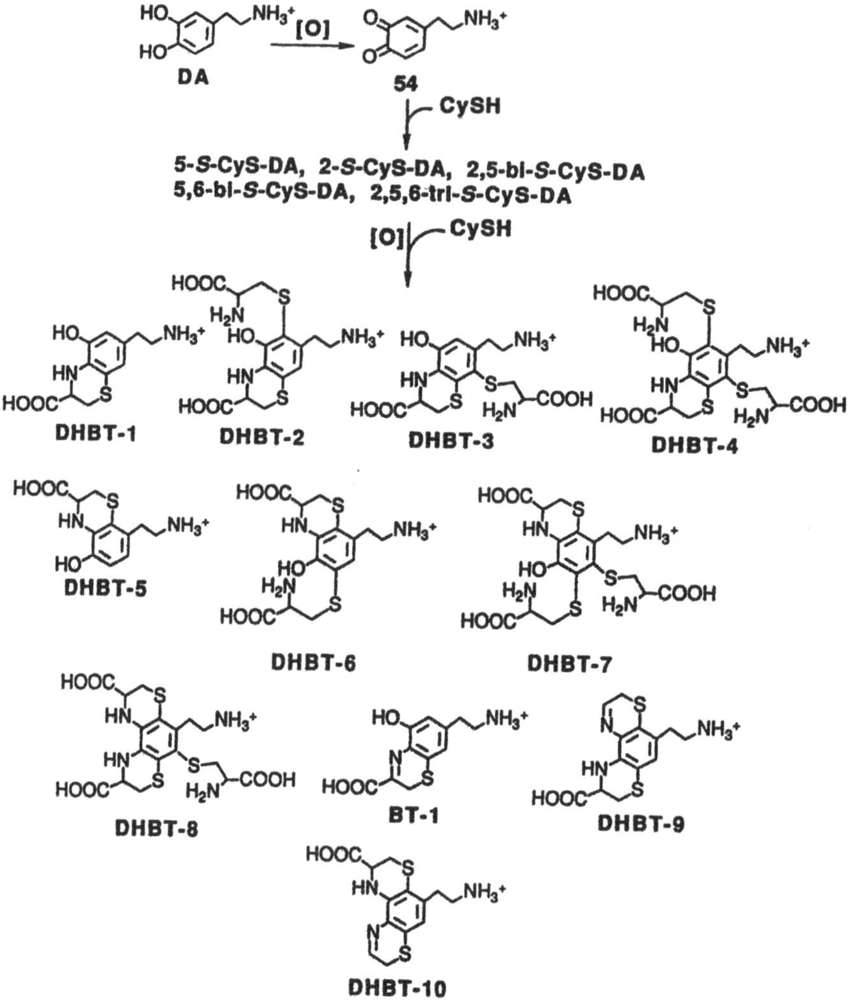

presence of CySH at pH 7.4 is presented in Scheme 14 (Zhang and Dryhurst, 1994; Shen and Dryhurst, 1996a, 1997). The HO·−, and O$_2$·− mediated oxidations of DA in the presence of CySH initially yield 5-S-CyS-DA as the major initial product with lower yields of more complex cysteinyldopamines. At the point when free CySH is virtually exhausted, DHBT-1 then becomes the major product.

5.3 *In vitro* oxidation chemistry of norepinephrine (NE)

The autoxidation (Graham, 1978) and electrochemically-driven oxidation (Tse et al., 1976; Shen and Dryhurst, 1996b) of NE generate NE-*o*-quinone 74 (probably via a phenoxyl radical intermediate) that deprotonates to 75 which then cyclizes to 3,5,6-trihydroxyindoline (76) (Scheme 15). Oxidation of 76 by *o*-quinone 74 then yields *p*-quinone imine 77 that

Scheme 15

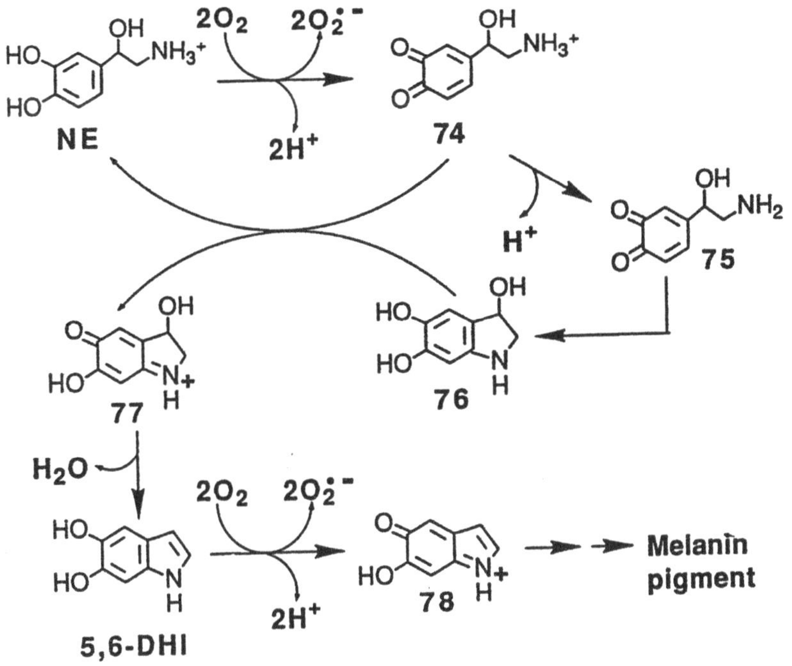

rearranges and loses the elements of water to generate 5,6-DHI. Oxidation of 5,6-DHI generates *p*-quinone imine 78 that polymerizes to black, insoluble melanin. Both GSH and CySH divert this pathway by scavenging *o*-quinone 74 to give glutathionyl and cysteinyl conjugates of NE, respectively. Cysteinyl conjugates of NE are very easily oxidized to *o*-quinone intermediates that can cyclize to DHBTs by reaction pathways similar to cysteinyl conjugates of DA (Shen and Dryhurst, 1996b). A summary of the identified products formed when NE is oxidized in the presence of CySH is presented in Scheme 16. This scheme represents only the initial stages of a very complex reaction and is based upon an electrochemically-driven process. However, oxidations of NE by $O_2-\cdot$ and HO· appear to yield similar initial products.

6. *In Vivo* Oxidation Chemistry of the Biogenic Amine Neurotransmitters

6.1   *In vivo* oxidation of 5-HT

Based on results of *in vitro* studies, the metabolites resulting from the *in vivo* oxidation of 5-HT in AD or as a result of ischemia-reperfusion or MA administration would depend upon the oxidant involved (i.e., $O_2-\cdot$, HO·, other chemical oxidants, or enzyme system). The first experimental results to suggest that 5-HT might be oxidized *in vivo* came when it

Scheme 16

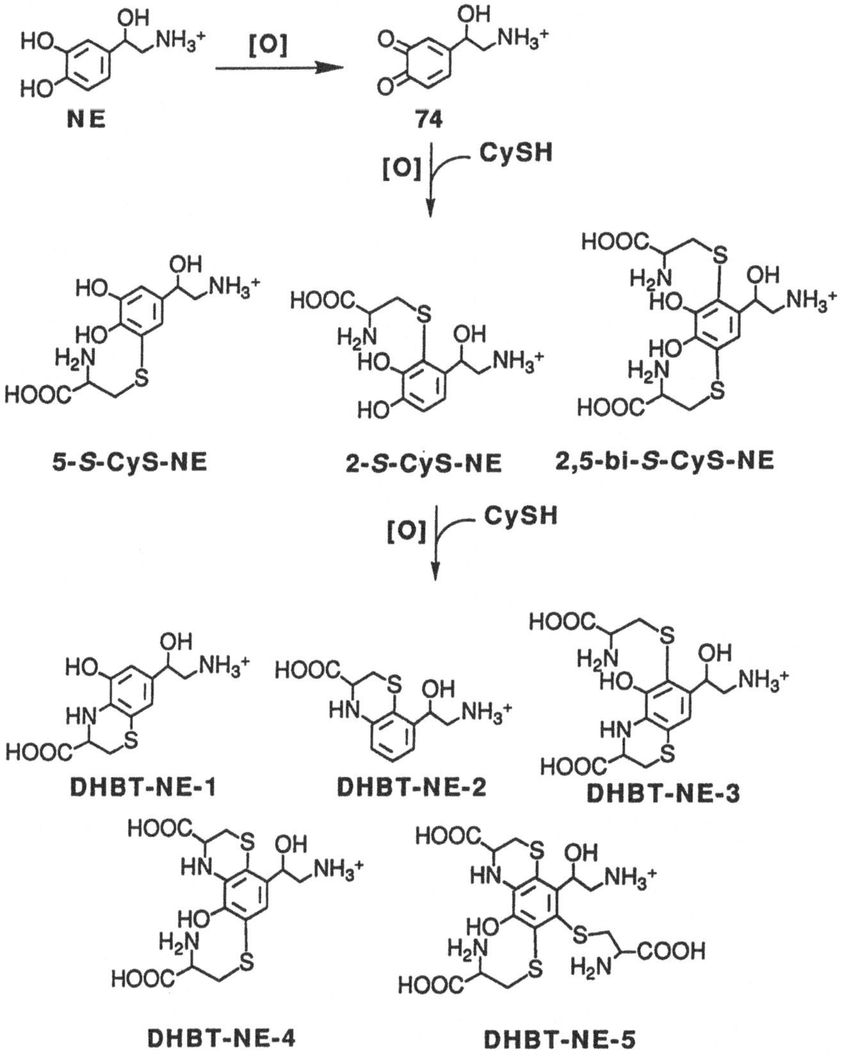

NE →[O]→ **74**

5-*S*-CyS-NE   2-*S*-CyS-NE   2,5-bi-*S*-CyS-NE

DHBT-NE-1   DHBT-NE-2   DHBT-NE-3

DHBT-NE-4   DHBT-NE-5

was reported that shortly after administering a single large subcutaneous (sc) dose of MA (100 mg/kg) to the rat 5,6-DHT could be detected in homogenates of the hippocampus and cortex (Commins et al., 1987a). 5,6-DHT was identified by HPLC-EC$_{ox}$. This observation led to the hypothesis (Commins et al., 1987a) that under conditions of elevated 5-HT release and MAO inhibition (Suzuki et al., 1980) caused by MA, non-enzymatic oxidation of 5-HT occurs in the vicinity of presynaptic serotonergic terminals to form 5,6-DHT that is then transported into and destroys these neurons. This is an attractive hypothesis and, from a number of perspectives, appears to provide a plausible explanation for many of the neurodegenerative effects evoked by MA. To illustrate, the deficits evoked by both MA and

5,6-DHT include long-term depletion of 5-HT (Baumgarten et al., 1971; Gerson et al., 1974; Ricaurte et al., 1980) in various brain regions, decreased TPH activity (Victor et al., 1974; Bakhit and Gibb, 1981), loss of 5-HT uptake sites (Gerson et al., 1974; Ricaurte et al., 1980), in addition to serotonergic terminal degeneration. Furthermore, the protective effects of 5-HT uptake inhibitors against MA-induced damage to serotonergic terminals (Ricaurte et al., 1983) can be expected if 5-HT is indeed oxidized to 5,6-DHT in the synaptic cleft because the latter neurotoxin is believed to express its neurodegenerative properties only following uptake by the 5-HT transporter (Tabatabaie and Dryhurst, 1997). Interestingly, 5,6-DHT is thought to evoke neurodegeneration as a result of its facile intraneuronal autoxidation, that might be catalyzed by mitochondria, in reactions that generate cytotoxic levels of ROS, and electrophilic intermediates that alkylate and crosslink vital cellular proteins and redox cycle depleting antioxidants (Baumgarten et al., 1978; Creveling and Rotman, 1978; Cohen and Heikkila, 1978; Singh and Dryhurst, 1990; Singh et al., 1990; Singh and Dryhurst, 1991; Tabatabaie and Dryhurst, 1997). Administration of the related serotonergic neurotoxin *p*-chloroamphetamine (PCA) to the rat has also been reported to result in formation of 5,6-DHT in the brain (Commins et al., 1987b). However, levels of 5,6-DHT measured in rat brain following MA or PCA administration were low and somewhat sporadic (Commins et al., 1987a,b). Indeed, efforts to replicate detection of 5,6-DHT in rat brain following MA administration have been unsuccessful (Yang et al., 1997) or difficult (Seiden and Sabol, 1995). Furthermore, a role for low levels of 5,6-DHT (and 6-OHDA, see later discussion) in the neurotoxic effects evoked by MA or PCA has been questioned (Evans and Cohen, 1989). However, 5,6-DHT is extremely unstable at physiological pH because of its very facile autoxidation. Thus, detection of this neurotoxin in rat brain tissue by HPLC-EC$_{ox}$, or indeed other analytical methods, in response to MA administration represents a significant analytical challenge. *In vitro* studies indicate that 5,6-DHT is formed only in the HO·-mediated oxidation of 5-HT (Wrona et al., 1995). Formation of elevated levels of dihydroxybenzoic acids in the brains of salicylic acid pretreated mice after MA administration also points to HO· generation (Kondo et al., 1992, 1993). However, a more stable and (usually) major product of the *in vitro* HO·-mediated oxidation of 5-HT is 5-HEO that, similar to 5,6-DHT, appears to be a product unique to this reaction (Scheme 4) (Wrona et al., 1995).

Thus, it has been suggested that 5-HEO might represent a better marker compound for the MA-mediated generation of HO· that oxidizes 5-HT. Recent studies have demonstrated that 5-HEO is slowly transformed into one major but unidentified metabolite in rat brain (Yang et al., 1997). Both 5-HEO and this metabolite can be readily detected and measured at very low concentrations when added to homogenates of rat brain tissue by HPLC-EC$_{ox}$. However, 1 h following a single large dose of MA (100 mg/kg, sc) neither 5-HEO, its unknown metabolite, nor 5,6-DHT could be detected in any region of the brains of rats (Yang et al., 1997). These results argue against the hypothesis that MA mediates HO· and hence 5,6-DHT formation and that the latter neurotoxin is responsible for degeneration of serotonergic terminals and, perhaps, certain cell body populations in the somatosensory cortex. Several other experimental observations are also poorly rationalized by this hypothesis. To illustrate, 5,6-DHT is a rather selective neurotoxin that evokes damage to other neurons only at very high doses (Tabatabaie and Dryhurst, 1997). Furthermore, mechanisms that underlie the protective effects of elevated GABA levels, NMDA, and DA receptor antagonists against MA-induced neurodegeneration are not easily reconciled with the proposition that 5,6-DHT is a major contributor to the neuronal damage evoked by this drug.

The protective effects of increased cytoplasmic Cu-Zn SOD activity against MA-induced neurodegeneration (Cadet et al., 1994; Hirato et al., 1995, 1996) and the fact that SOD inhibition exacerbates the damage evoked by this drug (De Vito and Wagner, 1989) point to $O_2-\cdot$ rather than $HO\cdot$ as the oxygen radical that in some way mediates the neurotoxic effects of MA, oxidation of sulfhydryl residues of TPH (Stone et al., 1989) and, perhaps, oxidation of 5-HT, DA and NE. The fact that Cu-Zn SOD transgenic mice are also protected against the neurodegenerative effects of ischemia-reperfusion (Kinouchi et al., 1991; Yang et al., 1994) similarly implies an important role for $O_2-\cdot$ rather than $HO\cdot$. Indeed, the generation of $O_2-\cdot$ during reperfusion of ischemic brain has been demonstrated in cats (Kontos and Wei, 1986). Studies in this laboratory have revealed that the *in vitro* oxidation of 5-HT by $O_2-\cdot$ at pH 7.4 gives T-4,5-D as the major identified initial product. This reaction does not yield significant levels of either 5-HEO or 5,6-DHT. These observations, therefore, raise the possibility that T-4,5-D, its glutathionyl conjugates such as 7-*S*-Glu-T-4,5-D (Scheme 6), or other compounds derived from reactions of this dione (Schemes 3 and 5) might be aberrant oxidative metabolites of 5-HT formed as a result of the $O_2-\cdot$-mediated oxidation of this neurotransmitter, mediated by MA or ischemia-reperfusion. Of possible relevance to this suggestion are reports that the CSF of patients with AD, but not age-matched control patients, contain substances that can be detected by HPLC-EC$_{ox}$ analysis (Matson et al., 1984; Volicer et al., 1985, 1989). These HPLC-EC$_{ox}$ signals were proposed to be due to *partially* oxidized forms of 5-HT and 5-HTPP based on the fact that solutions obtained from electrochemical oxidations of these indoles (*ca.* 5 μM) contained (unknown) products that exhibited similar chromatographic and electrochemical properties. The subsequent discovery of T-4,5-D as a major product of electrochemical oxidation of very dilute solutions of 5-HT (Wrona and Dryhurst, 1987) led to an unsuccessful search for this dione in the CSF of AD patients (Volicer et al., 1989). The reactivity of T-4,5-D, however, is such that it is extremely unlikely it could survive in the brain for significant periods of time. Nevertheless, *in vitro* and *in vivo* studies of the neurochemical and neurobiological properties of T-4,5-D and related putative metabolites that would result from the $O_2-\cdot$-mediated oxidations of 5-HT and 5-HTPP provide some support for the possible involvement of these compounds in the neurodegenerative processes in AD and, perhaps, following ischemia-reperfusion, and MA administration.

6.2 *In vivo* oxidation of DA and NE

The nigrostriatal dopaminergic system of rats is particularly susceptible to the neurodegenerative effects of MA (Seiden and Vosmer, 1984; Axt et al., 1994). Furthermore, as reviewed earlier, oxidative stress appears to play an important role in mediating the neurodegenerative properties of this drug. In view of the fact that 6-OHDA is a catecholaminergic neurotoxin (Kostrzewa and Jacobowicz, 1974) that *in vitro* can be formed by the $HO\cdot$-mediated oxidation of DA (Slivka and Cohen, 1985), it is not surprising that suspicion fell on this compound as a mediator of the neurodegenerative effects of MA. Indeed, 1 h after administration of a large dose of MA (100 mg/kg, sc), 6-OHDA has been detected in the rat striatum (Seiden and Vosmer, 1984). Thus, it has been proposed that following the MA-induced release of DA, this neurotransmitter is non-enzymatically oxidized to 6-OHDA and that carrier-mediated uptake of this neurotoxin accounts for the degeneration of dopaminergic terminals (Marek et al., 1990a,b). Support for this hypothesis derives from the fact that DA uptake inhibitors protect dopaminergic neurons against MA-induced damage (Marek et al., 1990a). There is evidence that MA participates in an exchange diffusion process (Raiteri et al., 1979) that releases DA from its intraneuronal (cytoplasmic) storage sites resulting in elevated levels of free or unbound neurotransmitter with subsequent efflux from the cell through the uptake carrier sites (Marek et al., 1990b). Thus, it is of interest that pharmacologic manipulations that increase the cytoplasmic pool of DA potentiate MA-induced damage to dopaminergic neurons (Wagner et al., 1983) and elevate levels of 6-OHDA formed (Marek et al., 1990c). By contrast, agents that decrease the cytoplasmic pool of DA attenuate long-lasting depletions of DA induced by MA (Wagner et al., 1983) and formation of 6-OHDA (Axt et al., 1990).

Taken together, these lines of evidence suggest that increased cytoplasmic levels of unbound DA evoked by MA might predispose this neurotransmitter to intraneuronal oxidation to 6-OHDA. However, attempts to replicate the detection of 6-OHDA in rat brain following neurotoxic doses of MA have been either unsuccessful (Rollema et al., 1986; Karoum et al., 1993) or difficult (Seiden and Sabol, 1995). Furthermore, it is unlikely that the low levels of 6-OHDA claimed to have been measured in the rat striatum following MA administration could evoke profound degeneration of dopaminergic terminals (Evans and Cohen, 1989). Thus, a role for 6-OHDA, formed as a result of the $HO\cdot$-mediated oxidation of DA (Slivka and Cohen, 1985), in the neurodegenerative effects of MA based on the preceding information appears somewhat questionable.

Nevertheless, many lines of evidence strongly support MA-induced formation of ROS (DeVito and Wagner, 1989; Stone et al., 1989; Kondo et al., 1993; Cadet et al., 1994; Hirata et al., 1995, 1996) and an important role for either DA itself or an aberrant metabolite of this neurotransmitter in the neurodegenerative effects evoked by MA in many (but not all) parts of the brain (Wagner et al., 1983; Sonsalla et al., 1986). Regardless of the oxidizing species formed in the brain as a result of MA administration, the proximate product of oxidation of DA must be DA-*o*-quinone (54), perhaps preceded by a phenoxyl radical intermediate. Oxidation of cytoplasmic DA would necessarily expose 54 to GSH and CySH, major constituents of dopaminergic axon terminals (Slivka et al., 1987; Philbert et al., 1990), and the cysteinyl residues of proteins. Thus, it is of particular interest that administration of MA (15 mg/kg, sc; every 2 h, four injections) to rats results in a significant increase of protein-bound 5-*S*-CyS-DA and formation of a glutathionyl conjugate of DA that was not present in the brains of control animals (LaVoie et al., 1996). These results provide support for the MA-induced oxidation of DA and reaction of DA-*o*-quinone with CySH and GSH in rat brain.

7. Properties of Putative Aberrant Oxidative Metabolites of the Biogenic Amine Neurotransmitters

HPLC-EC$_{ox}$ of the CSF from AD patients indicate the presence of unusual oxidized forms of 5-HT and 5-HTPP (Matson et al., 1984; Volicer et al., 1985, 1989). Similarly, HPLC-EC$_{ox}$ analysis of brain tissue from rats administered neurotoxic doses of MA reveal the presence of apparently oxidized forms of 5-HT (Commins et al., 1987a,b) and DA (Seiden and Vosmer, 1984; LaVoie et al., 1996). The aberrant metabolites detected in the CSF of AD patients are unknown. Considerable uncertainty now surrounds claims that MA mediates formation of 5,6-DHT and 6-OHDA in rat brain. However, more recent evidence supports the idea that MA does indeed evoke oxidation of DA based upon formation of glutathionyl and cysteinyl conjugates of the neurotransmitter (LaVoie et al., 1996). Interestingly, increased 5-*S*-CyS-DA/DA and 5-*S*-CyS-DA/homovanillic acid concentration ratios have been measured in the *striatum* and *substantia nigra* (Fornstedt et al., 1989) and CSF (Cheng et al., 1996) of PD patients. Increased 5-*S*-CyS-DA/DA ratios have been interpreted to implicate increased oxidative stress in the nigrostriatal pathway as a cause of the selective degeneration of these neurons in PD (Fornstedt et al., 1989). Strong evidence for oxidative stress in the degeneration of certain serotonergic and catecholaminergic pathways in the brain in AD, and following ischemia-reperfusion and MA administration, coupled with the ease of oxidation of 5-HT, DA, and NE together provide *prima facie* support for the hypothesis that unusual oxidative metabolites should indeed be formed in these brain disorders. However, *in vitro* studies suggest that aberrant metabolites such as 5-*S*-CyS-DA, for example, should represent only markers for the initial step in oxidation reactions that should lead to a plethora of products. A key question, therefore, is whether such putative metabolites might be implicated in neurodegenerative and other neurobiological alterations. Evidence, summarized below, is beginning to emerge that such compounds might indeed be involved in such alterations.

7.1   Redox properties of putative aberrant oxidative metabolites of 5-HT and 5-HTPP

A summary of relevant redox properties of 5-HT, 5-HTPP, and various compounds identified as in vitro oxidation products of these indoles is presented in Table 1. The formal potential ($E^{\circ\prime}$), peak oxidation, and peak reduction potentials were all measured using cyclic voltammetry at a pyrolytic graphite electrode at a pH value at or close to 7.4. $E^{\circ\prime}$ data are provided only for those compounds that exhibit reversible behavior in cyclic voltammetry experiments. All compounds that exhibit reversible electrochemical behavior have $E^{\circ\prime}$ values that correspond to *o*-quinone/*o*-dihydroxy (e.g., 5,6-DHT, T-4,5-D, 21, 23), *o*-quinone imine/*o*-hydroxyamine (e.g., 10, 31, 45–47) and/or *p*-quinone/*p*-dihydroxy (e.g., 13, 14) couples, *i.e.*, $2H^+$, $2e$ redox systems. The peak oxidation potentials, for example, for 5-HT, dimers 3 and 4, and 5-HEO are probably close to $E^{\circ\prime}$ values and permit an easy assessment of the relative ease of oxidation of these compounds. In the case of compounds 21 and 23 the $E^{\circ\prime}$ values correspond to the T-4,5-D residues (*i.e.*, T-4,5-D/4,5-DHT couple) whereas the peak oxidation potential corresponds to the irreversible oxidation of the 5-HEO residue. While the chemistry associated with the latter peaks is unknown, the relatively low oxidation potentials suggest that both 21 and 23 should be readily detected using HPLC-EC$_{ox}$ methods. Preliminary results from the author's laboratory indicate that T-4,5-D and other compounds containing this residue can be detected and quantitated at submicromolar concentrations in solution using HPLC-EC in the reductive mode at detector potentials at which dissolved molecular oxygen does not interfere.

A number of interesting conclusions can be drawn from the data presented in Table 1. Thus, with the exception of dimers 3 and 36, virtually all other major *in vitro* oxidation products of 5-HT and 5-HTPP are either more easily oxidized at pH 7.4 than these endogenous indoles (e.g. 5,6-DHT, 5-HEO, 4-*S*-CyS-5-HT) or are easily reduced species (e.g., T-4,5-D, 7-*S*-Glu-T-4,5-D). The former compounds, particularly 5,6-DHT and 4-*S*-CyS-5-HT, would therefore be expected to undergo further oxidation reactions under conditions where 5-HT is oxidized. The $E^{\circ\prime}$ values for cellular reductants/antioxidants have been estimated to extend to approximately –400 mV *vs.* NHE at physiological pH (Frank et al., 1987). The $E^{\circ\prime}$ values for the T4,5-D/4,5-DHT (2 mV), 7-*S*-Glu-T4,5-D/7-*S*-Glu-4,5-DHT

Table 1. Redox Properties of Putative Aberrant Oxidative Metabolites of 5-HT and 5-HTPP at pH 7.4[a,b]

Compound	$E^{\circ\prime c}$ mV *vs.* SCE (NHE)	Peak Potential[d]	
		Ox[e]	Red[f]
		mV *vs.* SCE[g] (NHE[h])	
5-HT		295 (537) at pH 7.3	
3		380 (622) at pH 7.2	
4		260 (502) at pH 7.2	
5-HEO			220 (462)
5,6-DHT	38 (280)		
T-4,5-D	−240 (2)		
21	−495 (−253)		240 (482)
23	−495 (−253)		290 (532)

(continued)

Table 1. Redox Properties of Putative Aberrant Oxidative Metabolites of 5-HT and 5-HTPP at pH 7.4[a,b] *(continued)*

Compound	$E^{o\prime c}$ mV *vs.* SCE (NHE)	Peak Potential[d]	
		Ox[e]	Red[f]
		mV *vs.* SCE[g] (NHE[h])	

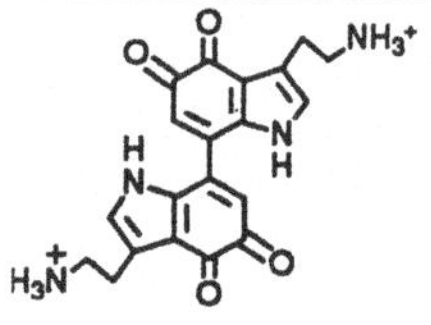

7,7'-T-4,5-D

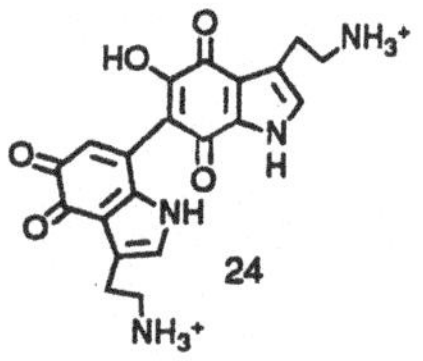

24

−280 (−38); −540 (−298)

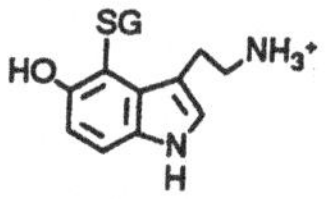

4-*S*-Glu-5-HT

275 (517) at pH 7.3

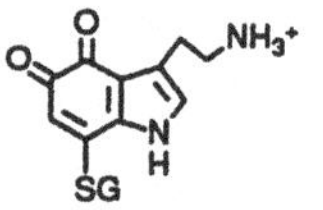

7-*S*-Glu-T-4,5-D

−248 (−6)

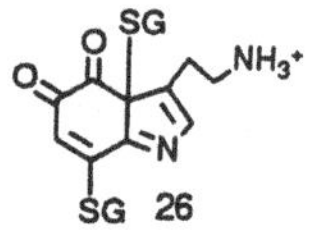

SG **26**

−510 (−268)

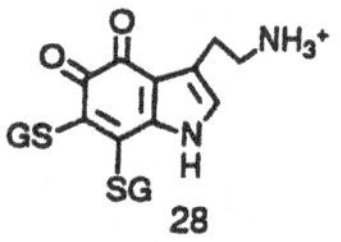

28

−570 (−328)

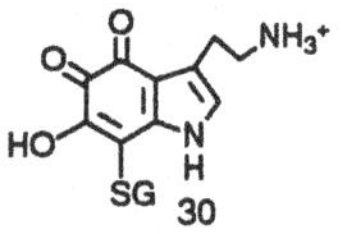

30

−500 (−258)

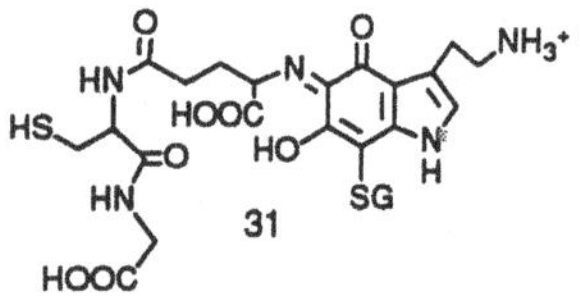

31

−484 (−242)

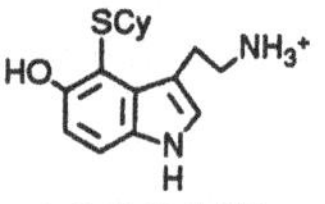

4-*S*-CyS-5-HT

170 (412)

(continued)

Table 1. Redox Properties of Putative Aberrant Oxidative Metabolites of 5-HT and
5-HTPP at pH 7.4[a,b] *(continued)*

| Compound | $E^{o'c}$ mV *vs.* SCE (NHE) | Peak Potential[d] | |
		Ox[e]	Red[f]
		mV *vs.* SCE[g] (NHE[h])	
10	−495 (−253)		
13	−473 (−231)		
14	−470 (−228)		
5-HTPP		253 (495)	
36			
37		147 (389)	
38		257 (499)	
42	−216 (8)		
43			−456 (−214)
44	−549 (−307)		

(continued)

Table 1.   Redox Properties of Putative Aberrant Oxidative Metabolites of 5-HT and 5-HTPP at pH 7.4[a,b] *(continued)*

Compound	$E^{\circ\prime c}$ mV *vs.* SCE (NHE)	Peak Potential[d]	
		Ox[e]	Red[f]
		mV *vs.* SCE[g] (NHE[h])	
45	−433 (−191)		
46	−386 (−144)		
47	−395 (−153)		
48	−616 (−374)		
49	−651 (−409)		

[a]Peak potential and E°′ values were measured using cyclic voltammetry at a pyrolytic graphite electrode in buffered aqueous solution. Typically, concentrations of each compound were 0.2–1.0 mM and a sweep rate of 200 mVs^{-1} was employed.
[b]pH values other than 7.4 are specified in the Table.
[c]E°′ values were calculated from the equation: $E^{\circ\prime} = [(E_p)_{Red} + (E_p)_{ox}]/2$ where $(E_p)_{Red}$ and $(E_p)_{ox}$ are peak potentials for the reduction and oxidation peaks observed in cyclic voltammetry. E°′ values are shown only for compounds that exhibit reversible behavior in cyclic voltammetry at a sweep rate of 200 mVs^{-1}.
[d]Peak potentials were determined by cyclic voltammetry at a sweep rate of 200 mVs^{-1}.
[e]Peak oxidation potential.
[f]Peak reduction potential.
[g]Saturated calomel reference electrode.
[h]Normal hydrogen electrode.

(−6 mV) couples and many other quinonoid compounds formed as a result of the *in vitro* oxidations of 5-HT and 5-HTPP are such, therefore, that in the presence of cellular reductants/antioxidants and molecular oxygen they should efficiently redox cycle. Indeed, when incubated with ascorbic acid, GSH, or NADPH, 7-*S*-Glu-T-4,5-D, for example, undergoes redox cycling reactions that catalyze oxidation of these reductants forming the H_2O_2 as a byproduct in almost quantitative yield (Scheme 6) (Wong et al., 1993). Reduction of 7-*S*-

Glu-T-4,5-D and related *o*-quinones, *o*-quinone imines, and *p*-quinones by ascorbate, GSH, or NADPH almost certainly proceeds by two one-electron steps via radical intermediates. Similarly, oxidation of the reduced (dihydro) form of these compound by dissolved molecular oxygen probably proceeds by two one-electron oxidation steps with resultant formation of $O_2-\cdot$ that subsequently dismutes into H_2O_2 and oxygen. The presence of trace, catalytic levels of iron or certain other transition metal ions mediate conversion of $O_2-\cdot$ and H_2O_2 to $HO\cdot$.

7.2 Redox properties of putative aberrant oxidative metabolites of DA and NE

Damage to dopaminergic neurons mediated by MA and to both dopaminergic and noradrenergic neurons following ischemia-reperfusion is localized to nerve terminals that are rich in GSH and CySH (Slivka et al., 1987; Philbert et al., 1990). Thus, the terminal regions of these neurons are presumably the sites where ROS are generated. Oxidation of DA and NE in the presence of CySH initially generates a number of cysteinyl conjugates of these neurotransmitters (Schemes 12, 14, 16). Table 2 presents voltammetric peak oxidation potentials for these cysteinyl conjugates and reveals that all are more easily oxidized than DA and NE. These peak oxidation potentials can be taken as rough approximations of $E^{\circ\prime}$ values for these cysteinyl conjugates and their *o*-quinone proximate product couples. Indeed, the peak oxidation potentials for 5-*S*-CyS-DA, 2,5-bi-*S*-CyS-DA, 5-*S*-CyS-NE, and 2,5-bi-*S*-CyS-NE (Table 2) approach that of 5,6-DHT (Table 1), a compound that is neurotoxic as a consequence of its intraneuronal autoxidation to toxic products and ROS (Tabatabaie and Dryhurst, 1997). Accordingly, intraneuronal formation of cysteinyl conjugates of DA and NE might be expected to be followed by their autoxidation forming ROS and a number of DHBTs (Schemes 13,14,16). Many of these DHBTs are also rather easily oxidized compounds (Table 2).

8. Neurochemical and Neurobiological Properties of Putative Aberrant Oxidative Metabolites of 5-HT, DA and NE

T-4,5-D is an intermediate or product of all *in vitro* oxidations of 5-HT that have been studied. Several investigations suggest that T-4,5-D, or secondary products derived from this dione, possess significant neurobiological activities. To illustrate, *in vitro* superfusion experiments demonstrate that T-4,5-D evokes a selective, dose-dependent (10^{-8}–10^{-5} M) increase of basal 5-HT efflux from rat hippocampal and striatal fragments (Chen et al., 1989). This effect has been proposed to result from binding of T-4,5-D to sulfhydryl residues of G-proteins (Fishman et al., 1991). Intracerebroventricular (icv) injections of T-4,5-D (2.5–80 μg) to the rat evoke dose-dependent degeneration of nerve terminals notably in layers 1 and 3 of the insular cortex, layer 1 of the cingulate cortex, and the molecular layer of the dentate cortex. Direct injections of T-4,5-D (5–20 μg) into the rat hippocampus also evoke a dose-dependent degeneration of axon terminals particularly in the CA1 and CA3 sectors of the dentate gyrus. Argyrophilic neurons were also observed in layers 2, 3

Table 2.   Voltammetric Peak Oxidation Potentials at pH 7.4. for
Cysteinyl Conjugates of DA and NE and Dihydrobenzothiazines[a,b]

Compound[c]	Peak Oxidation Potential mV *vs.* SCE[d] (NHE)[e]
DA	125 (367)
5-*S*-CyS-DA	69 (311)
2-*S*-CyS-DA	79 (321)
2,5-bi-*S*-CyS-DA	57 (299)
2,5,6-tri-*S*-CyS-DA	*ca.* 100 (342)
DHBT-1	68 (310)
DHBT-2	66 (308)
DHBT-4	*ca.* 100 (342)
DHBT-5	77 (319)

(continued)

Table 2. Voltammetric Peak Oxidation Potentials at pH 7.4. for
Cysteinyl Conjugates of DA and NE and
Dihydrobenzothiazines[a,b] *(continued)*

Compound[c]	Peak Oxidation Potential mV *vs.* SCE[d] (NHE)[e]
DHBT-6	50 (292)
DHBT-7	112 (354)
DHBT-8	122 (364)
DHBT-9	128 (370)
DHBT-10	155 (397)
BT-1	590 (832)
NE	136 (378)
5-*S*-CyS-NE	66 (308)
2-*S*-CyS-NE	72 (314)

(continued)

Table 2. Voltammetric Peak Oxidation Potentials at pH 7.4. for
Cysteinyl Conjugates of DA and NE and
Dihydrobenzothiazines[a,b] *(continued)*

Compound[c]	Peak Oxidation Potential mV *vs.* SCE[d] (NHE)[e]
2,5-bl-*S*-CyS-NE	53 (295)
DHBT-NE-1	84 (326)
DHBT-NE-2	84 (326)
DHBT-NE-3	64 (306)
DHBT-NE-4	58 (300)
DHBT-NE-5	88 (330)

[a]E_p values measured in pH 7.4 phosphate buffer at a pyrolytic graphite electrode using a sweep rate of 10 mVs^{-1}.
[b]Data from Shen and Dryhurst (1996).
[c]Concentrations of all compounds were 0.5 mM.
[d]Saturated calomel reference electrode.
[e]Normal hydrogen reference electrode.

and 4 of ipsilateral and contralateral entorhinal cortices. Injections of T-4,5-D into the anterior and posterior cingulate cortices produce degeneration in the caudate and anterior thalamic nuclei and contralateral cortex (Crino et al., 1989). These results suggest that T-4,5-D is a neurotoxin that targets medial limbic brain structures receiving projections from multiple neurotransmitter systems including several that degenerate in AD (Crino et al., 1989). Icv injections of T-4,5-D (80 µg/20 µL vehicle; 21 mM) to the rat evoke long-term (7–14 days) decrements (≥60 percent) of 5-HT and 5-HIAA in the hippocampus, striatum and prefrontal cortex along with decreased TPH activity, although apparently without elimination of serotonergic nerve terminals (Chen et al., 1992). However, *in vitro,* T-4,5-D has no inhibitory effect on TPH leading to the suggestion that *in vivo* the dione stimulates release of the latter enzyme from vesicles. T-4,5-D has no effect on noradrenergic or dopaminergic neurons in the rat hippocampus, corpus striatum, or prefrontal cortex (Chen et al., 1992). These are intriguing observations that point to aberrant oxidation of 5-HT and a potential role for T-4,5-D in at least some aspects of the pathogenesis of AD and, perhaps the neurodegeneration evoked by ischemia-reperfusion and MA. However, it is questionable whether all the neurobiological effects attributed to T-4,5-D are in fact evoked by this compound. To illustrate, under the experimental conditions employed to synthesize solutions of T-4,5-D at concentrations as high as 21 mM (Crino et al., 1989), the dione is initially transformed into 7,7'-D (in 0.5 M HCl solution) and upon adjustment to pH 7-7.3, this dimer is oxidized to 7,7'-T-4,5-D (Scheme 5) that subsequently polymerizes. Accordingly, the neurodegenerative properties attributed to T-4,5-D (Crino et al., 1989; Chen et al., 1992) were probably evoked by 7,7'-T-4,5-D and/or polymeric materials derived from this dimer. Nevertheless, it has more recently been demonstrated that multiple daily infusions of more dilute solutions of T-4,5-D (1.2 µg/5 µL of isotonic saline; 1.26 mM) into the rat hippocampus results in a small but significant decrease of 5-HT levels (Wrona et al., 1996). Whether such 5-HT decrements reflect the T-4,5-D-mediated degeneration of serotonergic terminals is presently unknown.

In the event that T-4,5-D is indeed formed as a result of oxygen radical-mediated oxidation of 5-HT, it is unlikely that it would survive in brain tissue principally because of its facile reactions with available nucleophiles, particularly GSH, CySH and cysteinyl residues of proteins. Indeed, when incubated with perchloric acid-soluble extracts of rat brain homogenate T-4,5-D reacts to give 7-S-Glu-T-4,5-D (Chen et al., 1989). This bright purple compound is lethal when administered into the brains of mice ($LD_{50} = 21$ µg, free base) and evokes a neurobehavioral response that includes hyperactivity and seizures (Wong et al., 1993). During this hyperactivity phase 7-S-Glu-T-4,5-D evokes release and elevated turnover of particularly NE, but also 5-HT and DA (Wong et al., 1993) that might be related to its ability to act as an inverse $GABA_B$ receptor agonist (Wrona et al., 1996). However, a single dose of 7-S-Glu-T-4,5-D does not cause long-lasting decrements of whole mouse brain levels of the biogenic amine neurotransmitters or acetylcholine.

Tryptophan-4,5-dione (35) is much more unstable at pH 7.4 than T-4,5-D (Wu and Dryhurst, 1996) and hence the biochemical properties of this compound are not known. However, its glutathionyl conjugate 42 is, similar to 7-S-Glu-T-4,5-D, lethal when administered into mouse brain ($LD_{50} = 23$ µg) and evokes a hyperactivity syndrome (Wu and Dryhurst, 1996). Ether-linked dimer 37, formed as a result of several oxidation reactions of 5-HTPP, is even more toxic in mouse brain ($LD_{50} = 3.3$ µg) and causes hyperactivity (Wu et al., 1995). During this neurobehavioral response 37 evokes elevated release and turnover of DA, NE, and 5-HT. The hyperactivity evoked by 37 is similar to that produced by pharmacologic manipulations that increase 5-HT synthesis in mouse and rat brain (Grahame-Smith, 1971; Modigh, 1972) suggesting that this dimer might be metabolized to metabolites that interact with 5-HT and perhaps other receptor populations. Dimer 37 exhibits a weak but selective affinity for 5-HT_1 receptors (Wu et al., 1995).

Preliminary screening experiments also suggest that other putative aberrant oxidative metabolites of 5-HT and 5-HTPP interact with a number of brain receptors. To illustrate, at the 10 μM concentration level, significant binding to the $GABA_B$ (7-S-Glu-T-4,5-D, 24, 42), NMDA (7-S-Glu-T-4,5-D), 5-HT_1 (7,7'-T-4,5-D, 4, 37), 5-HT_2 (4), bombesin (7,7'-T-4,5-D, 24), and calcium N-type or ω-conotoxin (24, 7,7'-T-4-5-D) receptors has been observed (unpublished results). However, these results must be viewed with caution because of the experimental difficulties in obtaining highly pure compounds and their instability in solution.

Investigations into the neurobiological and neurobehavioral effects of putative metabolites resulting from *in vitro* oxidations of DA and NE in the presence of CySH and GSH are at a very early stage. However, a rather remarkable number of DHBTs formed in these reactions are toxic (lethal) when administered into the brains of mice (Table 3). Furthermore, 5-S-Glu-DA is rapidly metabolized in rat brain to 5-S-CyS-DA in reactions mediated by γ-glutamyltranspeptidase (γ-GT) and cysteinyl glycine dipeptidase (Scheme 17) (Shen et al., 1996). 5-S-CyS-DA is more slowly metabolized to 5-S-(N-acetylcysteinyl)dopamine by cysteine conjugate N-acetyltransferase. The latter 5-S-N-acetylcysteinyl conjugate of DA and its 2-S- and 2,5-bi-S-congeners are also toxic in mouse brain (Table 3) (Shen et al., 1996). The various toxic DHBTs derived from DA and NE, and N-acetylcysteinyl conjugates of DA all evoke a similar neurobehavioral response that includes episodes of rapid running, jumping and rolling, and severe tremor (shivering). This neurobehavioral response develops very rapidly after drug administration. By contrast, following intracerebral administration of 2,5-bi-S-CyS-DA, mice exhibit no unusual behavioral response for 10–30 min and only after this lag time does the hyperactivity/tremor syndrome develop (Shen and Dryhurst, 1996a). Because of the very facile oxidation of 2,5-bi-S-CyS-DA (Table 2), it is conceivable that *in vivo* oxidation occurs generating toxic DHBT-6 (major product) and DHBT-2. Recent studies have demonstrated that DHBT-1 can cross the membrane of intact rat brain mitochondria and evoke a time-dependent irreversible inhibition of complex I ($NADH\text{-}CoQ_1$ reductase) respiration (Li and Dryhurst, 1997). Intramitochondrial antioxidants such as GSH and AA are unable to fully protect mitochondrial complex I against irreversible inhibition by DHBT-1 under conditions where they provide complete protection against the inhibition evoked by 1-methyl-4-pyridinium (MPP^+), a widely-used dopaminergic neurotoxin (Cleeter et al., 1992). Thus, DHBT-1 appears to damage complex I by mechanisms that are only partially related to ROS generation.

9. Serotonin Binding Proteins (SBPs)

Emerging evidence suggests that serotonergic and catecholaminergic neurons possess an endogenous defense mechanism designed to provide protection against toxic insults by electrophilic intermediates and products formed by intraneuronal oxidation of 5-HT, DA and NE in the form of so-called serotonin binding proteins (SBPs). Found in the brains of mammals, including humans, SBPs were long believed to participate in the storage, protection and/or transport of the biogenic amine neurotransmitters (Tamir et al., 1976; Tamir and Gershon, 1979; Jimenez Del Rio et al., 1992, 1993a). The binding of 5-HT and DA to

Table 3. LD$_{50}$ Values for Putative Aberrant Oxidative
Metabolites of DA and NE in Mice[a]

Compound[b]	LD$_{50}$ μg
2,5-bi-*S*-CyS-DA	37
DHBT-1	14
DHBT-2	70
DHBT-5	5
DHBT-6	17
DHBT-8	88
DHBT-9	18
DHBT-10	1.5
5-*S*-(*N*-acetylcysteinyl)DA	14

(continued)

Table 3. LD$_{50}$ Values for Putative Aberrant Oxidative
Metabolites of DA and NE in Mice[a] *(continued)*

Compound[b]	LD$_{50}$ μg
 2-S-(N-acetylcysteinyl)DA	25
 2,5-bi-S-(N-acetylcysteinyl)DA	42
 DHBT-NE-1	18
 DHBT-NE-2	23

[a]Compounds, dissolved in 5 μL of isotonic saline, left lateral ventricle of male
Sprague Dawley albino mice weighing approximately 30 g.
[b]Data from Zhang and Dryhurst (1994), Shen and Dryhurst (1996a,b; 1997) and
Shen et al., (1996).

SBPs is greatly enhanced by Fe^{2+}. Accordingly, until recently it was believed that Fe^{2+} initially binds to sulfhydryl residues at or near the binding site of SBPs and then the monoamines form coordinate bonds with the trapped iron (Tamir and Liu, 1982). More recent studies, however, have demonstrated that Fe^{2+} reacts with dissolved molecular oxygen to form O$_2$–· that oxidizes 5-HT or DA to electrophilic intermediates that bind covalently (and irreversibly) to the sulfhydryl residues of SBPs (Jimenez Del Rio et al., 1993b). These observations imply that SBPs are present in neurons to scavenge and presumably detoxify intraneuronal oxidation products of 5-HT, DA and NE.

10. Discussion

Cerebral ischemia-reperfusion evokes degeneration of serotonergic, noradrenergic, and dopaminergic terminals (Weinberger et al., 1983) and a number of other cells in the selected regions of the cortex and hippocampus (Pulsinelli and Brierley, 1979; Pulsinelli et al., 1982; Volpe et al., 1984; Ginsberg et al., 1985; Sapolsky and Pulsinelli, 1985). Neurotoxic doses of MA also evoke damage to serotonergic and dopaminergic terminals (Gibb et al., 1994; Bowyer and Holson, 1995; Seiden and Sabol, 1995), noradrenergic neurons apparently being spared (Wagner et al., 1980; Ricaurte et al., 1984), and a subpopulation of unknown cell bodies in the somatosensory cortex (Commins and Seiden, 1986). Many lines of evi-

Scheme 17

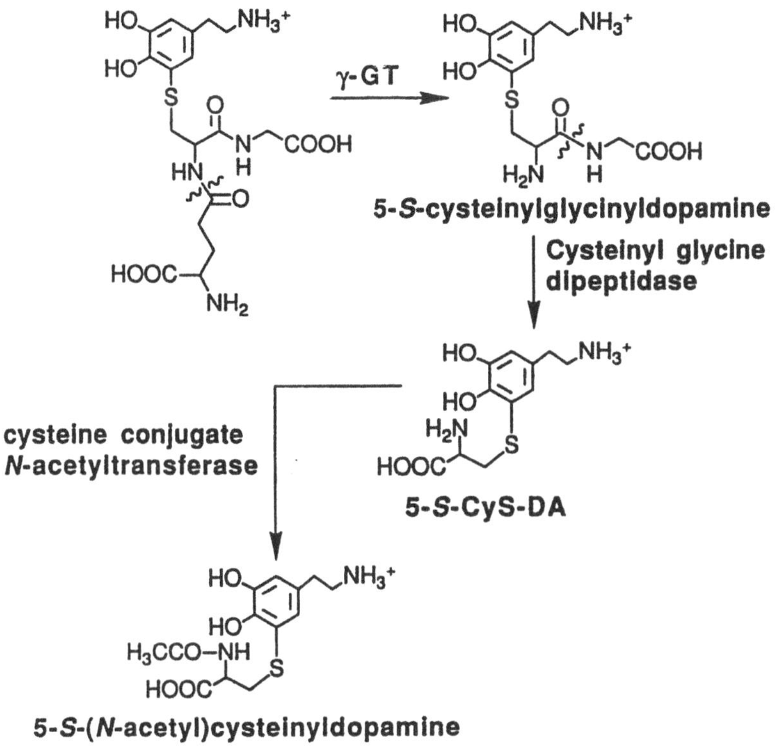

5-*S*-cysteinylglycinyldopamine

γ-GT

Cysteinyl glycine
dipeptidase

5-*S*-CyS-DA

cysteine conjugate
***N*-acetyltransferase**

5-*S*-(*N*-acetyl)cysteinyldopamine

dence strongly suggest that ROS are directly or indirectly involved in the neurodegeneration evoked by ischemia-reperfusion (Yoshida et al., 1984; Kontos and Wei, 1986; Hall et al., 1988; Floyd, 1990; Oliver et al., 1990; Sakomoto et al., 1991; Hyslop et al., 1995), particularly $O_2^-\cdot$ (Kinouchi et al., 1991; Yang et al., 1994).

Similarly, oxidative stress is clearly associated with MA-induced neurodegeneration (DeVito and Wagner, 1989; Stone et al., 1989; Kondo et al., 1993), and again $O_2^-\cdot$ appears to play the major role (Cadet et al., 1994; Hirata et el., 1995, 1996). There are potentially several sources of the oxygen radicals formed upon reperfusion of ischemic regions of the brain. These include a Ca^{2+} influx that mediates proteolysis of xanthine dehydrogenase to XOD and subsequent oxidation of xanthine (Onadera et al., 1986; Kinuta et al., 1989) either in nerve terminals or more probably in blood capillaries with subsequent damage to the BBB (Del Maestro et al., 1981; Chan et al., 1984; Betz, 1985) and resultant release of iron into the brain. Additionally, released 5-HT, NE and DA (Pulsinelli et al., 1982; Brannan et al., 1987; Globus et al., 1989; Phebus and Clemens, 1989) during the ischemic insult should, upon reoxygenation, be metabolized by MAO and perhaps undergo autoxidation in reactions that generate H_2O_2 and $O_2^-\cdot$, respectively (Kontos and Wei, 1986; Hyslop et al., 1995). However, there are far fewer obvious mechanisms that might account for MA-induced formation of ROS. Thus, MA is an MAO inhibitor (Suzuki et al., 1980) and hence it is unlikely that metabolism of the biogenic amines by this enzyme would provide damaging levels of H_2O_2. Furthermore, MAO inhibitors exacerbate MA-induced damage

(Marek et al., 1990c). This therefore might point to autoxidation of 5-HT, DA and perhaps NE as a source of MA-induced $O_2^-\cdot$ and ROS.

A number of lines of evidence suggest that ROS formation by one or more of these mechanisms cannot be solely responsible for the neurodegeneration evoked by ischemia-reperfusion or MA. For example, the protective effects of NMDA receptor antagonists (Gill et al., 1987), other Ca^{2+} channel blockers (Nakayama et al., 1988), ω-conotoxin receptor antagonists (Ooboshi et al., 1992), and pharmacologic agents that elevate brain GABA levels (Sternau et al., 1989) against ischemia-reperfusion are not easily reconciled with ROS being the sole mediators of neurodegeneration. The facts that NMDA receptor antagonists (Sonsalla et al., 1991; Farfel et al., 1992) and elevated GABA levels (Hotchkiss and Gibb, 1980) also protect against MA-induced neurodegeneration lead to the same conclusion and, indeed, might point to similar mechanisms underlying the neurotoxic effects evoked by both MA and ischemia-reperfusion.

One possibility is that the biogenic amines themselves directly mediate the neurodegeneration caused by ischemia-reperfusion and MA, i.e., are endotoxins under certain conditions. Indeed, administration of relatively massive doses of DA or NE into rat corpus striatum are neurotoxic (Filloux and Townsend, 1993), particularly when MAO is inhibited (Ben-Shachar et al., 1995), and evidence for autoxidation of the administered neurotransmitter has been obtained (Hastings et al., 1996). However, analysis of rat brain several hours after injection of large doses of DA or NE reveals no increases of lipid or protein peroxidation or other indices of oxidative stress (Ben-Shachar et al., 1995). Thus, it has been proposed that DA and NE are mitochondrial complex I toxins (Ben-Shachar et al., 1995). This suggestion is based on the ability of micromolar concentrations of DA or NE to inhibit mitochondrial NADH ferricyanide reductase, although their ability to inhibit the physiologically relevant NADH coenzyme Q reductase (complex I) has not been examined.

It seems a somewhat remote possibility that very low concentrations of DA or NE would in fact inhibit the latter system because other mitochondrial complex I inhibitors (rotenone, MPP^+) enhance the production of oxygen free radicals by the respiratory chain with resultant oxidative damage (Turrens and Bovaris, 1980; Hasegawa et al., 1990; Cleeter et al., 1992), which was not observed after injection of these neurotransmitters into rat brain (Ben-Shachar et al., 1985). Nevertheless, it seems clear that in some way DA and/or NE are involved in the neurodegeneration evoked by both ischemia-reperfusion and MA. To illustrate, surgical procedures or pharmacological manipulations that deplete DA or NE in certain brain regions provide significant protection against neuronal damage caused by ischemia-reperfusion (Busto et al., 1985; Weinberger et al., 1985; Globus et al., 1987; Siesjö, 1988) and MA (Schmidt et al., 1985; Commins and Seiden, 1986; Axt et al., 1990). Furthermore, DA uptake inhibitors protect striatal dopaminergic terminals (Schmidt and Gibb, 1985; Schmidt et al., 1985) and 5-HT uptake inhibitors protect serotonergic terminals in various brain regions (Ricaurte et al., 1983) against MA-induced damage.

These observations point to the conclusion that DA (and perhaps NE) and 5-HT, or other extraneuronal compounds that can utilize the uptake mechanisms for these neurotransmitters, must be transported into nerve terminals in order to evoke their neurodegenerative effects. It has been proposed that MA induces the release of DA and 5-HT that are then oxidized in the synaptic cleft to 6-OHDA and 5,6-DHT and then transported into and destroy dopaminergic and serotonergic terminals, respectively (Vosmer and Seiden, 1984; Commins et al., 1987a). However, the failure of other investigators to detect either 6-OHDA (Rollema et al., 1986; Karoum et al., 1993) or 5,6-DHT (Yang et al., 1997) in rat brain following MA administration argues against a role for these neurotoxins.

Nevertheless, it seems plausible that mechanisms that occur in the cytoplasm of serotonergic, dopaminergic, and perhaps noradrenergic axon terminals might be responsible, at least in part, for the degeneration of these neurons induced by MA. For example, studies on the dopaminergic system have demonstrated that pharmacologic agents that elevate the cytoplasmic pool of DA, such as reserpine or the MAO inhibitor pargyline, potentiate MA-induced damage to dopaminergic neurons (Wagner et al., 1983; Marek et al., 1990c). Conversely, agents that deplete the cytoplasmic pool of DA, such as the DA (and NE) synthesis inhibitor α-methyl-p-tyrosine (AMT), attenuate long-lasting MA-induced depletions of DA (Wagner et al., 1983; Axt et al., 1990). Furthermore, the protection afforded by increased Cu-Zn SOD activity against the neurodegeneration evoked by MA (Cadet et al., 1994; Hirata et al., 1995, 1996) and ischemia-reperfusion (Kinouchi et al., 1991; Yang et al., 1994), and the oxidation of sulfhydryl residues of TPH induced by MA (Stone et al., 1989) again point to cytoplasmic rather than extraneuronal generation of O_2–· and other ROS. Of potential relevance to this discussion is the fact that MA appears to displace both DA (Raiteri et al., 1979) and perhaps 5-HT (Kuczenski and Sabol, 1994) from cytoplasmic storage sites leading to increased cytoplasmic concentrations of the free or unbound neurotransmitters prior to their release. Perhaps, therefore, elevated cytoplasmic levels of DA and 5-HT (and NE) resulting from MA administration or ischemia-reperfusion in some way results in their intraneuronal oxidation. Oxidation of DA in the cytoplasm of dopaminergic nerve terminals would necessarily expose DA-o-quinone (54) to CySH and GSH (Slivka et al., 1987; Philbert et al., 1990). Thus, it is of considerable significance that treatment of guinea-pigs with reserpine, a drug that disrupts biogenic amine storage vesicles and greatly increases the cytoplasmic pool of these neurotransmitters, results in a marked and sustained elevation of striatal levels of 5-S-CyS-DA (Fornstedt and Carlsson, 1989). Similarly, neurotoxic doses of MA evoke increased formation of striatal 5-S-Glu-DA and 5-S-CyS-DA in the rat (La Voie et al., 1996). Presumably, reuptake of DA and 5-HT (and NE) released by MA and ischemia-reperfusion would serve to maintain greatly elevated cytoplasmic concentrations of these neurotransmitters with resultant intraneuronal oxidation.

It is also of considerable relevance that studies with cortical and hippocampal neuronal cultures, that did not contain biogenic aminergic neurons, have demonstrated that the uptake of DA, NE, or 5-HT followed by intraneuronal oxidation of these neurotransmitters by an unknown enzyme, possibly prostaglandin synthase (Hastings and Zigmond, 1992; Zigmond and Hastings, 1992; Hastings, 1995), is a key step in mediating glutamate oxidative neurotoxicity (Maher and Davis, 1996). Such intraneuronal oxidation of the biogenic amines has been proposed to generate cytotoxic levels of ROS (Maher and Davis, 1996). However, oxidation of DA, NE, or 5-HT in *any* type of nerve terminals would be expected to result in the reaction of electrophilic intermediates/products with intraneuronal CySH and GSH or protein sulfhydryl residues. These reactions, therefore, might provide an explanation for the depletion of cortical GSH without any increase in GSSG evoked by ischemia-reperfusion (Cooper et al., 1980; Rehncrona et al., 1980) following reoxygenation (Folbergrová et al., 1979).

Taken together, the preceding lines of evidence permit formulation of an hypothesis, many aspects of which might be tested by experiment. Consider first the vulnerability of dopaminergic and serotonergic terminals to the degenerative effects of both MA and ischemia-reperfusion and, in addition, the degeneration of noradrenergic terminals by the latter insult. Both MA and ischemia-reperfusion should evoke elevated cytoplasmic levels of free or unbound DA, NE, and 5-HT by displacing these neurotransmitters from storage sites (Small et al., 1982) and as a result of reuptake of released neurotransmitters. Under these conditions, 5-HT, NE, and DA undergo intraneuronal oxidation by molecular oxygen, perhaps in an enzyme-mediated reaction and/or transition metal ion-catalyzed reaction. Such reactions should generate $O_2^-\cdot$ and other ROS.

In vitro studies indicate that almost regardless of the oxidation mechanism, 5-HT would be oxidized to T-4,5-D as a major if not the major product. Several important and relevant consequences would flow from intraneuronal formation of T-4,5-D at levels exceeding the scavenging capacity of SBPs. It is virtually certain that T-4,5-D would react with cytoplasmic GSH (Scheme 6) and CySH (Scheme 3) to give a plethora of putative metabolites. Virtually all such putative metabolites have the proven (e.g., 7-S-Glu-T-4,5-D) or potential (Table 1) ability to redox cycle in the presence of intraneuronal antioxidants and molecular oxygen in reactions that would potentiate $O_2^-\cdot$ and ROS formation. Such a sequence of reactions involving only known constituents of serotonergic axon terminals provides a plausible rationale for the vulnerability of these neurons to degeneration as a result of MA administration and ischemia-reperfusion by oxygen radical-mediated peroxidation, and the protection against such brain insults by increased cytoplasmic Cu-Zn SOD activity and other antioxidants.

It is not hard to imagine that the redox cycling reactions of putative endotoxins derived from T-4,5-D might generate sufficiently high fluxes of $O_2^-\cdot$ and ROS that not only are lipids, proteins, and DNA oxidized but also 5-HT, hence potentiating additional T-4,5-D formation. The protection afforded by 5-HT uptake inhibitors might be rationalized by their ability to attenuate cytoplasmic levels of the neurotransmitter. The intraneuronal chemistry proposed could also account, in part, for the irreversible loss of cortical GSH that occurs following reoxygenation of the ischemic brain. There is also evidence that T-4,5-D or compounds derived from this dione are lethal in mouse and rat brain (e.g., 7-S-Glu-T-4,5-D) and may even be neurotoxic. Thus, release or leakage of these putative toxins from damaged or dying serotonergic terminals might contribute to the degeneration of, for example, connected cell bodies in the rat somatosensory cortex following MA administration, and pyramidal and other cells in the cortex and hippocampus that are connected to serotonergic terminals following ischemia-reperfusion. Interactions of such putative aberrant oxidative metabolites of 5-HT with, for example, various Ca^{2+} channel receptors could potentiate additional neurotransmitter release, such as glutamate, altered Ca^{2+} homeostasis, excitotoxic processes and $O_2^-\cdot$ formation, and account for the protective effects of NMDA and other Ca^{2+} channel receptor antagonists and elevated extracellular GABA levels against neurodegeneration mediated by MA and ischemia-reperfusion.

Intraneuronal oxidation of DA and NE, again almost regardless of the oxidant, would generate electrophilic o-quinones that must react avidly with CySH to give cysteinyl conjugates of these neurotransmitters (Schemes 12 and 16) or with GSH to give glutathionyl conjugates (Scheme 11). Detection of 5-S-CyS-DA and 5-S-Glu-DA in rat brain following MA administration (LaVoie et al., 1996) and 5-S-CyS-DA following reserpine administration to the guinea-pig (Fornstedt and Carlsson, 1989) together provide strong evidence for elevated cytoplasmic DA levels potentiating oxidation of this neurotransmitter. These reactions could again contribute to the massive irreversible loss of GSH following ischemia-reperfusion (Cooper et al., 1980; Rehncrona et al., 1980) and predict a similar loss as a result of MA administration. However, cysteinyl conjugates of DA and NE are more easily oxidized than the neurotransmitters (Table 2). Under intraneuronal conditions where DA and NE are oxidized, particularly when CySH (and GSH) levels are depleted, these cysteinyl conjugates must also be oxidized in reactions that generate DHBTs (Schemes 13, 14, and 16) and $O_2^-\cdot$ as a byproduct. A remarkable number of these DHBTs are toxic when administered into animal brains (Table 3). The biochemical mechanisms underlying the lethal properties of these DHBTs remain to be elucidated. However, at least one such compound, DHBT-1, is an irreversible inhibitor of mitochondrial complex I that, either by binding with this enzyme system and/or by its autoxidation, evokes oxygen radical formation. Whether other DHBTs, formed as a result of the *in vitro* oxidation of DA or NE in the presence of CySH, are also mitochondrial complex I toxins remains to be determined. Furthermore, there is presently no experimental evidence that DHBT-1 is indeed formed in dopaminergic terminals as a result of ischemia-reperfusion or MA administration. Nevertheless, MA does result in formation of its immediate precursor 5-*S*-Cys-DA.

Experimental evidence might point to formation of an irreversible mitochondrial complex I toxin, such as DHBT-1, in dopaminergic terminals with resultant ATP depletions as a result of ischemia-reperfusion. To illustrate, upon reoxygenation of ischemic rat brain ATP, phosphocreatine and lactate levels rapidly recover to near control values in the dopamine terminal-rich corpus striatum (Pulsinelli and Duffy, 1983). However, over the course of the subsequent 6–24 h, ATP and phosphocreatine concentrations fall significantly and lactate levels rise. The 6–24 h period during which ATP levels decline coincides with the onset and progression of morphological injury. Such a sequence of events might reflect the intraneuronal oxidation of elevated cytoplasmic levels of DA during reperfusion resulting from uptake of ischemia-mediated released neurotransmitter, to DA-*o*-quinone (54) that reacts with CySH and GSH to give 5-*S*-CyS-DA, other cysteinyl dopamines (Scheme 12) and glutathionyl dopamines (Scheme 11). Upon depletion of CySH and GSH further oxidation of 5-*S*-CyS-DA and other cysteinyl dopamines would, based on *in vitro* studies, generate DHBT-1 and other DHBTs (Schemes 13,14). Transport of DHBT-1 and perhaps other DHBTs into mitochondria with resultant inhibition of and irreversible oxygen radical-mediated damage to complex I might account for the progressive decline of ATP production.

Such a reduction of energy stores in dopaminergic terminals would evoke a reduced transmembrane potential that relieves the voltage-sensitive Mg^{2+} block of NMDA receptors, thereby permitting persistent excitotoxic effects by even normal extracellular levels of glutamate (Novielli et al., 1988; Beal et al., 1993). Activation of NMDA receptors under such conditions evokes an influx of Ca^{2+} and intraneuronal $O_2-\cdot$ and other ROS formation (Coyle and Puttfarcken, 1993; Lafon-Cazal et al., 1993), thus perhaps further potentiating DA oxidation, DHBT formation, and mitochondrial damage in a self-perpetuating cycle leading to cell peroxidative death. Together, these events could also provide an explanation for the protective effects of NMDA (Gill et al., 1987), other Ca^{2+} channel (Nakayama et al., 1988) and ω-conotoxin (Ooboshi et al., 1992) receptor antagonists, increased GABA levels (Sternau et al., 1989), increased Cu-Zn SOD activity (Kinouchi et al., 1991; Yang et al., 1994) and other antioxidants (Hall et al., 1988; Clemens et al., 1993) against neurodegeneration caused by ischemia-reperfusion. Exactly parallel processes might account for MA-induced degeneration of striatal dopaminergic terminals. In the event that intraneuronal oxidation of NE generates DHBTs that are also mitochondrial toxins, then a similar sequence of processes might account for the degeneration of noradrenergic terminals following ischemia-reperfusion (Weinberger et al., 1983). Because of the very many similarities between the neurodegeneration evoked by ischemia-reperfusion and MA, it is rather surprising that the latter drug does not induce the degeneration of noradrenergic terminals, at least in regions of the brain that have been studied (Wagner et al., 1980; Ricaurte et al., 1984).

Pharmacologic agents, such as AMT, that deplete both DA and NE synthesis (Spector et al., 1965) attenuate not only MA-induced damage to dopaminergic terminals in the corpus striatum and serotonergic terminals in cortex and hippocampus, but also a subpopulation of unknown cell bodies in the somatosensory cortex (Commins and Seiden, 1980; Axt et al., 1990). The fact that the cortex and particularly the hippocampus and somatosensory cortex have little or no dopaminergic input points to NE rather than DA mediating the neurotoxic effects of MA in these brain regions. Similarly, AMT protects dopaminergic, serotonergic and glutamatergic neurons against degeneration by ischemia-reperfusion (Weinberger and Cohen, 1983; Weinberger et al., 1985; Clemens and Phebus, 1988). Again, the degeneration of serotonergic and glutamatergic neurons evoked by ischemia-reperfusion often occurs in brain regions in the cortex and hippocampus containing little or no dopaminergic innervation. That released NE might mediate damage in these areas is also supported by the observation that severing noradrenergic projections from the LC to hippocampal CA1 cells and various cortical regions, that are normally severely degenerated by forebrain ischemia-reperfusion (Pulsinelli and Brierley, 1979; Volpe et al., 1984; Sapolsky and Pulsinelli, 1985), protects these cells (Pulsinelli, 1985; Clemens and Phebus, 1988).

In view of the fact that uptake of biogenic amines mediates oxidative glutamate toxicity in hippocampal and cortical neuronal cultures (Maher and Davis, 1996), it thus becomes plausible that NE plays the key role in mediating degeneration in regions of the cortex and hippocampus having little dopaminergic input caused by both MA and ischemia-reperfusion. This is further supported by the fact that ischemia-reperfusion (Benveniste et al., 1994) and possibly MA (Sonsalla et al., 1991) also evoke glutamate release in these regions. Oxidation of NE in the cytoplasm of cortical and hippocampal neurons, perhaps mediated by an unknown enzyme (Maher and Davis, 1996) would generate NE-o-quinone (74) that would react with CySH and GSH forming ultimately DHBTs (Scheme 16). Such reactions would account for the loss of cortical GSH following ischemia-reperfusion (Cooper et al., 1980; Rehncrona et al., 1980).

Assuming that one or more DHBTs derived from NE are irreversible mitochondrial complex I toxins, then an explanation for peroxidative damage evoked by both MA and ischemia-reperfusion ensues. Interestingly, upon reoxygenation of ischemic rat brain, ATP, phosphocreatine, and lactate levels rapidly return to control values in the cortex and CA1 zone of the hippocampus (Pulsinelli and Duffy, 1983). However, only after 24–72 h do ATP and phosphocreatine concentrations fall and lactate levels rise accompanied by the onset and progression of morphological injury. Together, these observations clearly point to intraneuronal processes that oxidize NE, consume CySH and/or GSH and interfere with mitochondrial respiration. However, the fall of ATP levels in cortex and hippocampus is appreciably delayed compared to similar changes in the corpus striatum. This difference could simply reflect the much higher concentrations of DA, the precursor of DHBT mitochondrial complex I toxins in the corpus striatum, compared to much lower concentrations of NE, the precursor of similar putative DHBT toxins in the hippocampus and cortex.

In summary, the preceding hypothesis proposes that the degeneration of dopaminergic and serotonergic terminals (ischemia-reperfusion and MA) and noradrenergic terminals (ischemia-reperfusion) can be traced to intraneuronal oxidation of their neurotransmitters. The common factor connecting the neurodegeneration of biogenic aminergic terminals evoked by ischemia-reperfusion and MA is the release and reuptake of their neurotransmitters with resultant major increases in their free or unbound cytoplasmic concentrations. Intraneuronal oxidation of 5-HT in serotonergic terminals would generate T-4,5-D at concentrations that exceed the scavenging capacity of SBPs. This putative intraneuronal metabolite and secondary metabolites formed by its reactions with GSH and CySH are proposed to undergo redox cycling reactions to generate ROS that potentiate further oxidation of 5-HT and lipid, protein and DNA oxidation leading to cell death. Interactions of these putative metabolites with connected neurons might contribute to the degeneration of other neurons in the cortex and hippocampus that receive extensive serotonergic innervation, perhaps involving interactions with a number of receptors. Released 5-HT might also be taken up by connected neurons potentiating oxidative glutamate toxicity. This hypothesis proposes that the degeneration of dopaminergic and noradrenergic terminals is initiated by intraneuronal oxidation of DA and NE, respectively, to *o*-quinones again at levels that exceed the protective capacity of SBPs.

Reactions of these *o*-quinones with CySH and GSH ultimately leads to DHBTs that are possibly mitochondrial toxins, thus accounting for reduced ATP production, oxidative damage, and excitotoxicity mediated by glutamate. Released DA and particularly NE in the cortex and hippocampus and uptake by connected serotonergic, glutamatergic and perhaps other neurons followed by their intraneuronal oxidation provides a mechanism for formation of DHBT mitochondrial toxins in non-catecholaminergic neurons with resultant energy depletion, oxidative damage, excitotoxicity, and cell death. Thus, this hypothesis advances the proposition that ischemia-reperfusion and MA both evoke system neurodegenerations of certain serotonergic, catecholaminergic and connected neurons by processes in which the biogenic amine neurotransmitters, because of their ease of oxidation, are the precursors of endotoxins.

The system neurodegenerations evoked by both MA and ischemia-reperfusion are massive and occur very rapidly following the brain insult. By contrast, the system neurodegeneration that occurs in AD is almost certainly very slow. Clinical symptoms of this brain disorder probably appear many years or decades after the degenerative processes were initiated. However, as noted by other investigators (Hardy et al., 1985; Saper et al., 1987), regions of the brain that exhibit the most profound neurodegeneration are innervated with serotonergic and noradrenergic neurons that project from subcortical cell bodies. Furthermore, these neurons innervate microvessels in the cortex and hippocampus (Edvinsson et al., 1983; Kaleria et al., 1989). Several lines of evidence suggest that an early event in the pathogenesis of AD might be an increased BBB permeability (Wisniewski and Kozlowski, 1982; Alafuzoff et al., 1983; Mann et al., 1982; Mann, 1988), perhaps caused by head trauma (French et al., 1985; Mortimer et al, 1985; Shalat et al., 1986), exposure to certain chemical toxicants in the environment (Hardy et al., 1985), and/or genetic factors, resulting in the release of low molecular weight iron species into the brain. Intraneuronal and extracellular antioxidants would maintain such species in the Fe^{2+} state, a form that mediates oxygen radical formation in the presence of molecular oxygen and H_2O_2. Within or in the vicinity of serotonergic and noradrenergic terminals that innervate blood microvessels in the cortex and hippocampus, Fe^{2+}-mediated oxygen radical formation might also be expected to evoke oxidation of 5-HT and NE to the same putative aberrant oxidative metabolites that are proposed to evoke neurodegeneration caused by ischemia-reperfusion and MA. Indeed, detection of trace levels of unknown but apparently oxidized forms of 5-HT and 5-HTPP in the CSF of AD patients (Volicer et al., 1985, 1989) provides some support for formation of such metabolites in this disorder. Although iron released in this fashion might mediate the oxygen radical oxidation of 5-HT and NE, perhaps with neurodegenerative consequences to selected serotonergic and noradrenergic terminals, such a mechanism fails to adequately rationalize the system degeneration that occurs in AD, i.e., the degeneration of non-aminergic neurons connected to specific noradrenergic and serotonergic neurons in the cortex and hippocampus.

By analogy with the hypothesis proposed for the system neurodegeneration evoked by ischemia-reperfusion and MA, the release of low molecular weight iron from microvessels in the vicinity of serotonergic and noradrenergic terminals in specific regions of the cortex and hippocampus should evoke elevated release of 5-HT and NE (and perhaps glutamate). Subsequent uptake of these neurotransmitters with resulting increase of cytoplasmic levels of 5-HT and NE in serotonergic and noradrenergic terminals and other connected neurons followed by their intraneuronal oxidation to endotoxins that mediate degeneration of these cells by oxygen radicals and mitochondrial damage should then ensue. It is of potential importance, therefore, that using brain microdialysis, we have found that perfusion of Fe^{2+} into the rat hippocampus evokes a massive increase of extracellular 5-HT and decreased 5-HIAA levels (unpublished observations). The effects of Fe^{2+} on the release of NE or other transmitters remain to be studied. Nevertheless, these results may indicate that an increased permeability of the BBB and release of Fe^{2+} into the brain might evoke release of 5-HT and NE with consequent intraneuronal oxidation of these neurotransmitters and a very anatomically selective system neurodegeneration by processes that include oxidative stress and mitochondrial damage as discussed earlier in connection with ischemia-reperfusion and MA. These mechanisms might in turn account for lipid peroxidation (Hajimohammadadreza and Brammer, 1990; Subbarao et al., 1990; Palmer and Burns, 1994) with resultant crosslinking of apolipoprotein E by low molecular weight products (Martine et al., 1996), increased levels of heme oxygenase-1 (Smith et al., 1994; Schipper et al., 1995), mitochondrial 8-hydroxydeoxyguanosine (Mecocci et al., 1996), and decreased mitochondrial ATP production (Sims et al., 1987; Blass et al., 1990) that occur in selected regions of the AD brain.

While mechanistically the neurodegenerative processes in AD might be similar to those that occur as a result of ischemia-reperfusion and MA, they are undoubtedly much slower and occur over years or decades. This might be expected if only minor elevations of low molecular weight iron occur with small releases of 5-HT and NE so that putative endotoxic metabolites formed by intraneuronal oxidation of these neurotransmitters are generated in lower concentrations than are proposed to occur following ischemia-reperfusion and MA administration. Thus, relatively minor elevations of ROS over long periods of time in brain regions innervated by serotonergic and noradrenergic neurons might contribute to the transformation of soluble βAP into its aggregated state (Koh et al., 1990; Yanker et al, 1990; Dyrks et al., 1992; Pike et al., 1993) that serves as point sources of yet another neurotoxin in the AD brain that kills surrounding neurons of diverse neurotransmitter content (Walker et al., 1988) in a centrifugal fashion (Selkoe, 1989) accounting for the remarkably spherical form of SPs. Similarly, oxygen radical-mediated polymerization of tau protein might contribute to NFT formation (Troncoso et al., 1993).

Mitochondrial damage and decreased ATP production (Mecocci et al., 1994; Sims et al., 1987; Blass et al., 1990), perhaps mediated by intraneuronal oxidation of NE and formation of DHBTs, might as noted previously, relieve the voltage-sensitive Mg^{2+} blockade of NMDA receptors, thereby permitting excitotoxic effects even by normal extracellular levels of glutamate (Novielli et al., 1988; Beal et al., 1993) potentiating an influx of Ca^{2+}, intraneuronal ROS formation, NE oxidation, DHBT formation, and further mitochondrial damage in a self-perpetuating and progressive cycle of cell death. Indeed, there are profound losses of glutamate and NMDA receptors in certain regions of the hippocampus and cortex in AD (Hyman et al., 1987; Proctor et al., 1988; Greenamyre and Young, 1989). However, the most severe pathology in AD affects regions with relatively low NMDA receptor populations while other regions rich in this receptors are spared (Greenamyre et al., 1985; Greenamyre and Young, 1989), suggesting that it is their anatomical location rather than their density that is important in the degenerative processes.

11. Summary

One or more of the biogenic amine neurotransmitters appear to play key roles in the neurodegeneration caused by ischemia-reperfusion and neurotoxic doses of MA. Based on many lines of evidence, it is suggested that the massive release of the biogenic amines evoked by ischemia-reperfusion and MA followed by uptake into both their parent terminals and connected neurons is a key step in the system degenerations that occur. Elevated cytoplasmic levels of free or unbound biogenic amines is proposed to permit their intraneuronal oxidation to electrophilic intermediates/products that react with CySH and GSH. The resulting aberrant oxidative metabolites are proposed to include endotoxins that evoke neuronal death by redox cycling reactions and irreversible inhibition of mitochondrial respiration, processes that potentiate $O_2-\cdot$ and other ROS formation. The energy crisis evoked by inhibition of mitochondrial respiration is further proposed to relieve voltage-sensitive Mg^{2+} blockade of NMDA receptors thereby potentiating excitotoxic effects of even normal extracellular levels of glutamate. This, in turn, would potentiate elevated intraneuronal Ca^{2+} levels, ROS formation, biogenic amine oxidation, and endotoxin formation in a self-perpetuating cycle of neuronal death. Similar processes might also contribute to the anatomically-selective degeneration that occurs in certain regions of the cortex and hippocampus in AD that affects neurons connected to serotonergic and noradrenergic pathways projecting from cell bodies in the brain stem. The terminals of these monoaminergic neurons innervate microvessels in the cortex and hippocampus. The apparent permeability of the BBB in the AD brain might release low molecular weight iron that initiates a similar system neurodegeneration mediated by intraneuronal oxidation of 5-HT and NE. While this, and earlier hypotheses, are clearly speculative, they might provide a plausible rationale for the anatomic selectivity of the neurodegeneration of many neurotransmitter systems that occurs in AD.

Acknowledgements

Supported by grants from the United States National Institutes of Health (GM32363 and NS29886). The author would like to express his appreciation to Drs. Monika Z. Wrona, Fu-Chou Cheng, Keith Humphries, Kit-Sum Wong, Tahereh Tabatabataie, Zheng Wu, Xue-Ming Shen, Hong Li, Bing Xia, Zhaoliang Yang, and Xiang-Rong Jiang for their contributions to studies of the oxidation chemistry of the biogenic amine neurotransmitters and their metabolites and the neuropharmacology/neurotoxicology of the resulting products.

References

Alafuzoff I., Adolfsson R., Bucht G., and Winblad B. (1983) Albumin and immunoglobin in plasma and cerebrospinal fluid and blood-cerebrospinal fluid barrier function in patients with dementia of the Alzheimer-type and multiinfarct dementia. J. Neurol. Sci. 60:465–472.

Alvisatos S.G.A., and Williams-Ashman H.G. (1964) Serotonin-mediated oxidation of dihydronicotinamide derivatives by cytochrome c. Biochim. Biophys. Acta 86:392–395.

Annarén G., Gardner A., and Lundin T. (1986) Increased glutathione peroxidase activity in erythrocytes in patients with Alzheimer's disease/senile dementia of Alzheimer type. Acta Neurol. Scand. 73:586–589.

Arai H., Moroji T., and Kosaka K. (1984) Somatostatin and VIP in *post-mortem* brain from patients with senile dementia of the Alzheimer type. Neurosci. Lett. 52:73–78.

Aust S.D. (1988) Sources of iron for lipid peroxidation in biological systems. In: Oxygen Radicals and Tissue Injury (Halliwell B., ed.), Federation of American Societies for Experimental Biology, Bethesda, MD, pp. 27–33.

Axt K.J., Commins D.L., Vosmer G., and Seiden L.S. (1990) α-Methyl-p-tyrosine pretreatment partially prevents methamphetamine-induced neurotoxin formation. Brain Res. 515:269–276.

Axt K.J., Mamounas L.A., and Molliver M.E. (1994) Structural features of amphetamine neurotoxicity in the brain. In: Amphetamine and Its Analogs: Psychopharmacology, Toxicology, and Abuse (Cho A.K., and Segal D.S., eds.), pp. 315–367, Academic Press, New York.

Bakhit C., and Gibb J.W. (1981) Methamphetamine-induced depression of tryptophan hydroxylase following acute treatment. Eur. J. Pharmacol. 76:229–233.

Ball M.J. (1977) Neuronal loss, neurofibrillary tangles and granovacuolar degeneration in the hippocampus with aging and dementia. Acta Neuropath. 37:111–118.

Barrass B.C., Coult D.B., Pinder R.M., and Skells M. (1973) Substrate specificity of ceruloplasmin indoles and indole isosteres. Biochem. Pharmacol. 22:2891–2895.

Baumgarten H.G., Björklund A., Lachenmeyer L., Nobin A., and Stenevi U. (1971) Long-lasting selective depletion of brain serotonin by 5,6-dihydroxytryptamine. Acta Physiol. Scand. Suppl. 373:1–15.

Baumgarten H.G., Björklund A., Nobin A., Rosengren E., and Schlossberger H.G. (1975) Neurotoxicity of hydroxylated tryptamines: Structure-Activity Relationships: 1. Long-term effects on monoamine content and fluorescence morphology of central monoamine neurons. Acta Physiol. Scand. Suppl. 429:6–27.

Baumgarten H.G., and Björklund A. (1976) Neurotoxic indoleamines and monoamine neurons. Annu. Rev. Pharmacol. 16:101–111.

Baumgarten H.G., Klemm H.P., Lachenmayer L., Björklund A., Lovenberg W., and Schlossberger H.G. (1978) Mode and mechanism of action of neurotoxic indoleamines: A review and a progress report. Ann. N.Y. Acad. Sci. USA 305:3–24.

Beal M.F., Mazurek M.F., Svendsen C.N., Bird E.D., and Martin J.B. (1986) Widespread reduction of somatostatin-like immunoreactivity in the cerebral cortex in Alzheimer's disease. Ann. Neurol. 20:489–495.

Beal M.F., Hyman B.T., and Koroshetz W. (1993) Do defects in mitochondrial energy metabolism underlie the pathology of neurodegenerative diseases? Trends Neurosci. 16:125–131.

Ben-Shachar D., Zuk R., and Glinka Y. (1995) Dopamine neurotoxicity: Inhibition of mitochondrial respiration. J. Neurochem. 64:718–723.

Benveniste H., Drejer J., Schouboe A., and Diemer N.H. (1984) Elevation of extracellular concentrations of glutamate and aspartate in rat hippocampus during transient cerebral ischemia monitored by intracerebral microdialysis. J. Neurochem. 43:1369–1374.

Betz A.L. (1985) Identification of hypoxanthine transport and xanthine oxidase activity in brain capillaries. J. Neurochem. 44:574–579.

Blashko H., and Hellman K. (1953) Pigment formation from tryptamine and 5-hydroxytryptamine in tissues: A contribution to the histochemistry of amine oxidase. J. Physiol. (London) 122:419–427.

Blass J.P., Baker A.C., Ko L.-W., and Black R.S. (1990) Induction of Alzheimer antigens by an uncoupler of oxidative phosphorylation. Arch. Neurol. 47:864–869.

Borg D.C. (1965) Transient free radical forms of hormones: EPR spectra from iodothyronines, indoles, estrogens, and insulin. Proc. Nat. Acad. Sci. USA 53:829–836.

Bowen D.M., Allen S.J., Benton J.S., Goodhart M.J., Haan E.A., Palmer A.M., Sims N.R., Smith C.C.T., Spillane J.A., Esiri M.M., Neary D., Snowden J.S., Wilcock G.K., and Davison A.N. (1983) Biochemical assessment of serotonergic and cholinergic dysfunction in cerebral atrophy in Alzheimer's disease. J. Neurochem. 41:266–272.

Bowyer J.F., Gough B., Slikker W., Lipe G.W., Newport G.D., and Holson R.R. (1993) Effects of a cold environment or age on methamphetamine-induced dopamine release in the caudate putamen of female rats. Pharmacol. Biochem. Behav. 44:87–98.

Bowyer J.F., and Holson R.R. (1995) Methamphetamine and amphetamine neurotoxicity. In: Handbook of Neurotoxicology (Chang L.W., and Dyer R.S., eds.), Marcel Dekker, New York, pp. 845–870.

Brannan T., Weinberger J., Knott P., Taff I., Kaufman H., Tagaski D., Nieves-Rosa J., and Maker H. (1987) Direct evidence for acute massive striatal dopamine release in gerbils with unilateral stroke. Stroke 18:108–110.

Brumback R.A., and Leech R.W. (1994) Alzheimer's disease: Pathophysiology and hope for therapy. J. Okla. State Med. Assoc. 87:103–111.

Buening M.K., and Gibb J.W. (1974) Influence of methamphetamine and neuroleptic drugs on tyrosine hydroxylase activity. Eur. J. Pharmacol. 26:30–34.

Busto R., Harik S.I., Yoshida S., Scheinberg P., and Ginsberg M.D. (1985) Cerebral norepinephrine depletion enhances recovery after brain ischemia. Ann. Neurol. 18:329–336.

Cadet J.L., Sheng P., Ali S., Rothman R., Carlson E., and Epstein C. (1994) Attenuation of methamphetamine-induced neurotoxicity in copper/zinc superoxide dismutase transgenic mice. J. Neurochem. 62:380–383.

Chan P.H., Schmidley J.W., Fishman R.A., and Longar S.M. (1984) Brain injury, edema, and vascular permeability changes induced by oxygen-derived free radicals. Neurology 34:315–320.

Chen J.-C., Crino P.B., Schnepper P.W., To A.C.S., and Volicer L. (1989) Increased serotonin efflux by a partially oxidized serotonin: tryptamine-4,5-dione. J. Pharmacol. Exp. Therap. 250:141–148.

Chen J.-C., Schnepper P.W., To A., and Volicer L. (1992) Neurochemical changes in the rat brain after intraventricular administration of tryptamine-4,5-dione. Neuropharmacology 31:215–219.

Cheng F.-C., Kuo J.-S., Chia L.-G., and Dryhurst G. (1996) Elevated 5-S-cysteinyl-dopamine/homovanillic acid ratio and reduced homovanillic acid in cerebrospinal fluid: Possible markers for and potential insights into the pathoetiology of Parkinson's disease. J. Neural Transm. 103:433–446.

Choi D.W. (1988) Glutamate neurotoxicity and diseases of the nervous system. Neuron 1:623–634.

Choi D.W. (1992) Excitotoxic cell death. J. Neurobiol. 23:1261–1276.

Chu D.C., Penney J.B., and Young A.B. (1987). Cortical $GABA_B$ and $GABA_A$ receptors in Alzheimer's disease: A quantitative autoradiographic study. Neurology 37:1454–1459.

Cleeter M.W.J., Cooper J.M., and Schapira A.H.V. (1992) Irreversible inhibition of mitochondrial complex I by 1-methyl-4-pyridinium: Evidence for free radical involvement. J. Neurochem. 58:786–789.

Clemens J.A., and Phebus L.A. (1988) Dopamine depletion protects striatal neurones from ischemia-induced cell death. Life Sci. 42:707–713.

Clemens J.A., Saunders R.D., Ho P.P., Phebus L.A., and Panetta J.A. (1993) The antioxidant LY231617 reduces global ischemic insult neuronal injury in rats. Stroke 24:716–723.

Cohen G. (1994) Enzymatic/nonenzymatic sources of oxyradicals and regulation of antioxidant defenses. Ann. N.Y. Acad. Sci. USA 738:8–14.

Cohen G., and Heikkila R.E. (1978) Mechanisms of action of hydroxylated phenylethylamine and indoleamine neurotoxins. Ann. N.Y. Acad. Sci. USA. 305:74–84.

Colvin R.A., Bennet J.W., Colvin S.L., Allen R.A., Martinez J., and Miner G.D. (1991) Na^+/Ca^{2+} exchange activity is increased in Alzheimer brain tissue. Brain Res. 543:139–147.

Commins D.L., and Seiden L.S. (1986) α-Methyltyrosine blocks methamphetamine-induced degeneration in the rat somatosensory cortex. Brain Res. 365:15–20.

Commins D.L., Axt K.J., Vosmer G., and Seiden L.S. (1987a) 5,6-Dihydroxytryptamine, a serotonergic neurotoxin, is formed endogenously in the rat brain. Brain Res. 403:7–14.

Commins D.L., Axt K.J., Vosmer G., and Seiden L.S. (1987b) Endogenously produced 5,6-dihydroxytryptamine may mediate the neurotoxic effects of para-chloroamphetamine. Brain Res. 419:253–261.

Cooper J.L., Pulsinelli W.A., and Duffy T.E. (1980) Glutathione and ascorbate during ischemia and postischemic reperfusion in rat brain. J. Neurochem. 35:1242–1245.

Coyle J.T, and Puttfarcken P. (1993) Oxidative stress, glutamate and neurodegenerative disorders. Science 262:689–695.

Creveling C.R., and Rotman A. (1978) Mechanism of action of dihydroxytryptamines. Ann. N.Y. Acad. Sci. USA 305:57–73.

Crino P.B, Vogt B.A., Chen J.-C., and Volicer L. (1989) Neurotoxic effects of partially oxidized serotonin: Tryptamine-4,5-dione. Brain Res. 504:247–257.

D'Amato R.J., Zweig R.M., Whitehouse P.J., Wenk G.L., Singer H.S., Mayeux R., Price D.L., and Snyder S.H. (1987) Aminergic systems in Alzheimer's disease and Parkinson's disease. Ann. Neurol. 22:229–236.

Davies P., and Maloney A.F.J. (1976) Selective loss of cerebral cholinergic neurones in Alzheimer's disease. Lancet 2:1403.

Del Maestro R.F., Bjork J., and Arfors K.E. (1981) Increase in microvascular permeability induced by enzymatically generated free radicals. Microvasc. Res. 22:239–254.

DeVito M.J., and Wagner G.C. (1989) Methamphetamine-induced neuronal damage: A possible role for free radicals. Neuropharmacology 28:1145–1150.

Dyrks T., Dyrks E., Hartmann T., Masters C., and Beyreuther K. (1992) Amyloidogenicity of βA4 and βA4-bearing amyloid protein precursor fragments by metal-catalyzed oxidation. J. Biol. Chem. 267:18210–18217.

Edvinsson L., Degueurce A., Duverger D., McKenzie E.T., and Scatton B. (1983) Central serotonergic nerves project to the pial vessels of the brain. Nature 306:85–87.

Eriksen N., Martin G.M, and Benditt E.P. (1960) Oxidation of the indole nucleus of 5-hydroxytryptamine and the formation of pigments: Isolation and partial characterization of a dimer of 5-hydroxytryptamine. J. Biol. Chem. 235:1662–1667.

Evans J.M., and Cohen G. (1989) Can trace amounts of neurotoxins destroy dopamine neurons? Neurochem. Int. 15:127–129.

Farfel G.M., Vosmer G.L., and Seiden L.S. (1992) The N-methyl-D-aspartate antagonist MK-801 protects against serotonin depletions by methamphetamine, 3,4-methylenedioxy-methamphetamine and p-chloroamphetamine. Brain Res. 595:121–127.

Filloux F., and Townsend J.J. (1993) Pre- and postsynaptic neurotoxic effects of dopamine demonstrated by intrastriatal injection. Exp. Neurol. 119:79–88.

Fishman J.B., Rubins J.B., Chen J.-C., Dickey B.F., and Volicer L. (1991) Modification of brain guanine nucleotide-binding regulatory proteins by tryptamine-4,5-dione, a neurotoxic derivative of serotonin. J. Neurochem. 56:1851–1854.

Floyd R.A. (1990) Role of oxygen free radicals in carcinogenesis and brain ischemia. FASEB J. 4:2587–2597.

Folbergrová J., Rehncrona S., and Siesjö B. (1979) Oxidized and reduced glutathione in the rat brain under normoxic and hypoxic conditions. J. Neurochem. 32:1621–1627.

Fornstedt B., and Carlsson A. (1989) A marked rise in 5-S-cysteinyldopamine levels in guinea-pig striatum following reserpine treatment. J. Neural Transm. 76:155–161.

Fornstedt B., Rosengren E., and Carlsson A. (1986) Occurrence and distribution of 5-S-cysteinyl derivatives of dopamine, DOPA and DOPAC in the brains of eight mammalian species. Neuropharmacology 25:451–454.

Fornstedt B., Brun A., Rosengren E., and Carlsson A. (1989) The apparent autoxidation rate of catechols in dopamine-rich regions of human brains increases with the degree of depigmentation of substantia nigra. J. Neural Transm. 1:279–295.

Frank D.M., Arora P.K., Blumer J.L., and Sayre L.M. (1987) Model study on the bioreduction of paraquat, MPP$^+$, and analogs. Evidence against a "redox cycling" mechanism in MPTP neurotoxicity. Biochem. Biophys. Res. Commun. 147:1095–1104.

Frautshy S.A., Baird A., and Cole G.M. (1991) Effects of injected Alzheimer β-amyloid cores in rat brain. Proc. Nat. Acad. Sci. USA 88:8362–8366.

Freeman B.A., and Crapo J.D. (1982) Free radicals and tissue injury. Lab. Invest. 47: 412–426.

French L.R., Schuman L.M., Mortimer J.A., Hutton J.T., Boatman R.A., and Christians B. (1985) A case-control study of dementia of the Alzheimer-type. Am. J. Epidemiol. 121:414–421.

German D.C., White C.L., and Sparkman D.R. (1987) Alzheimer's disease: Neurofibrillary tangles in nuclei that project to the cerebral cortex. Neuroscience 21:305–312.

Gerson S., Baldessarini R.J., and Wheeler S.C. (1974) Biochemical effects of dihydroxylated tryptamines on central indoleamine neurons. Neuropharmacology 13:987–1004.

Gibb J.W., Hanson G.R., and Johnson M. (1994) Neurochemical mechanisms of toxicity. In: Amphetamine and Its Analogs: Psychopharmacology, Toxicology, and Abuse (Cho A.K., and Segal D.S., eds.), pp. 269–295, Academic Press, New York.

Gill R., Foster A.C., and Woodruff G.N. (1987) Systematic administration of MK-801 protects against ischemia-induced hippocampal degeneration in the gerbil. J. Neurosci. 7:3343–3349.

Ginsberg M.D., Graham D.I., and Busto R. (1985) Regional glucose utilization and blood flow following graded forebrain ischemia in the rat: Correlation with neuropathology. Ann. Neurol. 18:470–481.

Good P.F., Perl D.P., Bierer L.M., and Schmeidler J. (1992) Selective accumulation of aluminum and iron in the neurofibrillary tangles of Alzheimer's disease: A laser microprobe (LAMMA) study. Ann. Neurol. 31:286–292.

Globus M.Y.-T., Ginsberg M.D., Dietrich W.D., Busto R., and Scheinberg P. (1987) Substantia nigra lesion protects against ischemic damage to the striatum. Neurosci. Lett. 80, 251–256.

Globus M.Y.-T., Busto R., Dietrich W.D., Martinez E., Valdés I., and Ginsberg M.D. (1989) Direct evidence for acute and massive norepinephrine release in hippocampus during transient ischemia. J. Cereb. Blood Flow Metab. 9, 842–846.

Graham D.G. (1978) Oxidation pathways for catecholamines in the genesis of neuromelanin and cytotoxic quinones. Mol. Pharmacol. 14, 633–643.

Grahame-Smith D.G. (1971) Studies in vivo on the relationship between brain tryptophan, brain 5-HT synthesis and hyperactivity in rats treated with a monoamine oxidase inhibitor and L-tryptophan. J. Neurochem. 18, 1053–1066.

Greenamyre J.T., Penney J.B., Young A.B., D'Amato C.J., Hicks S.P., and Shoulson I. (1985) Alterations in L-glutamate binding in Alzheimer's and Huntington's disease. Science 227, 1496–1499.

Greenamyre J.T. and Young A.B. (1989) Excitatory amino acids and Alzheimer's disease. Neurobiol. Aging 10, 593–602.

Gutteridge J.M.C. (1986) Iron promoters of the Fenton reaction and lipid peroxidation can be released from haemoglobin by peroxides. FEBS Lett. 201, 291–295.

Hajimohammadadreza I., and Brammer M. (1990) Brain membrane fluidity and lipid peroxidation in Alzheimer's disease. Neurosci. Lett. 112, 333–337.

Hall E.D., and Braughler J.M. (1988) The role of oxygen radical-induced lipid peroxidation in acute central nervous system trauma. In: Oxygen Radicals and Tissue Injury (Halliwell B., ed.), pp. 92–98, Federation of American Societies for Experimental Biology, Bethesda, MD.

Hall E.D., Pazara K.E., and Braughler J.M. (1988) 21-Aminosteroid lipid peroxidation inhibitor U74006F protects against cerebral ischemia in gerbils. Stroke 19, 997–1002.

Hall E.D., Andrus P.K., Yonkers P.A., Smith S.L., Zhang J.-R., Taylor B.M., and Sun F.F. (1994) Generation and detection of hydroxyl radical following experimental head injury. Ann. N.Y. Acad. Sci. USA 738, 15–24.

Halliwell B. (1992a) Reactive oxygen species and the central nervous system. J. Neurochem. 59, 1609–1623.

Halliwell B. (1992b) Oxygen radicals as key mediators in neurological disease: Fact or fiction? Ann. Neurol. 32, S10–S15.

Halliwell B., and Gutteridge J.M.C. (1987) Free Radicals in Biology and Medicine. Clarendon Press, Oxford.

Hardy J., Adolfssun R., Alafuzoff L., Bucht G., Marcusson J., Nyberg P., Perdahl E., Wester P., and Winblad B. (1985) Transmitter deficits in Alzheimer's disease. Neurochem. Int. 7, 545–563.

Hasegawa E., Takeshige K., Oishi T., Murai Y., and Minikami S. (1990) 1-Methyl-4-pyridinium (MPP^+) induces NADH-dependent lipid peroxidation in bovine heart submitochondrial particles. Biochem. Biophys. Res. Commun. 170, 1049–1055.

Hastings T.G. (1995) Enzymatic oxidation of dopamine: The role of prostaglandin H synthase. J. Neurochem. 64, 919–924.

Hastings T.G., and Zigmond M.J. (1992) Prostaglandin synthase-catalyzed oxidation of dopamine. Soc. Neurosci. Abstr. 18, 1444.

Hastings T.G., Lewis D.A., and Zigmond M.J. (1996) Role of oxidation in the neurotoxic effects of intrastriatal dopamine injections. Proc. Nat. Acad. Sci. USA 93, 1956–1961.

Heikkila R.E., and Cohen G. (1973) 6-Hydroxydopamine: Evidence for superoxide radical as an oxidative intermediate. Science 181, 456–457.

Hensley K., Carney J.M., Mattson M.P., Aksenova M., Harris M., Wu J.F., Floyd R.A., and Butterfield D.A. (1994) A model for β-amyloid aggregation and neurotoxicity based on free radical generation by the peptide: Relevance to Alzheimer's disease. Proc. Nat. Acad. Sci. USA 91, 3270–3274.

Hirata H., Ladenheim B., Rothman R.B., Epstein C., and Cadet J.L. (1995) Methamphetamine-induced serotonin neurotoxicity is mediated by superoxide radicals. Brain Res. 677, 345–347.

Hirata H., Ladenheim B., Carlson E., Epstein C., and Cadet J.L. (1996) Autoradiographic evidence for methamphetamine-induced striatal dopaminergic loss in mouse brain: attenuation in CuZn-superoxide dismutase transgenic mice. Brain Res. 714, 95–103.

Hotchkiss A.J., and Gibb J.W. (1980a) Blockade of methamphetamine-induced depression of tyrosine hydroxylase by GABA-transaminase inhibitors. Eur. J. Pharmacol. 66, 204–205.

Hotchkiss A.J., and Gibb J.W. (1980b) Long-term effects of multiple doses of methamphetamine on neostriatal tryptophan hydroxylase and tyrosine hydroxylase activity in rat brain. J. Pharmacol Exp. Therap. 214, 257–262.

Hubbard B.M., and Anderson J.M. (1985) Age-related variation in the neuron content of the cerebral cortex in senile dementia of the Alzheimer-type. Neuropath. Appl. Neurobiol. 11, 369–382.

Humphries K.A., and Dryhurst G. (1987) Electrochemical oxidation of 5-hydroxytryptophan. J. Pharm. Sci. 76, 839–847.

Humphries K.A., and Dryhurst G. (1990) Biomimetic electrochemistry. A study of the electrochemical and peroxidase-mediated oxidation of 5-hydroxytryptophan. J. Electrochem. Soc. 137, 1144–1149.

Humphries K.A., Wrona M.Z., and Dryhurst G. (1993) Electrochemical and enzymatic oxidation of 5-hydroxytryptophan. J. Electroanal. Chem. 346, 377–403.

Hyman B.T., Van Hoesen G.W., and Damasio A. (1987) Alzheimer's disease: glutamate depletion in the hippocampal perforant pathway zone. Ann. Neurol. 22, 37–40.

Hyslop P.A., Zhang Z., Pearson D.V., and Phebus L.A. (1995) Measurement of striatal H_2O_2 by microdialysis following global forebrain ischemia and reperfusion in the rat: Correlation with the cytotoxic potential of H_2O_2 in vitro. Brain Res. 671, 181–186.

Ito E., Oka K., Etcheberrigaray R., Nelson T.J., McPhie D.L., Tofel-Grehl B., Gibson G.E., and Alkon D.E. (1994) Internal Ca^{2+} mobilization is altered in fibroblasts from patients with Alzheimer's disease. Proc. Nat. Acad. Sci. USA 91, 534–538.

Jacoby J.H., and Lytle L.D. (1978) Serotonergic Neurotoxins. Ann. N.Y. Acad. Sci. USA 305, 1–702.

Jimenez Del Rio M., Pinxteren J., De Potter W.P., Ebinger G., and Vauquelin G. (1992) Serotonin-binding proteins in the bovine cerebral cortex: Interaction with serotonin and catecholamines. Eur. J. Pharmacol. 225, 225–234.

Jimenez Del Rio M., Pinxteren J., De Potter W., Ebinger G., and Vauquelin G. (1993a) Serotonin binding proteins in bovine retina: Binding of serotonin and catecholamines. Neurochem. Int. 22, 111–119.

Jimenez Del Rio M., Pardo C.V., Pinxteren J., De Potter W., Ebinger G., and Vauquelin G. (1993b) Binding of serotonin and dopamine to 'serotonin binding proteins' in bovine frontal cortex: Evidence for iron-induced oxidative mechanisms. Eur. J. Pharmacol. 247, 11–21.

Kaleria R.N., Stockmeier C.A., and Harik S.I. (1989) Brain microvessels are innervated by locus ceruleus noradrenergic neurons. Neurosci. Lett. 97, 203–208.

Karoum F., Chrapusta S.J., Egan M.F., and Wyatt R.J. (1993) Absence of 6-hydroxydopamine in the rat brain after treatment with stimulants and other dopaminergic agents: A mass fragmentographic study. J. Neurochem. 61, 1369–1375.

Kinouchi H., Epstein C.J., Mizui T., Carlson E.J., Chen S.F., and Chan P.H. (1991) Attenuation of focal cerebral ischemic injury in transgenic mice overexpressing CuZn superoxide dismutase. Proc. Nat. Acad. Sci. USA 88, 11158–11162.

Kinuta Y., Kimura M., Itokawa Y., Ishikawa M., and Kikuchi H. (1989) Changes in xanthine oxidase in ischemic rat brain. J. Neurosurg. 71, 417–420.

Klemm H.P., Baumgarten H.G., and Schlossberger H.G. (1980) Polarographic measurements of spontaneous and mitochondria-promoted oxidation of 5,6- and 5,7-dihydroxytryptamine. J. Neurochem. 35, 1400–1408.

Koh J.-Y., Yang L-L., and Cotman C.W. (1990) β-Amyloid protein increases the vulnerability of cultured cortical neurons to excitotoxic damage. Brain Res. 533, 315–320.

Kondo T., Sugita Y., Kanazawa A., Ito T., and Mizuno Y. (1992) Free dopamine and iron contribute to the hydroxyl radical generation in the methamphetamine induced experimental parkinsonism. Movement Disord. 17 (Suppl. 1), 73–79.

Kondo T., Ito T., Kanazawa A., and Mizuno Y. (1993) Degeneration of dopaminergic nerve terminals induced by methamphetamine: Study of mechanism. Clin. Neurol. 33, 1474–1479.

Kontos H.A., and Wei E.P. (1986) Superoxide production in experimental brain injury. J. Neurosurg. 64, 803–807.

Kostrzewa R.M., and Jacobowicz D.M. (1974) Pharmacological actions of 6-hydroxydopamine. Pharmacol. Rev. 26, 199–288.

Lafon-Cazal M., Pletri S., Culcasi M., and Bockaert J. (1993) NMDA-dependent superoxide production and neurotoxicity. Nature 364, 535–537.

LaVoie M.J., Zigmond M.J., and Hastings T.G. (1996) Methamphetamine induced neurotoxicity is associated with the formation of cysteinyl-dopamine. Soc. Neurosci. Abstr. 22, 221.

Li H., and Dryhurst G. (1997) Irreversible inhibition of mitochondrial complex I by 7-(2-aminoethyl)-3,4-dihydro-5-hydroxy-2N-1,4-benzothiazine-3-carboxylic acid (DHBT-1): A putative nigral endotoxin of relevance to Parkinson's disease. J. Neurochem. 69, 1530–1541.

Maher P., and Davis J.B. (1996) The role of monoamine metabolism in oxidative glutatmate toxicity. J. Neurosci. 16, 6394–6401.

Mann D.M.A. (1988) Neuropathological and neurochemical aspects of Alzheimer's disease. In: Psychopharmacology of the Aging Nervous System (Iversen L.L., Iversen S.D., and Snyder, S.H., eds.), pp. 1–67, Plenum Press, New York.

Mann D.M.A., Yates P.O., and Hawkes J. (1982) The noradrenergic system in Alzheimer and multi-infarct dementias. J. Neurol. Neurosurg. Psychiatry 45, 113–119.

Marcyniuk B., Mann D.M.A., and Yates P.O. (1986) The topography of cell loss from locus ceruleus in Alzheimer's disease. J. Neurol. Sci. 76, 335–345.

Marek G.J., Vosmer G., and Seiden L.S. (1990a) Dopamine uptake inhibitors block long-term neurotoxic effects of methamphetamine upon dopaminergic neurons. Brain Res. 513, 274–279.

Marek G.J., Vosmer G, and Seiden L.S. (1990b) The effects of monoamine uptake inhibitors and methamphetamine on neostriatal 6-hydroxydopamine (6-OHDA) formation, short-term monoamine depletions and locomotor activity in the rat. Brain Res. 516, 1–7.

Marek G.J., Vosmer G., and Seiden L.S. (1990c) Pargyline increases 6-hydroxydopamine levels in neostriatum of methamphetamine-treated rats. Pharmacol. Biochem. Behav. 36, 187–190.

Martin G.M., Benditt E.P., and Eriksen N. (1960) Enzymic oxidation of the indole nucleus of 5-hydroxytryptamine: Properties of an enzyme in human serum and of the products of oxidation. Arch. Biochem. Biophys. 90, 208–217.

Martins R.N., Harper C.G., Stokes G.B., and Masters C.L. (1986) Increased cerebral glucose-6-phosphate dehydrogenase activity in Alzheimer's disease may reflect oxidative stress. J. Neurochem. 46, 1042–1045.

Matson W.R., Langlais P., Volicer L., Gamache P.H., Bird E., and Mark K.A. (1984) n-Electrode three-dimensional liquid chromatography with electrochemical detection for determination of neurotransmitters. Clin. Chim. 30, 1477–1488.

Mattson M.P. (1992) Calcium as sculptor and destroyer of neural circuitry. Exp. Gerontol. 27, 29–49.

Mecocci P., MacGarvey U., and Beal M.F. (1994) Oxidative damage to mitochondrial DNA is increased in Alzheimer's disease. Ann. Neurol. 36, 747–751.

Meldrum B. (1993) Amino acids as dietary excitotoxins: a contribution to understanding neurodegenerative disorders. Brain Res. Rev. 18, 293–314.

Miyakawa T., Shimoji A., Kuramoto R., and Higuchi Y. (1982) The relationship between senile plaques and cerebral blood vessels in Alzheimer's disease and senile dementia. Virchows Arch. B40, 121–129.

Modigh K. (1972) Central and peripheral effects of 5-hydroxytryptophan on motor activity in mice. Psychopharmacologica 23, 48–54.

Montine J.J., Huang D.Y., Valentine W.M., Amarnath V., Saunders A., Weisgraber K.H., Graham D.G., and Strittmatter W.J. (1996) Crosslinking of apolipoprotein E by products of lipid peroxidation. J. Neuropath. Exp. Neurol. 55, 202–210.

Mortimer J.A., French L.R., Hutton J.T., and Schuman L.M. (1985) Head injury as a risk factor for Alzheimer's disease. Neurology 35, 264–267.

Murphy T.H., Miyamoto M., Sastre A., Schnaar R.L., and Coyle J.T. (1989) Glutamate toxicity in a neuronal cell line involves inhibition of cystine transport leading to oxidative stress. Neuron 2, 1547–1558.

Nakayama H., Ginsberg M.D., and Dietrich W.D. (1988) (S)-Emopil, a novel calcium channel blocker and serotonin S_2 antagonist, markedly reduces infarct size following middle cerebral artery occlusion in the rat. Neurology 38, 1667–1673.

Nelson D.R., and Huggins A.K. (1975) The interaction of 5-hydroxytryptamine and related hydroxyindoles with horseradish and mammalian peroxidase systems. Biochem. Pharmacol. 24, 181–192.

Novielli A., Reilly J.A., Lysko P.G., and Henneberry R.C. (1988) Glutamate becomes neurotoxic when intracellular energy levels are reduced. Brain Res. 451, 205–212.

O'Dell S.J., Weihmuller F.B., and Marshall J.F. (1991) Multiple methamphetamine injections induce marked increases in extracellular striatal dopamine which correlate with subsequent neurotoxicity. Brain Res. 564, 256–260.

Oliver C.N., Starke-Reed P.E., Stadtman E.R., Liu G.J., Carney J.M., and Floyd R.A. (1990) Oxidative damage to brain proteins, loss of glutamine synthetase activity, and production of free radicals during ischemia/reperfusion-induced injury in gerbil brain. Proc. Nat. Acad. Sci. USA 87, 5144–5147.

Onodera H., Iijima K., and Kogure K. (1986) Mononucleotide metabolism in the rat brain after transient ischemia. J. Neurochem. 46, 1704–1710.

Ooboshi H., Sadoshima S., Yao H., Nakahara T., Uchimura H., and Fujishima M. (1992) Inhibition of ischemia-induced dopamine release by ω-conotoxin, a calcium channel blocker, in the striatum of spontaneously hypertensive rats: *In vivo* brain dialysis study. J. Neurochem. 58, 298–303.

Palmer A.M., Francis P.T., Bowen D.M., Benton J.S., Neary D., Mann D.M.A., and Snowden J.S. (1987a) Catecholaminergic neurones assessed ante-mortem in Alzheimer's disease. Brain Res. 414, 365–375.

Palmer A.M., Francis P.T., Benton J.S., Sims N.R., Mann D.M.A., Neary D., Snowden J.S., and Bowen D.M. (1987b) Presynaptic serotonergic dysfunction in patients with Alzheimer's disease. Brain Res. 48, 8–15.

Palmer A.M. and Bowen D.M. (1990) Neurochemical basis of dementia of the Alzheimer type: Contribution of postmortem and antemortem studies. In: Biological Markers in Dementia of Alzheimer Type: Proceedings of the Stiftelsen Gamla Jjanarinnor Symposium on Aging and Aging Disorders No 1. (Fowler C., Carlson L.A., Gottfries C.G., and Winblad B., eds). Smith-Gordon, London.

Palmer A.M. (1991) Excitatory amino acid neurons and receptors in Alzheimer's disease. In: Neurobiology of the NMDA Receptor: From Chemistry to the Clinic (Kozikowski A.P., and Barrionuevo G., eds.), pp. 203–237, VCH Publisher, New York.

Palmer A.M., and Burns M. (1994) Selective increase in lipid peroxidation in the inferior temporal cortex in Alzheimer's disease. Brain Res. 645, 338–342.

Pappolla M.A., Omar R.A., Kim K.S., and Robakis N.K. (1992) Immunohistochemical evidence of antioxidant stress in Alzheimer's disease. Am. J. Pathol. 140, 621–628.

Pearson R.C.A., Esiri M.M., Hiorns R.W., Wilcock G.K., and Powell T.P.S. (1985) Anatomical correlates of the distribution of the pathological changes in the neocortex in Alzheimer's disease. Proc. Nat. Acad. Sci. USA 82, 4531–4534.

Peat M.A., Warren P.F., Bakhit C., and Gibb J.W. (1985) The acute effects of methamphetamine, amphetamine and p-chloroamphetamine on the cortical serotonergic system of the rat brain: Evidence for difference in the effects of methamphetamine and amphetamine. Eur. J. Pharmacol. 116, 11–16.

Perez-Reyes E., and Mason R.P. (1981) Characterization of the structure and reactions of free radicals from serotonin and related indoles. J. Biol. Chem. 256, 2427–2432.

Perry E.K., Perry R.H., Blessed G., and Tomlinson B.E. (1977) Necropsy evidence of cerebral cholinergic defects in senile dementia. Lancet 1, 189.

Perry R.H., Candy J.M., Perry E.K., Irving D., Blessed G., Fairburn F., and Tomlinson B.E. (1982) Extensive loss of choline acetyl transferase activity is not related to neuronal loss in the nucleus basalis of Meynert in Alzheimer's disease. Neurosci. Lett. 33, 311–315.

Phebus L.A., and Clemens J.A. (1989) Effects of transient global cerebral ischemia on striatal extracellular dopamine, serotonin and their metabolites. Life Sci. 44, 1335–1342.

Philbert M.A., Beiswanger C.M., Waters D.K., Reuhl K.R., and Lowndes H.E. (1990) Cellular and regional distribution of reduced glutathione in the nervous system of the rat: Histochemical localization by mercury orange and o-phthalaldehyde-induced histofluorescence. Toxicol. Appl. Pharmacol. 107, 215–227.

Pike C.J., Burdick D., Walencewicz A.J., Glabe C.G., and Cotman C.W. (1993) Neurodegeneration induced by β-amyloid peptides in vitro: The role of peptide assembly state. J. Neurosci. 13, 1676–1687.

Pinxteren J., Jimenez Del Rio M., Velez-Pardo C., Ebinger G., Vauquelin G., and De Potter W. (1993) Soluble serotonin and catecholamine binding proteins in the bovine adrenal medulla. Neurochem. Int. 23, 343–350.

Porter C.C., Titus D.C., Saunders B.E., and Smith E.V.C. (1957) Oxidation of serotonin in the presence of ceruloplasmin. Science 126, 1014–1015.

Proctor A.W., Palmer A.M., Francis P.T., Lowe S.L., Neary D., Mann D.M.A., and Bowen D.M. (1988) Evidence of glutamatergic denervation and possible abnormal metabolism in Alzheimer's disease. J. Neurochem. 50, 790–802.

Pryor W. (1986) Oxy-radicals and related species: Their formation, lifetimes, and reactions. Annu. Rev. Physiol. 48, 657–667.

Pulsinelli W.A. (1985) Deafferation of the hippocampus protects CA1 pyramidal neurons against ischemic injury. Stroke 16, 144.

Pulsinelli W.A., and Brierley J.B. (1979) A new model of bilateral hemispheric ischemia in the unanesthetized rat. Stroke 10, 267–272.

Pulsinelli W.A., Brierley J.B., and Plum F. (1982) Temporal profile of neuronal damage in a model of transient forebrain ischemia. Ann. Neurol. 11, 491–498.

Pulsinelli W.A., and Duffy T.E. (1983) Regional energy balance in rat brain after transient forebrain ischemia. J. Neurochem. 40, 1500–1503.

Puppo A., and Halliwell B. (1988) Formation of hydroxyl radicals from hydrogen peroxide in the presence of iron. Is haemoglobin a biological Fenton catalyst? Biochem. J. 249, 185–190.

Raiteri M., Cerrito F., Cervoni A.M., and Levi G. (1979) Dopamine can be released by two mechanisms differentially affected by the dopamine transport inhibitor nomifensine. J. Pharmacol. Exp. Therap. 208, 195–202.

Rehncrona S., Folbergrová J., Smith D.B., and Siesjö B.K. (1980) Influence of complete and pronounced incomplete cerebral ischemia and subsequent recirculation on cortical concentrations of oxidized and reduced glutathione in the rat. J. Neurochem. 34, 477–486.

Ricaurte G.A., Schuster C.R., and Seiden L.S. (1980) Long-term effects of repeated methylamphetamine administration on dopamine and serotonin neurons in the rat brain: A regional study. Brain Res. 193, 153–163.

Ricaurte G.A., Fuller R.W., Perry K.W., Seiden L.S., and Schuster C.R. (1983) Fluoxetine increases long-lasting neostriatal dopamine depletion after administration of d-methamphetamine and d-amphetamine. Neuropharmacology 22, 1165–1169.

Ricaurte G.A., Seiden L.S., and Schuster C.R. (1984) Further evidence that amphetamines produce long-lasting dopamine neurochemical deficits by destroying dopamine nerve fibers. Brain Res. 303, 359–364.

Richards D.A. (1983) Use of high performance liquid chromatography to study the ceruloplasmin-catalyzed oxidation of biogenic amines. J. Chromatogr. 256, 71–79.

Roberts G.W., Gentleman S.M., Lynch A., and Graham D.I. (1991) βA4 Amyloid protein deposition in brain after head trauma. Lancet 338, 1422–1423.

Rollema H., De Vries J.B., Westerink B.H.C., Van Putten F.M., and Horn A.S. (1986) Failure to detect 6-hydroxydopamine in rat striatum after the dopamine releasing drugs dexamphetamine, methylamphetamine and MPTP. Eur. J. Pharmacol. 132, 65–69.

Rudelli R., Strom J.O., Welch P.T., and Ambler M.W. (1982) Post-traumatic premature Alzheimer's disease. Arch. Neurol. 39, 570–575.

Sakamoto A., Ohnishi S.T., Ohnishi T., and Ogawa R. (1991) Relationship between free radical production and lipid peroxidation during ischemia-reperfusion injury in rat brain. Brain Res. 554, 186–192.

Saper C.B., Wainer B.H., and German D.C. (1987) Axonal and transneuronal transport in the transmission of neurobiological disease: Potential role in system degenerations, including Alzheimer's disease. Neuroscience 23, 389–398.

Sapolsky R.M., and Pulsinelli W.A. (1985). Glucocorticoids potentiate ischemic injury to neurons: therapeutic implications. Science 229, 1397–1400.

Scheulen M., Wollenberg P., Bolt H.M., Kappus H., and Remmer H. (1975) Irreversible binding of DOPA and dopamine metabolites to protein by rat liver microsomes. Biochem. Biophys. Res. Commun. 66, 1396–1400.

Schipper H., Cisse S., and Stopa E. (1995) Expression of heme oxygenase-1 in the senescent and Alzheimer-diseases brain. Ann. Neurol. 37, 758–768.

Schmidt C.J., and Gibb J.W. (1985) Role of the dopamine uptake carrier in the neurochemical response to methamphetamine: Effects of amfonelic acid. Eur. J. Pharmacol. 109, 73–80.

Schmidt C.J., Ritter J.K., Sonsalla P.K., Hanson G.R., and Gibb J.W. (1985) Role of dopamine in the neurotoxic effects of methamphetamine. J. Pharmacol. Exp. Therap. 233, 539–544.

Seiden L.S., and Vosmer G. (1984) Formation of 6-hydroxydopamine in caudate nucleus of the rat brain after a single large dose of methylamphetamine. Pharmacol. Biochem. Behav. 21, 29–31.

Seiden L.S., and Sabol K.E. (1995) Neurotoxicity of methamphetamine-related drugs and cocaine. In: Handbook of Neurotoxicology (Chang L.W., and Dyer R.S., eds), pp. 825–843, Marcel Dekker, New York.

Selkoe D.J. (1989) Biochemistry of altered brain proteins in Alzheimer's disease. Ann. Rev. Neurosci. 12, 463–490.

Shalat S.L., Seltzer B., Pidcock C., and Baker E.L. (1986) A case control study of medical and familial history and Alzheimer's disease. Am. J. Epidemiol. 124, 540–541.

Shen X.-M., and Dryhurst (1996a) Further insights into the influence of L-cysteine on the oxidation chemistry of dopamine: Reaction pathways of potential relevance to Parkinson's disease. Chem. Res. Toxicol. 9, 751–763.

Shen X.-M., and Dryhurst G. (1996b) Oxidation chemistry of (–)-norepinephrine in the presence of L-cysteine. J. Med. Chem. 39, 2018–2029.

Shen X.-M., Xia B., Wrona M.Z., and Dryhurst G. (1996) Synthesis, redox properties, *in vivo* formation and neurobehavioral effects of N-acetylcysteinyl conjugates of dopamine: Possible metabolites of relevance to Parkinson's disease. Chem. Res. Toxicol. 9, 1117–1126.

Shen X.-M., and Dryhurst G. (1997) Oxidation of dopamine in the presence of cysteine: Characterization of new toxic products. Chem. Res. Toxicol. 10, 147–155.

Siesjö B.K. (1988) Historical overview: Calcium, ischemia, and death of brain cells. Ann. N.Y. Acad. Sci., USA 522, 638–661.

Siesjö B. (1992) Pathophysiology and treatment of focal cerebral ischemia. Part II. Mechanisms of damage and treatment. J. Neurosurg. 77, 337–354.

Simonian N.A., and Coyle J.T. (1996) Oxidative stress in neurodegenerative diseases. Annu. Rev. Pharmacol. Toxicol. 36, 83–106.

Sims N.R., Finegan J.M., Blass J.P., Bowen D.M., and Neary D. (1987) Mitochondrial function in brain tissue in degenerative dementia. Brain Res. 436, 30–38.

Singh S., and Dryhurst G. (1990) Further insights into the oxidation chemistry and biochemistry of the serotonergic neurotoxin 5,6-dihydroxytryptamine. J. Med. Chem. 33, 3035–3044.

Singh S., Jen J.-F., and Dryhurst G. (1990) Autoxidation of the indolic neurotoxin 5,6-dihydroxytryptamine. J. Org. Chem. 55, 1484–1489.

Singh S., and Dryhurst G. (1991) Reactions of the serotonergic neurotoxic 5,6-dihydroxytryptamine with glutathione. J. Org. Chem. 56, 1767–1773.

Singh S., Wrona M.Z., and Dryhurst G. (1992) Synthesis and reactivity of the putative neurotoxin tryptamine-4,5-dione. Bioorg. Chem. 20, 189–203.

Slivka A., and Cohen G. (1985) Hydroxyl radical attack on dopamine. J. Biol. Chem. 260, 15466–15472.

Slivka A., Mytilineou C., and Cohen G. (1987) Histochemical evaluation of glutathione in brain. Brain Res. 409, 275–284.

Small D.H., Ozaki Y., and Wurtman R.J. (1982) Isolation of a cytoplasmic serotonin storage protein from synaptosomes. Trans. Am. Soc. Neurochem. 13, 219.

Smith C.D., Carney J.M., Starke-Reed P.E., Oliver C.N., Stadtman E.R., and Markesbery W.R. (1991) Excess brain protein oxidation and enzyme dysfunction in normal aging and in Alzheimer's disease. Proc. Nat. Acad. Sci. USA 88, 10540–10543.

Smith M., Kutty R.K., Richey P.L., Yan S.-D., Stern D., Chader G.J., Wiggert B., Peterson R.B., and Perry G. (1994) Heme oxygenase-1 is associated with the neurofibrillary pathology of Alzheimer's disease. Am. J. Pathol. 145, 42–47.

Sonsalla P.K., Gibb J.W., and Hanson G.R. (1986) Roles of D_1 and D_2 dopamine receptor subtypes in mediating the methamphetamine-induced changes in monoamine systems. J. Pharmacol. Exp. Therap. 238, 932–937.

Sonsalla P.K., Riordan D.E., and Heikkila R.E. (1991) Competitive and noncompetitive antagonists of N-methyl-D-aspartate receptors protect against methamphetamine-induced dopaminergic damage in mice. J. Pharmacol. Exp. Therap. 256, 506–512.

Spector S., Sjoerdsma A., and Udenfriend S. (1965) Blockade of endogenous norepinephrine synthesis by alpha-methyl-tyrosine, an inhibitor of tyrosine hydroxylase. J. Pharmacol. Exp. Therap. 147, 86–95.

Sternau L.L., Lust W.D., Ricci A.J., and Racheson R. (1989) Role for γ-aminobutyric acid in selective vulnerability in gerbils. Stroke 20, 281–287.

Stone D.M., Johnson M., Hanson G.R., and Gibb J.W. (1989) Acute inactivation of tryptophan hydroxylase by amphetamine analogs involves the oxidation of sulfhydryl sites. Eur. J. Pharmacol. 172, 93–97.

Subbarao K.V., Richardson J.S., and Ang L.C. (1990) Autopsy samples of Alzheimer's cortex show increased peroxidation *in vitro*. J. Neurochem. 55, 342–345.

Suzuki O., Hattori H., Asano M., Oya M., and Katsumata Y. (1980) Inhibition of monoamine oxidase by D-methamphetamine. Biochem. Pharmacol. 29, 2071–2073.

Tabatabaie T., and Dryhurst G. (1997) Molecular mechanisms of action of 5,6- and 5,7-dihydroxytryptamine. In: Highly Selective Neurotoxins: Basic and Clinical Applications. Kostrzewa R.M., ed., (in press). Humana Press.

Tamir H., and Gershon M.D. (1979) Storage of serotonin and serotonin binding protein in synaptic vesicles. J. Neurochem. 33, 35–44.

Tamir H., and Liu K.P. (1982) On the nature of the interaction between serotonin and serotonin binding protein: Effect of nucleotides, ions, and sulfhydryl reagents. J. Neurochem. 38, 135–141.

Tamir H., Klein A., and Rapport M.M. (1976) Serotonin binding protein: Enhancement of binding by Fe^{++} and inhibition of binding by drugs. J. Neurochem. 26, 871–878.

Tejani-Butt S.M, Yang J., and Pawlyk A.C. (1995) Altered serotonin transporter sites in Alzheimer's disease raphe and hippocampus. NeuroReports 6, 1207–1210.

Tomlinson B.E., Irving D., and Blessed G. (1982) Cell loss in locus ceruleus in senile dementia of the Alzheimer type. J. Neurol. Sci. 49, 418–421.

Troncoso J., Costello A., Watson A., and Johnson G. (1993) *In vitro* polymerization of oxidized tau into filaments. Brain Res. 613, 313–316.

Tse D.C.S., McCreery R.L., and Adams R.N. (1976) Potential oxidative pathways of brain catecholamines. J. Med. Chem. 19, 37–40.

Turrens J.F., and Bovaris A. (1980) Generation of superoxide anion by the NADH dehydrogenase of bovine heart mitochondria. Biochem. J. 191, 421–427.

Udenfriend S., Titus E., Weissbach H., and Peterson R.E. (1956) Biogenesis and metabolism of 5-hydroxyindole compounds. J. Biol. Chem. 219, 335–344.

Uemura T., Shimazu T., Miura R., and Yamano T. (1980) NADPH-dependent melanin pigment formation from 5-hydroxyindoleamines by hepatic and cerebral microsomes. Biochem. Biophys. Res. Commun. 93, 1074–1081.

Van Woert M.H., and Ambani L.M. (1974) Biochemistry of neuromelanin. Adv. Neurol. 5, 215–233.

Van Woert M.H., Prasad K.N., and Borg D.C. (1967). Spectroscopic studies of substantia nigra pigment in human subjects. J. Neurochem. 14, 707–716.

Victor S.J., Baumgarten H.G., and Lovenberg W. (1974) Depletion of tryptophan hydroxylase by 5,6-dihydroxytryptamine in rat brain time-course and regional differences. J. Neurochem. 22, 541–546.

Volicer L., Langlais P.J., Matson W.R., Mark K.A., and Gamache P.H. (1985) Serotoninergic system in dementia of the Alzheimer type. Abnormal forms of 5-hydroxytryptophan and serotonin in cerebrospinal fluid. Arch. Neurol. 42, 1158–1161.

Volicer L., Chen J.-C., Crino P.B., Vogt B.A., Fishman J., Rubins J., Schnepper P.W., and Wolfe N. (1989) Neurotoxic properties of serotonin oxidation product: Possible role in Alzheimer's disease. In: Alzheimer Disease and Related Disorders (Iqbal K., Wisniewski H.M., and Winblad B., eds.) pp. 453–465, Alan R. Liss, New York.

Volpe B.T., Pulsinelli W.A., Tribuna J., and Davis H.P. (1984) Behavioral performance of rats following transient forebrain ischemia. Stroke 15, 558–562.

Wagner G.C., Ricaurte G.A., Seiden L.S., Schuster C.R., Miller R.J., and Westley J. (1980) Long-lasting depletions of striatal dopamine and dopamine uptake sites following repeated administration of methamphetamine. Brain Res. 181, 151–160.

Wagner G., Lucot J.B., Schuster C.R., and Seiden L.S. (1983) Alpha-methyltyrosine attenuates and reserpine increases methamphetamine-induced neuronal changes. Brain Res. 270, 285–288.

Walaas E., and Walaas O. (1961) Oxidation of reduced phosphopyridine nucleotides by p-phenylenediamines, catecholamines and serotonin in the presence of ceruloplasmin. Arch. Biochem. Biophys. 95, 151–162.

Walker L.C., Kitt C.A., Cork L.C., Struble R.G., Dellovade G.L., and Price D.L. (1988) Multiple transmitter systems contribute neurites to individual senile plaques. J. Neuropath. Exp. Neurol. 47, 138–144.

Wei E.P., and Kontos H.A. (1987) Oxygen radicals in cerebral ischemia. Physiologist 30, 122.

Weinberger J., Cohen G., and Nieves-Rosa J. (1983) Nerve terminal damage in cerebral ischemia: Greater susceptibility of catecholamine nerve terminals relative to serotonin nerve terminals. Stroke 14, 986–989.

Weinberger J., Nieves-Rosa J., and Cohen G. (1985) Nerve terminal damage in cerebral ischemia: Protective effects of alpha-methyl-para-tyrosine. Stroke, 16, 864–870.

Wisniewski H.M., and Kozlowski P.B. (1982) Evidence of blood-brain-barrier changes in senile dementia of the Alzheimer type. Ann. N.Y. Acad. Sci. USA 396, 119–129.

Wong K.-S., and Dryhurst G. (1990) Tryptamine-4,5-dione: Properties and reaction with glutathione. Bioorg. Chem. 18, 253–264.

Wong K.-S., Goyal R.N., Wrona M.Z., Blank C.L., and Dryhurst G. (1993) 7-S-Glutathionyl-tryptamine-4,5-dione: A possible aberrant metabolite of serotonin. Biochem. Pharmacol. 46, 1637–1652.

Wrona M.Z., and Dryhurst G. (1987) Oxidation chemistry of 5-hydroxytryptamine. I. Mechanisms and products formed at micromolar concentrations. J. Org. Chem. 52, 2817–2825.

Wrona M.Z., and Dryhurst G. (1988) Further insights into the oxidation chemistry of 5-hydroxytryptamine. J. Pharm. Sci. 77, 911–917.

Wrona M.Z., and Dryhurst G. (1989) Electrochemical oxidation of 5-hydroxytryptamine in acidic aqueous solution. J. Org. Chem. 54, 2718–2721.

Wrona M.Z., and Dryhurst G. (1990a) Oxidation chemistry of 5-hydroxytryptamine. Part II. Mechanisms and products formed at millimolar concentrations in acidic aqueous solution. J. Electroanal. Chem. 278, 249–267.

Wrona M.Z., and Dryhurst G. (1990b) Electrochemical oxidation of 5-hydroxytryptamine in aqueous solution at physiological pH. Bioorg. Chem. 18, 291–317.

Wrona M.Z., and Dryhurst G. (1991) Interactions of 5-hydroxytryptamine with oxidative enzymes. Biochem. Pharmacol. 41, 1145–1162.

Wrona M.Z., Goyal R.N., Turk D., Blank C.L., and Dryhurst G. (1992) 5,5′-Dihydroxy-4,4′-bitryptamine: A potentially aberrant neurotoxic metabolite of serotonin. J. Neurochem. 59, 1392–1398.

Wrona M.Z., Singh S., and Dryhurst G. (1994) Influence of L-cysteine on the oxidation chemistry of serotonin. Bioorg. Chem. 22, 421–445.

Wrona M.Z., Singh S., and Dryhurst G. (1995a) Influence of glutathione on the electrochemical and enzymatic oxidation of serotonin. J. Electroanal. Chem. 382, 41–51.

Wrona M.Z., Yang Z., McAdams M., O'Connor-Coates S., and Dryhurst G. (1995b) Hydroxyl radical-mediated oxidation of serotonin: Potential insights into the neurotoxicity of methamphetamine. J. Neurochem. 64, 1390–1400.

Wrona M.Z., Yang Z, Waskiewicz J., and Dryhurst G. (1996) Oxygen radical-mediated oxidation of serotonin: Potential relationship to neurodegenerative diseases. In: Neurodegenerative Diseases (Fiskum G., ed.), pp. 285–297, Plenum Press, New York.

Wu Z., and Dryhurst G. (1996) 7-S-Glutathionyltryptophan-4,5-dione: Formation from 5-hydroxytryptophan and reactions with glutathione. Bioorg. Chem. 24, 127–149.

Wu, Z., Shen X-M., and Dryhurst G. (1995) Oxidation chemistry of 5-[[3-(2-amino-2-carboxyethyl)-5-hydroxy-1H-indol-4-yl]oxy]-[3-(2-amino-2-carboxyethyl)]-1H-indole: A putative aberrant metabolite of 5-hydroxytryptophan. Bioorg. Chem. 23, 227–255.

Yamamoto T., and Hirano A. (1985) Nucleus raphe dorsalis in Alzheimer's disease: Neurofibfillary tangles and loss of large neurones. Ann. Neurol. 17, 573–577.

Yang G.Y., Chan P.H., Chen J., Carlson E., Chen S.F., Weinstein P., Epstein C.J., and Kamii H. (1994) Human copper-zinc superoxide dismutase transgenic mice are highly resistant to reperfusion injury after focal cerebral ischemia. Stroke 25, 165–170.

Yang Z., Wrona M.Z., and Dryhurst G. (1997) 5-Hydroxy-3-ethylamino-2-oxindole is not formed in rat brain following a neurotoxic dose of methamphetamine: Evidence that methamphetamine does not induce hydroxyl radical mediated oxidation of serotonin. J. Neurochem. 68, 1929–1941.

Yanker B.A., Duffy L.K., and Kirschner K.A. (1990) Neurotrophic and neurotoxic effects of amyloid-β-protein: Reversal by tachykinin neuropeptides. Science 250, 279–282.

Young T.E., and Babbitt B.W. (1983) Electrochemical study of the oxidation of α-methyldopamine, α-methylnoradrenaline, and dopamine. J. Org. Chem. 48, 562–566.

Yoshida S., Busto R., Watson B.K.D., and Ginsberg M.D. (1984) Postischemic cerebral lipid peroxidation *in vitro:* Modification by dietary vitamin E. J. Neurochem. 42, 1593–1601.

Yoshida T., Tanaka M., Sotomatsu A., and Hirai S. (1995) Activated microglia cause superoxide-mediated release of iron from ferritin. Neurosci. Lett. 190, 21–24.

Zemlan F.P., Thienhaus O.J., and Bosman H.B. (1989) Superoxide dismutase activity in Alzheimer's disease: Possible mechanism for paired helical formation. Brain Res. 476, 160–162.

Zhang F., and Dryhurst G. (1993) Oxidation chemistry of dopamine: Possible insights into the age-dependent loss of dopaminergic nigrostriatal neurons. Bioorg. Chem. 21, 392–410.

Zhang F., and Dryhurst G. (1994) Effects of L-cysteine on the oxidation chemistry of dopamine: New reaction pathways of potential relevance to idiopathic Parkinson's disease. J. Med. Chem. 37, 1084–1098.

Zhang F., and Dryhurst G. (1995) Influence of glutathione on the oxidation chemistry of the catecholaminergic neurotransmitter dopamine. J. Electroanal. Chem. 398, 117–128.

Zigmond M.J., and Hastings T.G. (1992) A method for measuring dopamine-protein conjugates as an index of dopamine oxidation. Soc. Neurosci. Abstr. 18, 1443.

β-Carboline Derivatives as Neurotoxins

Michael A. Collins and Edward J. Neafsey

Contents in Brief

Carbolines (pyrido-indoles) are relatively omnipresent indole alkaloid constituents in our ecosystem and most diets (Robinson, 1981). They are often present in α-, β-, γ- and δ-forms in pyrolyzed/broiled proteinaceous materials and foods, industrial wastes and various types of smoke, with the structurally "simple" β-carboline (βC; 9H-pyrido[3,4-b] indole or *harmala*) alkaloids represented mainly by norharman and harman (Sugimura and Nagao, 1979; Felton and Knize, 1990). Furthermore, many plants and fungi, while containing the above-mentioned βC's along with oxygenated *harmala* alkaloid constituents such as harmine, harmol and harmaline (Allen and Holmstedt, 1980), are also a source of more complex, medicinally important βC-based alkaloids—for example, reserpine and yohimbine (Saxton, 1960). Ibogaine, another indole alkaloid of current topical interest in addiction research, is often pharmacologically associated with harmaline, but it is not in the carboline subclass. Figure 1 shows the structures of the aforementioned simple βC's and several other natural derivatives that are the main focus of this review.

1. Biosynthetic and Organo-synthetic Routes to THβC's and βC's

The essential amino acid tryptophan or a related "open chain" indole such as tryptamine is the precursor that produces various carboline isomers depending on the environmental or plant catalyst(s), carbonyl reactants, temperature and milieu. There also is evidence suggesting that simple βC's, particularly the 1,2,3,4-tetrahydro-forms (described below), may be biosynthesized from tryptophan or its metabolites in animal cells, i.e., "mammalian" alkaloids (Airaksinen and Kari, 1981; Melchior and Collins, 1982; Bringmann et al., 1991). The key (bio)synthetic pathways are represented in Fig. 2. The initial products from open chain amine or amino acid precursor(s) cyclizing in a Pictet-Spengler (or Mannich) reaction with carbonyl-containing compounds (pathway A, shown with an aldehyde) are 1,2,3,4-tetrahydro-β-carbolines (THβC's) (Whaley and Govindachari, 1951a). Sometimes identified as tryptolines, THβC's can undergo two-electron oxidation to 3,4-dihydrogenated intermediates (3,4-dihydro-βC's or DHβC's) that can be dehydrogenated (and/or decarboxylated, if tryptophan is a precursor) to the heteroaromatic structure. In theory, an alternate pathway (B in Fig. 2) leading directly either to a DHβC or a βC entails cyclization of an N-acylated tryptamine or tryptophan *via* the Bischler-Napieralski reaction (Whaley and Govindachari, 1951b). However, this latter conversion typically requires organic synthetic conditions of strong Lewis acid with heat, and is not viewed as a "physiological" route, although it may well occur during pyrolysis. In general, the exact sequence of the specific steps in the pathways is yet to be established. Indeed, other, more complicated biosynthetic condensation routes are also plausible.

2. Overview of the Effects of βC's and Their Metabolic Derivatives on the Nervous System

Recognition of the environmental ubiquity of βC-based alkaloids accounts in part for a substantial body of knowledge about their neurophysiological and neuropharmacological actions. Considerable information is available about *harmala* alkaloids and monoamine

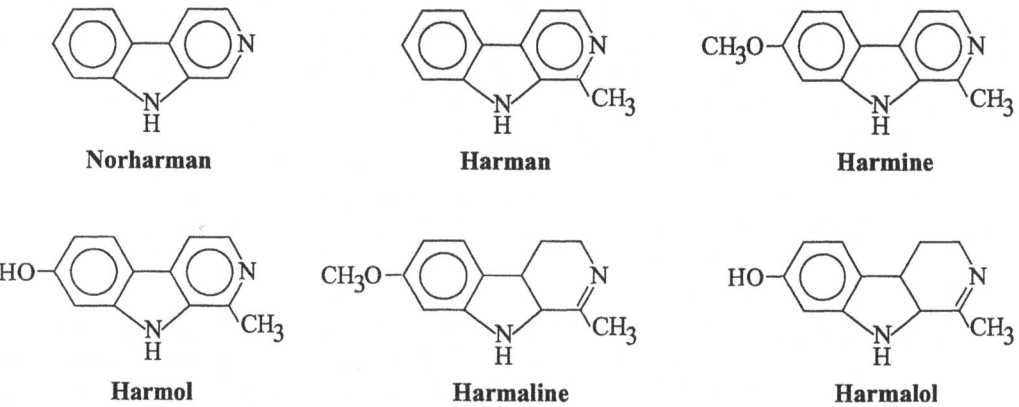

Fig. 1   Structures of relevant β-carbolines (βC's; *harmala* alkaloids).

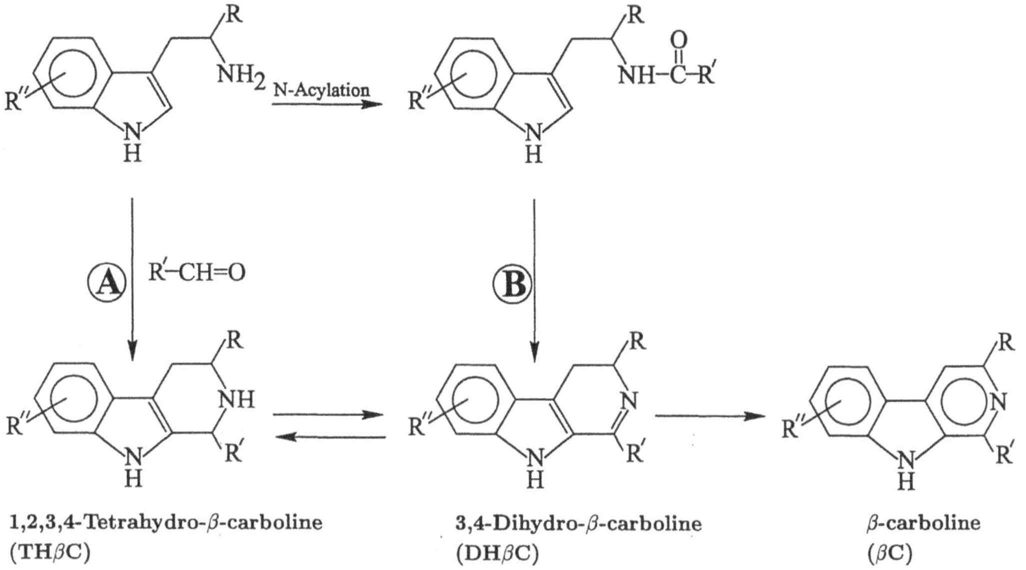

Fig. 2   Reaction pathways for the formation of 1,2,3,4,tetrahydro-β-carbolines (THβC's) or 3,4-dihydro-β-carbolines (DHβC's) *via* (A) the Pictet-Spengler condensation or (B) the Bischler-Napieralski cyclization. DHβC's can be dehydrogenated (oxidized) to heteroaromatic β-carbolines (βC's), and also can be reduced to THβC's.

oxidase (MAO) inhibition, effects on membrane ion transport, blockade of the serotonin transporter, and antagonism of the GABA/benzodiazepine receptor complex, for example, which is beyond the scope of this review (Buckholtz, 1980; Segonzac et al., 1985; Rommelspacher et al., 1991; Braestrup and Nielsen, 1993; Rommelspacher and Schmidt, 1995). And perhaps the earliest interest in natural βC's is reflected in their centuries of use and enjoyment by indigenous peoples for hallucinogenic, mind-altering and religious purposes (Allen and Holmstedt, 1980; Schultes, 1982). Furthermore, implicit in early studies of THβC's as possible *in vivo* products of alcohol-derived acetaldehyde and neuroactive indoleamines was that the alkaloidal compounds had some toxic or causative central role in human alcohol abuse (McIsaac, 1961; Holman et al., 1980; Melchior and Collins, 1982). Neurotoxic effects were inferred to underlie the persistent intake of high alcohol solutions that is induced in rats infused centrally with THβC (tetrahydro-norharman) or harman (Myers and Melchior, 1977; Adell and Myers, 1994), but the definite occurrence of neuronal loss remains to be established. There is convincing evidence of βC neurotoxicity in animal husbandry, where persistent neurological effects occur in lifestock that ingest forage containing certain indoles: the consumption of *Phalaris* grasses by sheep results in a dramatic nervous system syndrome that is linked to toxic forms of THβC's and tryptamine compounds (Cheeke,1995).

However, only recently have βC derivatives been experimentally linked with prevalent human neurodegenerative conditions. This linkage had its roots in the important discovery that the small heterocyclics, N-methyl-4-phenylpyridinium cation (MPP⁺) and its tetrahydro precursor/illicit drug contaminant, N-methyl-4-phenyl-1,2,3,6-tetrahydropyridine (MPTP), evoked profound nigrostriatal loss and irreversible parkinsonism in humans and primates (Burns et al., 1983; Langston et al., 1983). MPTP gave new to the idea that Parkin-

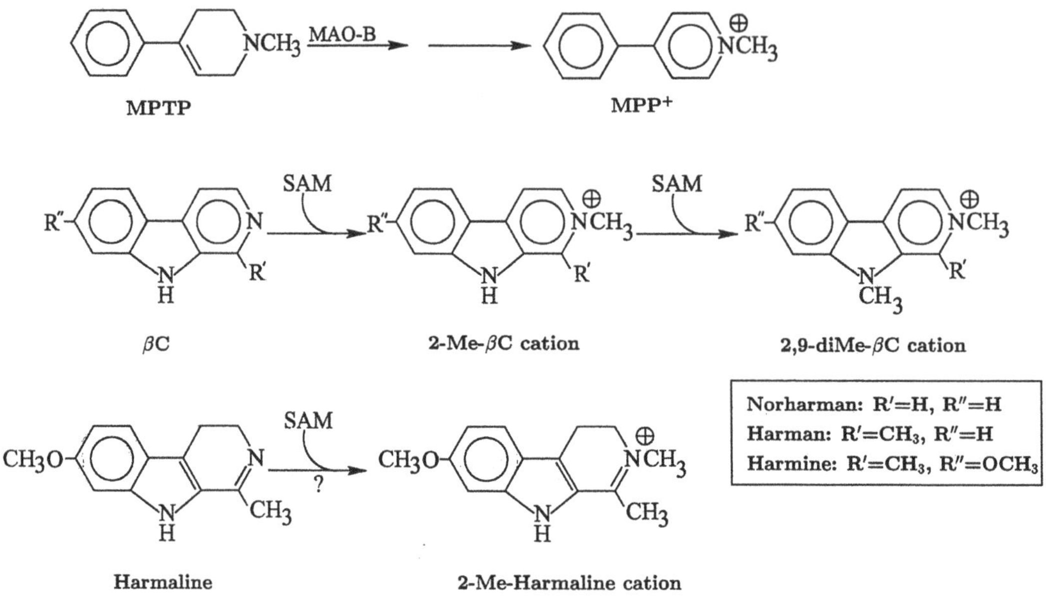

Fig. 3 (Top) Structure of N-methyl-4-phenyl-tetrahydropyridine (MPTP) and its MAO-catalyzed transformation to N-methyl-4-phenylpyridinium ion (MPP$^+$).

(Middle) S-Adenosylmethionine (SAM)-dependent N-methylation route from βC's such as norharman, harman or harmine that sequentially yields 2-Me-βC and 2,9-diMe-βC cations.

(Bottom) Hypothesized SAM-dependent N-methylation of the DHβC, harmaline, to produce the 2-Me-DHβC, 2-Me-harmaline cation.

son's disease, a neuropathological condition of multifactorial etiology that is associated with aging, might be linked to environmental (or endogenous) toxins (Tanner and Langston, 1990). The fact that MPP$^+$ and MPTP (shown in Fig. 3) are encompassed within the N-methylated THβC or βC cation structures provided initial impetus for hypotheses proposing simple N-methylated carbolines as causative factors in Parkinson's disease (Collins and Neafsey, 1985; Ohkubo et al., 1985; Ramsden and Williams, 1985; Testa et al., 1985; Collins et al., 1986).

Driven by recent results, these hypotheses have converged into the concept that the carboline-based neurotoxic entities possibly involved in Parkinson's disease might be quaternary, cationic βC's containing both 2[β]- and 9[indole]-N-methyl groups (e.g., 2,9-diMe-βC cations) (Collins et al., 1992; Collins et al., 1996). The charged molecules could form via sequential methyl transfer reactions within brain from hydrophobic, blood-brain barrier-permeable βC's and THβC's of environmental as well as endogenous biosynthetic origins. These pathways and the 2-Me- and 2,9-diMe-cationic products of the βC's, norharman, harman and harmine, and the DHβC, harmaline (solely 2-methylated), are shown in Fig. 3. The structural overlap of MPP$^+$ and N-methylated βC cations is readily apparent. Finally, a possibly more restricted hypothesis proposed by Bringmann et al. (1996) focuses on the 1-trichloromethyl-substituted THβC, termed TaClo, which may form *in vivo* from tryptamine and the occupationally associated aldehyde, chloral. TaClo has been shown to

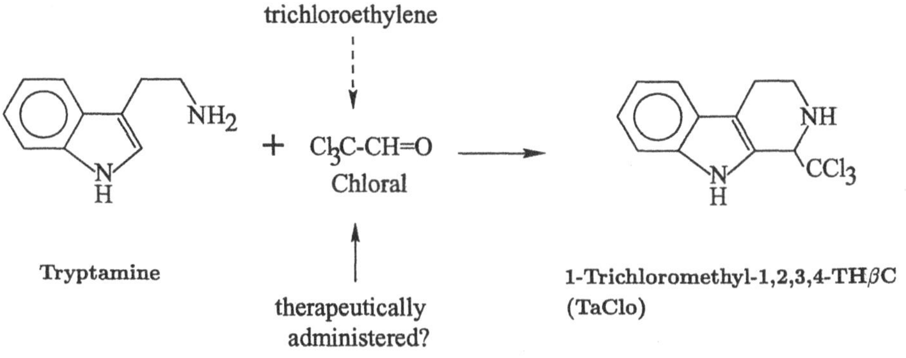

trichloroethylene

Fig. 4   Formation of TaClo from the Pictet-Spengler condensation of tryptamine and chloral.

have neurotoxic properties (*vide infra*) that in part could reflect the metabolite from N-methylation (2-Me-TaClo), which bears some structural resemblance to MPTP. The formation and structure of TaClo are shown in Fig. 4 (see Chapter 6).

3. Measurement and Analysis of THβC's, βC's and Their Derivatives

Assays of THβC's: Gas chromatography (GC) on capillary columns and high performance liquid chromatography (HPLC) have been the methods of choice for the separation and analysis of THβC's. By derivatizing the 2-nitrogen with trifluoroacetyl, heptafluorobutyryl or related acyl residues to increase the volatility of THβC's (and many other amines), separation and sensitive detection in GC-based systems is greatly-improved (Araiksinen and Kari, 1981; Barker et al., 1981; Johnson et al., 1985). Analyses often incorporate deuterated internal standards for more precise quantitation (e.g., Hayashi et al., 1990). The use of solid phase extraction (SPE) columns has made the extractive isolation of THβC's and βC's from complex matrices such as animal tissues and urine a much less complicated task.

The problem of artifactual production has been of concern for high sensitivity THβC assays, since, as aqueous condensation products, the THβC's could form during the assay procedure itself from traces of aldehydes and open chain amines. While various approaches have been used, the analysis of THβC and 1-MeTHβC by Tsuchiya et al. (1995b) appears to rigorously prevent artifactual condensations, while simultaneously derivatizing the THβC's that have a secondary pyridyl nitrogen for GC analysis. These researchers show that added fluorescamine reacts with possible traces of tryptamine precursor during the isolation procedure and prevents artifactual THβC production. An analogous "trapping" approach reported earlier by Bosin and Jarvis (1985) used methyl chloroformate for HPLC/fluorescence analysis of THβC's.

Concurrent analysis of 3-carboxylated THβC's and their N-nitroso derivatives in foods and beverages was done by HPLC-fluorescence detection and confirmed by HPLC with MS detection, following solid phase extraction with microcolumns (Sen et al., 1995). Fluorescence detection after HPLC separation was also used for the assay of a 3-carboxylated THβC in human lens (Manabe et al., 1996). An assay method for the highly non-polar

THβC, TaClo (Fig. 4), utilized heptafluorobutyryl-derivatization of the 2-nitrogen and analysis by GC/mass spectrometry (GC/MS) with selected ion monitoring and a deuterated TaClo internal standard (Bringmann et al., 1995). Because the multiple fluoro and chloro groups are excellent electron acceptors, high sensitivity detection of TaClo was also possible using GC/electron capture detection. Repeated peripheral administration of TaClo in rats resulted in its facile penetration of the blood-brain barrier and uninhibited brain distribution, as evidenced by readily detectable levels in many brain regions.

Analysis of βC's: Most βC's show very high native fluorescence, and this has facilitated their sensitive analysis by chromatographic means. Unlike THβC's, the artifactual production of βC's during isolation procedures is not considered a complicating factor. The early thin layer chromatography (TLC) and liquid chromatographic (LC) procedures for the analysis of norharman, harman, harmine and harmaline were often dependent on fluorescent detection, as summarized in Popl et al. (1990). The N-methylated βC cations, as strong fluorophores, are readily analyzed by fluorescence detection after HPLC separation (Matsubara et al., 1995). Also, GC/MS with 9-ethyl-substituted norharman internal standard was used to analyze the Me-βC cations after their extraction from a biological matrix, but they were first reduced to the tetrahydro-forms with sodium borohydride (Matsubara et al., 1993). Such a reductive derivatization approach is feasible, however, only if it is established that the reduction products, 2-Me-THβC's and 2,9-diMe-THβC's, are not detectable in the tissue being studied.

4. Enzymatic Formation of N-Methylated βC Cations From Nonpolar βC's

S-Adenosylmethionine (SAM)-dependent N-methyltransferases that utilize heterocyclic amine substrates are present in animals, and the activities in brain, when examined, are usually considerably less than in liver and other organs (Saavadra et al., 1973; Ansher and Jacoby, 1986; Crooks et al., 1988). Stimulated by the discovery of MPTP and MPP$^+$ was the idea that N-methyltransferases could be involved in the toxification of xenobiotic pyridine compounds (Ansher et al., 1986; Godin and Crooks, 1989; Williams et al., 1993). Probing possible carboline N-methylation in animals, Matsubara et al. (1992a,b) first reported the substrate capabilities of THβC's and βC's toward SAM-dependent N-methyltransferases in brain fractions from adult guinea pig and rat. 2-N-Methylation of THβC, 6-methoxy-THβC and 1-methyl-6-hydroxy-THβC was demonstrated with HPLC and radiochemical detection by utilizing tritium-labeled SAM cofactor. While THβC 2-methylation was solely cytosolic in guinea pig brain, significant nuclear activity was observed in rat brain (~20% of total; Matsubara et al., 1992a). Whether the THβC 2-methyltransferase, with its relatively low activity (V_{max}'s 1–3 pmoles/mg protein/hr), is identical to other cytosolic amine N-methyltransferases that methylate nonaromatic nitrogen atoms is not known (Saavedra et al., 1973; Ansher et al., 1986; Naoi et al., 1989).

In contrast to THβC's, heteroaromatic βC substrates may undergo considerable nuclear 2-N-methylation in both guinea pig and rat brain, apparently by a different enzyme than the THβC 2-methyltransferase (Matsubara et al., 1992b). However, βC's differ in a more significant way from THβC's in that the derived 2-methylated cationic products undergo subsequent methylation on the 9[indole] nitrogen, as shown in Fig. 3 (Collins et al., 1992; Matsubara et al., 1992b). The driving force for indole-N-methylation most likely resides in the resonance capability of the 2-methylated cation in Fig. 3, which markedly increases the basicity/nucleophilicity of the indole nitrogen. Such activation is not available to open chain indoles and simple (nonquaternary) βC's, and in that regard, an earlier report of indole-N-methylation of tryptamine by liver enzymes was found to be in error (Crooks et al., 1986). Indole-N-methylation is also precluded in 2-methyl-THβC's because of the tetrahydro structure—explaining the absence of 9-N-methyl products with these substrates (Matsubara et al., 1992a). Methylation of the indole nitrogen is thus highly substrate-specific. Parenthetically, 9[indole]-alkylated βC alkaloids are found plants and/or fungi, but their biosynthetic routes have not been clarified.

Unlike the initial finding of an extensive nuclear distribution, brain βC-2-N-methyltransferase activity isolated by Gearhart et al. (1995) was highly localized in the cell cytosol. The incongruity could be explained by subtle differences in procedure, or by translocation during or prior to the isolation procedure. There is evidence, for example, that glycine-N-methyltransferase is identical to an aromatic hydrocarbon-binding receptor-like protein, and as such, is a transactivation factor that is either nuclear or cytosolic, depending on factors such as the aromatic hydrocarbon content of the tissue preparation (Raha et al., 1994). A similar circumstance might pertain to βC 2-N-methyltransferase with heteroaromatic βC's. Regardless of its subcellular location, the βC 2-N-methylating activity would have an initial key role in trapping hydrophobic pyrido-indoles within the brain.

Gearhart et al. (1997) further found that βC 2-N-methylation (bovine brain) was inhibited like other methyltransferases by S-adenosyl-homocysteine (K_i, ~15 uM), the proximal reaction product of SAM. Also, the enzyme's maximum velocity with 9-methyl βC substrate was originally underestimated by a factor of 20 in earlier studies because the SAM concentrations used were well below its K_m for the enzyme. This also may explain the reportedly low *in vitro* activity of 9[indole]-N-methyltransferase. Furthermore, βC 2-N-methylation activity is increased 150% by addition of iron or manganese, two metals that have been associated with parkinsonism (Gearhart et al., 1997).

Perhaps of equal physiological significance are indications that βC 2-N- methyltransferase activity is due to phenylethanolamine-N-methyltransferase (PNMT) (Gearhart, 1997). This is indicated by the facts that: (a) the activity with 9-methyl βC substrate is enriched in the adrenal gland, and is completely inhibited (in brain or adrenal) by the PNMT substrate norepinephrine and by the selective PNMT inhibitor, LY134046; and (b) commercial PNMT carries out the 2-N-methylation of βC substrate, but not its subsequent 9-N-methylation (a further indication that the two βC N-methyltransferase activities are different). The exciting possibility that PNMT could conceivably initiate a bioactivation process that would introduce and trap toxicants within the brain is pertinent to PD. Limited epidemiological studies suggest that there is a relationship between the incidence of Parkinson's disease and "crucial life events" in childhood, apparently including stress (Eatough et al., 1990). Experimentally, PNMT is regulated by stress in adrenal and brain (Turner et al., 1978). Also, potential βC substrates for N-methylation may increase with forms of stress; Harrison (1982) demonstrated with GC/MS that rats subjected to both mild isolation stress and prolonged restraint stress had significant elevations in adrenal and brain contents of THβC and 6-methoxy-THβC.

Studying the two N-methylating processes in the substantia nigra, putamen and frontal cortex of postmortem human brain, Gearhart et al. (1996) found to significant differences in supernatant (cytosolic + microsomal) and particulate (mitochondrial + nuclear) βC 2-N-methylation activities between parkinsonian and control subjects. In assays with relatively low SAM, Matsubara et al. (1993) first reported the human brain presence of activity for 2-N-methyltransferase, but not βC 9[indole]-N-methyltransferase. However, Gearhart et al. (1996) obtained measurable βC 9-methyltransferase activity, and found that supernatant component, which constituted ~75% of total indole-N-methylation, was three-fold higher (p < 0.02), specifically in parkinsonian frontal cortex, a region of the brain neuropathologically spared by the disease process. Since other brain regions that are relatively unaffected in Parkinson's disease were not studied, the meaning of this provocative finding is unclear. One possibility is that indole-N-methylation is elevated throughout the brain for unknown reasons (and plays a role) in the early disease process, but it drops to normal nigrostriatal tissue activity as neurons are lost (Gearhart, 1997).

5. Uptake and Intracellular Actions of N-Methylated βC Cations

Selective neuronal uptake of MPP$^+$ by the dopamine transporter is considered critical for the high toxic specificity of this pyridinium cation toward nigrostriatal dopaminergic neurons and terminals (Javitch et al., 1985; Heikkila et al., 1989); however, the transporter's role is questioned in some studies (Hung et al., 1995). 2-N-Methylated βC cations have considerably lower affinities for this transporter than MPP$^+$ (Drucker et al., 1989). Their IC$_{50}$'s for inhibition of radioactive dopamine uptake in brain synaptosomes tended to be in the range of 12 μM to 80 μM or higher, compared ~0.5 μM for MPP$^+$, and only about 15–20% of synaptosomal uptake of labeled 2-Me-harmine cation was prevented by nomifensine, a potent antagonist of the dopamine transporter. However, results in primary cell cultures, discussed later, indicate that neurotoxic effects exerted by 2,9-diMe-βC cations may depend to a great extent on uptake by the dopamine transporter.

The neurotoxicity of MPP$^+$ is regarded the end result of inhibition of neuronal mitochondrial respiration by the pyridinium cation, specifically by blockade of NADH dehydrogenase activity within Complex I of the respiratory chain (Nicklas et al., 1985; Heikkila et al., 1989; Tipton and Singer, 1993). Intracellular generation of destructive free radicals also has been associated with MPP$^+$'s toxic actions (e.g., Cleeter et al., 1992). Free radical production as a neurotoxic mechanism is unexplored with N-Me-βC cations; in contrast, harmine and other βC's have been reported to trap free radicals in some systems. However, it is quite clear that a number of N-methylated βC cations mirror MPP$^+$ as potent inhibitors of Complex I (NADH-linked) mitochondrial respiration (Albores et al., 1990; Sayre et al., 1991; Fields et al., 1992; Krueger et al., 1993). Table 1 contains a comparison of their reported or estimated IC$_{50}$'s for inhibition of Complex I.

Although weaker, inhibition of Complex II (succinate-linked) respiration by selected N-Me-βC cations (Table 1) has been suggested to play a role in their neurotoxic actions (Fields et al., 1992). An in-depth study with 1-desmethyl analogs of 2-Me-harmine and 2-Me-harmol cations and MPP$^+$ by Sayre et al. (1991) reported inhibitory constants for Complex I that coincided with Albores et al. (1990), and noted inhibition of Complex II by the 2-Me-βC cations as well. Because of significant uncoupling of state 2 respiration at higher concentrations, the 2-methylated cations were considered inhibitors-uncouplers. Krueger et al. (1993) reported very weak inhibition at Complex II by 2,9-diMe-βC cations along with significant uncoupling (Table 1), and concluded that blockade of succinate oxidation at

Table 1. IC_{50}'s (μM) for inhibition of mitochondrial respiration by
N-methyl-β-carboline cations and MPP$^+$

Cation	Complex I	Complex II	Reference
MPP$^+$	170	—	Albores et al., 1990
	100	1500	Krueger et al., 1993
	—	>1200	Fields et al., 1992
2,9-diMe-harman	100	250	Fields et al., 1992
	29	725	Krueger et al., 1993
2,9-diMe-norharman	135	—	Collins (unpubl. data)
	80	830	Krueger et al., 1993
2-Me-harmaline	232	—	Albores et al., 1990
2-Me-harmine	185	—	Albores et al., 1990
	—	225	Fields et al., 1992
2-Me-harmol	209	—	Albores et al., 1990
	—	225	Fields et al., 1992
2-Me-harman	2850	—	Albores et al., 1990
	—	250	Fields et al., 1992
2-Me-norharman	1145	—	Albores et al., 1990

Complex II by the cations would be unimportant for neurotoxicity. However, the strong inhibition of Complex I by the 2,9-Me-βC cations (70–250% more potent than MPP$^+$, Table 1) appears to preclude arguments about the importance of Complex II inhibition.

Several relevant aspects of Complex I inhibition by N-methylated βC cations should be summarized. First, whereas the 2-methyl cations derived from norharman and harman were relatively innocuous inhibitors, their IC_{50} values dropped sharply upon introduction of a 7-oxygenated substituent (Table 1, 2-Me-harman cation versus 2-Me-harmol or 2-Me-harmine cations; also, compare 2-Me-norharman cation in Table 1 with the inhibition by the 7-hydroxy and 7-methoxy derivatives in Sayre et al., 1991). Why 7-oxygenated substitution should be so effective has not been elucidated, but it is worth noting that the *in vivo* neurotoxic actions of 2-Me-norharman or 2-Me-harman cations also increase markedly due to 7-hydroxy or 7-methoxy substitution (Neafsey et al., 1995; discussion of neurotoxic effects is in a subsequent section).

Second, the time-course of mitochondrial inhibition for the 2-methylated cations derived from harmine, harmol or harmaline was very rapid (Albores et al., 1990), whereas MPP$^+$'s inhibitory time-course was gradual, reflecting the slow accumulation of a pyridinium cation. This constitutes evidence that, to a substantial degree, the 2-Me-βC species entering the inner mitochondrial membrane are neutral, indole-N-deprotonated carbolines, or in chemical terms, anhydronium bases. This notion is strongly supported by the results with the 2,9-diMe-βC cationic derivatives of norharman and harman, which cannot deprotonate the indole nitrogen; accordingly they display relatively slow time-courses of inhibition that closely mimic that of MPP$^+$ (Albores et al., 1990; Fields et al., 1992). Furthermore, addition of triphenylborate anion, which facilitates transfer of cations across the mitochondrial membrane and their penetration into the hydrophobic regions, causes nearly immediate inhibition of respiration by MPP$^+$ and the 2,9-Me-βC cations, but only moderately potentiates the effects of 2-Me-βC species—again indicating that neutral uncharged forms of the 2-mono-methylated compounds are key inhibitory players. Thus, aromatic oxygenation (hydroxylation, methoxylation) transforms weakly inhibitory 2-Me-βC anhydronium bases into strong (but still mainly uncharged) inhibitors of mitochondrial respiration, while 9-N-indole methylation converts these anhydronium base species (either weak or strong uncharged inhibitors) into potent, MPP$^+$-like cationic inhibitors.

Mitochondrial respiratory inhibition by the trichlorinated THβC's, TaClo, N-Me-TaClo and several derivatives, has been examined as a possible mechanism for putative neurotoxic actions (Janetzky et al., 1995; Bringmann et al., 1996). TaClo appeared to act as a relatively strong inhibitor in submitochondrial particles, but because of its uncharged nature, accumulation by intact mitochondria was not significant, nor was it potentiated by triphenylborate. Its N-methyl derivative, a possible *in vivo* metabolite, was reported to be a stronger inhibitor at both Complex I and Complex II. An increase in the extent of mitochondrial inhibition with prolonged incubations of TaClo was suggested to indicate the toxic generation of free radical species (Janetzky et al., 1995).

Inhibition of key enzymes like MAO is also of possible importance to the purported neurotoxic actions of carboline-based compounds. It has long been known that *harmala*-related βC's - in particular, harmine and harmaline - are potent, selective and reversible inhibitors of monoamine oxidase A (MAO-A) (Buckholtz and Boggan, 1977). An earlier report by Ho et al. (1973) first described MAO inhibition by a 2,9-diMe-βC cation, but Hasegawa et al. (1995) and Kim et al. (1997) have systematically examined the effect of mono- and di-N-methylation of norharman and other *harmala* alkaloids on mitochondrial MAO inhibition. As is evident by the K_i's in Table 2, both studies concurred in finding that sequential (2- and 9-) N-methylation of norharman significantly reduced the K_i for inhibition of MAO-A. They differed, however, in regard to harmine and its derivatives. In one study, harmine was a surprisingly weak noncompetitive inhibitor, and harmine's 2-methylated and 2,9-dimethylated cations were very strong inhibitors (Hagasawa et al. 1995). In contrast, Kim et al. (1997) determined a very low K_i for harmine that agrees with previous experiments with this *harmala* alkaloid, but they found considerably less potent inhibition for the 2-methyl and 2,9-dimethyl forms. Differences in mitochondrial sources (human

Table 2. K_i values (μM) for inhibition of MAO-A by β-carboline derivatives

Compound	Hasegawa et al. (1995)	Kim et al. (1997)
norharman	2.67	3.34
2-Me-norharman cation	0.74	1.43
2,9-diMe-norharman cation	0.29	0.41
harman	0.12	0.26
2-Me-harman cation	0.25	0.68
2,9-diMe-harman cation	0.17	0.16
harmine	1.42	0.005
2-Me-harmine cation	0.19	0.069
2,9-diMe-harmine cation	0.15	0.015
harmaline	0.002	0.048
2-Me-harmaline cation	0.006	0.14

brain versus beef liver), preparation and experimental procedures may explain a portion of the disagreement in these studies.

6. Neurotoxicity *In Vitro* of N-Methylated βC Cations

Comparisons of the cytotoxicities of N-methyl βC cations and MPP$^+$ have been carried out in rat pheochromocytoma (PC12) cells and fetal rat mesencephalic cultures. In PC12 cells cultured in media with low glucose concentrations (0.22 mM), 2,9-diMe-norharman cation, 2,9-diMe-harman cation and 2-Me-harmaline cation (structures in Fig. 3) consistently displayed cytotoxicities that approached or surpassed MPP$^+$; in contrast, other 2-mono-N-methylated βC cations that were tested were negligibly cytotoxic when cell protein loss and lactate dehydrogenase release were used as criteria (Cobuzzi et al., 1995). At a higher media glucose concentration of 5.55 mM, however, PC12 cell killing by both MPP$^+$ and 2,9-diMe-βC cations (represented by 2,9-diMe-norharmanium cation) was greatly suppressed or even erased. This indicated that the principal cytotoxic mechanism of 2,9-diMe-βC cations, like MPP$^+$, is interference with (mitochondrial) energy metabolism, which is readily overcome in these glycolytic cells by the additional glycolytic energy source. However, the high glucose conditions failed to suppress potent cytotoxicity of the 2-methylated cation derived from harmaline, indicating that this carbolinium species may have a different mechanism of action (Cobuzzi et al., 1995).

In fetal rat primary mesencephalic cultures, the cations of 2,9-diMe-norharman, 2,9-diMe-harman and 2-Me-harmaline had EC$_{50}$'s for toxicity toward dopaminergic neurons (EC$_{50DA}$) of approximately 10 μM under the conditions utilized (48 hr exposures in 6 day-old cultures) (Collins et al., 1995; Collins et al., 1996). By comparison, MPP$^+$ was some 25-fold more effective as a dopaminergic neurotoxin in these primary cultures. Furthermore, the above cationic βC's did not display the remarkably high toxic selectivity of exogenous MPP$^+$ for dopaminergic versus GABA-ergic neurons, as manifested by a high EC$_{50GABA}$/EC$_{50DA}$ ratio for the pyridinium cation (Collins et al., 1996).

However, an aromatic methoxy group appeared to have a dramatic potentiating effect of the toxicity of the 2,9-dimethylated βC cations. Specifically, the EC$_{50DA}$ for 2,9-diMe-harmine cation was <2 μM in mesencephalic cultures, or nearly five times stronger than its non-methoxylated analog, 2,9-diMe-harman cation, and only several-fold less effective than MPP$^+$. Methoxylation of the 6-, 7- and/or 8-positions of βC's is a known metabolic pathway in animals and microbes (Melchior and Collins, 1982; Neef et al., 1982), and hydroxlated THβC's have been identified as metabolites in rats and humans by mass spectrometric analysis (Beck et al., 1986; Tsuchiya et al., 1995a). Methoxylation of the indole moiety could possibly be an additional toxification step, along with 2- and 9-N-methylation, for xenobiotic βC's.

Experiments with the primary mesencephalic cultures showed that inhibitors of nitric oxide synthase do not prevent the neuronal cell loss induced by MPP$^+$, 2,9-diMe-norharman cation or 2-Me-harmaline cation (Collins et al., 1995; 1996). The failure of nitric oxide synthase inhibitors to block killing action of MPP$^+$ on dopaminergic cells in these cultures is in contrast to reports that the inhibitors prevent MPTP's neurotoxic effects *in vivo* (Przedborski et al., 1996; Schulz et al., 1995). In further studies with primary cultures, specific blockade of the dopamine transporter with GBR 12909 or nomifensine largely prevented dopaminergic neurotoxicity caused by MPP$^+$ (in agreement with a number of published studies on MPP$^+$ uptake) or by 2,9-diMe-norharman cation, but did not diminish the neurotoxic actions of 2-Me-harmaline cation - again indicating comparable processes for 2,9-di-N-methylated βC cations and MPP$^+$, and a markedly dissimilar mechanism for the 2-Me-harmaline cation (Collins et al., 1995).

7. Neurotoxicity *In Vivo* of N-Methylated THβC's and βC Cations

Initial *in vivo* experiments attempting to relate carboline derivatives to nigrostriatal damage and parkinsonism in monkeys and mice involved peripheral administration of 2[N]-Me-THβC (2-Me-tetrahydronorharman) rather than N-methylated βC cations (Collins and Neafsey, 1985; Collins et al., 1986; Perry et al., 1986). 2-Me-THβC was utilized because of the presumption that the molecule would cross the blood-brain barrier and be oxidized to the 2-methyl cationic species, analogous to MPTP. Also, it was known that 2-methylated THβC occurs *in vivo* (Barker et al., 1981) and in plants (Agurell et al., 1968). Comparing the experiments with 2-Me-THβC in C57/BL mice, disparate results were obtained that may be due to different doses as well as times of sacrifice. The levels of striatal dopamine and its two acid metabolites were unaltered for 1 month after 4 days of subcutaneous treatment with a cumulative dose of 280 mg/kg (Perry et al. 1986), but they were as much as 60% below control values ($p < 0.05$)—suggesting neurotoxic effects—a week following 5 days of intraperitoneal treatment with a total of 900 mg/kg (Collins et al. 1986). A high dose of 2-Me-THβC may be needed to induce apparent neuronal loss because of possibly slow enzymatic dehydrogenation (oxidation) to 2-Me-βC cation—which, as reviewed in the following paragraph, is not a highly potent neurotoxin.

The nigrostriatal neurotoxic effects of the MPP$^+$-like N-methylated βC cations have been determined and compared with MPP$^+$ in rats. Central placement was done because the cationic structures were expected to impede brain entry from the periphery. Microdialyzed into the *corpus striatum* at relatively high concentrations, 2-Me-norharman cation exerted appreciable and apparently irreversible neurotoxicity (Rollema et al., 1988). Comparisons of the nigrostriatal toxicity following acute intranigral administration indicated that 2-Me-norharman cation was several orders of magnitude less potent than MPP$^+$ (Neafsey et al., 1989). Sayre and colleagues (Arora et al., 1990; Sayre et al., 1991) reported substantial neurotoxicity after intranigral placement of another 2-methylated species, 2-Me-harmine cation, but again its potency appeared to be ~30-fold less than MPP$^+$. With 2-Me-norharman cation, addition of a 9-[indole]-N-methyl group clearly resulted in a substantial increase in neurotoxic efficacy, such that the 2,9-dimethylated cationic derivative was only an order of magnitude less toxic than MPP$^+$ to nigrostriatal dopaminergic terminals (Collins et al., 1992).

In a systematic study that utilized a number of neutral, 2-Me- and 2,9-diMe-βC derivatives, the nigral lesion sizes and striatal neurotransmitter changes following acute intranigral administration revealed, consistent with cell culture results, that 2,9-diMe-βC cations and 2-Me-harmaline cation were the most neurotoxic βC compounds (Neafsey et al., 1995). The above N-methyl carboline cations caused nigral lesions after unilateral intranigral administration that approached the size of MPP$^+$-induced lesions, and significantly depleted striatal levels of both dopamine and its acid metabolite, dihydroxy-phenylacetic acid. Similar injections of neutral βCs and most 2-mono-N-methylated βC compounds other than 2-Me-harmaline cation caused little or no neurotoxic effects when histological and neurochemical endpoints were co-evaluated. Such findings again emphasize the unique and unexplained toxic potency of 2-Me-harmaline cation, in comparison to its 3,4-dehydrogenated product, 2-Me-harmine cation and other 2-Me-βC cations that have similar mitochondrial inhibitory potencies. In agreement with primary mesencephalic culture studies, the most cytotoxic N-methylated βC cations, the 2,9-diMe cations and 2-Me-harmaline cation, were not selective toxins for nigral dopaminergic neurons *in vivo* (Neafsey et al., 1995). However, the lack of neuronal specificity may be of less concern if the N-methylated products of xenobiotic carbolines tend to form/accumulate within specific brain regions. Indeed, there is evidence indicating that this might ensue *in vivo,* as discussed in the last section.

Correlations between the toxic strengths of selected N-methylated βC cations *in vivo* and their potencies in *in vitro* studies, namely, blockade of synaptosomal DA uptake, inhibition of mitochondrial respiration, toxicities in PC12 cells and inhibition of rat brain MAO-A, revealed unexpected relationships (Neafsey et al., 1995). For example, the ability of βC's and N-methylated βC cations to inhibit dopamine uptake in isolated brain synaptosomes correlated well with the size of nigral lesions ($r = +0.78$; $p < 0.05$) or the percent depletions of striatal dopamine ($r = -0.70$) obtained in *in vivo* experiments; however, the opposite correlations should have been observed if the neurotoxicities of the cations depended on affinity for the dopamine uptake system. Furthermore, in comparisons between *in vitro* studies only, there was a strong negative relationship ($r = -0.84$) between toxicities of N-methylated βC cations in PC12 cells and their inhibition constants with MAO-A. Such a correlation might indicate that MAO-A further "bioactivates" the βC cations to unknown species, in much the same way that MAO-B promotes bioactivation of MPTP (Tipton and Singer, 1993). Alternatively, the βC cations' primary toxic mechanism of mitochondrial respiratory inhibition could depend upon or be potentiated by an amine which accumulates as a result of the MAO-A blockade.

Behavioral and neurochemical indications for neurotoxicity have been determined in studies of TaClo and 2-Me-TaClo in rats, further emphasizing the degenerative potential of these possibly endogenous THβC's. Peripheral daily doses of TaClo over 7 weeks resulted in apparently permanent locomotor deficits (Sontag et al., 1995), and acute intranigral placement of TaClo (~35 ng) caused significant reductions in dopamine and DOPAC in the ipsilateral striatum (Grote et al., 1995).

8. Endogenous Presence of THβC's, βC's and Their N-Methylated Derivatives in Animals and Humans

The detection of norharman and harman and their tetrahydro forms in pioneering early and more recent experiments with animals and humans has been reviewed in detail elsewhere (Airaksinen and Kari, 1981; Melchior and Collins, 1982; Bringmann et al., 1991; Rommelspacher and Schmidt, 1995). Norharman was found to be elevated in the plasma of chronic alcoholics (Spies et al., 1995), but the results of Breyer-Pfaff et al. (1996) indicate that cigarette smoking rather than alcohol intake may explain the increased levels. Furthermore, the reported elevation of norharman in the plasma of individuals with Parkinson's disease (Kuhn et al., 1995) is obviously relevant to the hypothesis of βC N-methylation, but the contribution of smoking, if important in these patients, would appear inconsistent with the hypothesis, since epidemiological studies suggest that smoking is associated with a reduced incidence of Parkinson's disease (Jenner et al., 1992; Tanner and Langston, 1990). With regard to the endogenous presence of TaClo, to date there are no reports of the THβC in humans, but it has been detected by GC/MS in the blood and brain of some, but not all, rats treated with tryptamine and chloral (Bringmann et al., 1996).

Norharman has been called a normal body constituent (Fekkes et al., 1992), but whether it and its congener, harman, are truly endogenously biosynthesized is still subject to debate. Urinary measurements by Ushiyama et al. (1995) support endogenous biosynthesis as a contributor to the body βC content. Specifically, norharman and harman were found to be excreted by patients on parenteral diets apparently lacking the βC's, albeit at significantly lower levels than healthy volunteers on a normal diet (24-h urinary levels of norharman, 9-33 ng; harman levels were ~10-fold greater). However, the βC levels increased when the patients were switched to the normal diet, indicating a significant dietary contribution. In contrast, Tsuchiya et al. (1996) concluded from a study of βC excretion by drinking party-goers, with one subject given deuterated L-tryptophan in order to follow labeled indole excretion, that *in vivo* condensation was not a significant route.

The 3-carboxylated THβC's and βC's (R=COOH in Fig. 2), which most reasonably are cyclization/oxidation products of tryptophan, have received recent analytical attention. 3-Carboxy-THβC's are produced from reaction with aldehydes during brewing and fermentation processes (Bosin et al., 1986; Adachi et al., 1991; Herraiz and Ough, 1993; Sen et al., 1995), but they are found as well in various smoked foods and cheeses (Adachi et al., 1991; Papavergou and Clifford, 1992). They could be potential initiating factors in GI cancer, primarily because their N-nitroso products that may form *in vivo* from nitrite/acid reactions are highly mutagenic (Wakabayashi et al., 1983; Higashimoto et al., 1996). Although endogenous formation of 3-carboxylated THβC's and DHβC's from tryptophan has been implied (Dillon et al., 1976), an unequivocal demonstration is needed. Manabe et al. (1996) showed that human lens accumulation of a 3-carboxy-THβC was dependent on age, cataract state and lens tryptophan levels, suggestive of *in vivo* biosynthesis. However, brain levels of 1-methyl-3-carboxy-THβC in rats were not changed during ethanol treatment under conditions which would highly favor the carboline's formation (Fukushima et al., 1991).

The levels of endogenous N-methylated-βC cations have been estimated, in concert with their norharman and harman precursors, in human substantia nigra and parietal cortex (Matsubara et al., 1993; Matsubara, 1996). The 2-Me-norharman and 2,9-diMe-norharman cations, analyzed as their reduced derivatives by GC/MS, were detectable in most or all samples, as were norharman and harman using HPLC. The analogous N-Me cations derived from harman were undetectable in nigral samples and observed in only a few cortices. In general, the levels of the N-methylated norharman derivatives were lower than the precursor βC, consistent with knowledge about the slow rates for the sequential N-methylation process. An important finding was that the nigral levels of norharman, 2-Me-norharman cation and 2,9-diMe-norharman cation were appreciably higher than levels in cortex (factors of 28, 18 and 7.7, respectively; p < 0.01), implying differential accumulation, formation and/or metabolism in the principal region which generates in idiopathic parkinsonism. A smaller but nevertheless significant difference also was evident for harman.

Although comparative analyses of Parkinson's disease brain tissue are not yet available, lumbar cerebrospinal fluids (CSF) from patients in various Hoehn-Yahr stages of Parkinson's disease and control individuals have been assayed for norharman and its two N-methylated derivatives by HPLC (Matsubara et al. 1995). Approximately half of the patient—but none of the controls—had detectable CSF levels of the neurotoxic 2,9-diMe-norharman cation (mean level, ~50 pmoles/l), and the combined levels of N-methylated norharman derivatives were significantly greater in parkinsonian patients' CSF. It is not known at present whether these 2,9-diMe-cation levels are indicative of neurotoxic concentrations in the brains of the patients, or whether higher levels occurred at a much earlier stage. Despite that caveat, the CSF results represent strong support for the general idea that, in metabolically and genetically susceptible individuals, a range of MPP⁺-like neurotoxic agents may trigger the accelerated neurodegeneration characterizing idiopathic Parkinson's disease (Jenner et al., 1992), with N-methylated βC cations as prominent, endogenously bioactivated components in that potential group of agents.

Acknowledgments

We acknowledge the support of the USPHS NINDS and the Loyola University Neuroscience & Aging Institute, and the collaborative efforts of Dr. K. Matsubara in part of the research reviewed in this report.

References

Adachi H., Mizoi Y., Naito T., Ogawa Y., Uetani Y. and Ninomiya I. (1991) Identification of tetrahydro-β-carboline-3-carboxylic acid in foodstuffs, human urine and human milk. J. Nutr. 121:646–652.

Adell A., and Myers R.D. (1994) Increased alcohol intake in low drinking rats after chronic infusion of the β-carboline harman into the hippocampus. Pharmacol. Biochem. Behav. 49:949–953.

Airaksinen M.M., and Kari I. (1981) Beta-carbolines, psychoactive compounds in the mammalian body. Med. Biol. 59:21–34.

Albores R., Jr., Neafsey E.J., Drucker G., Fields J.Z., and Collins M.A. (1990) Mitochondrial respiratory inhibition by N-methyl-β-carboline derivatives structurally resembling MPP⁺. Proc. Natl. Acad. Sci. USA 87:9368–9372.

Allen Holmstedt B. (1980) The simple β-carboline alkaloids. Phytochem. 19:1573–1582.

Ansher S., and Jacoby W.B. (1986) Amine N-methyltransferases from rabbit liver. J. Biol. Chem. 261:3996–4001.

Ansher S., Cadet J., Jacoby W.B., and Baker J. (1986) Role of N-methyltransferases in the neurotoxicity associated with metabolites of MPTP and other 4-substituted pyridines in the environment. Biochem. Pharmacol. 35:3359–3363.

Arora P.K., Riachi N.J., Fiedler G.C., Singh M.P., Abdallah F., Harik S.I., and Sayre L.M. (1990) Structure-neurotoxicity trends of analogues of MPP⁺, the cytotoxic metabolite of dopaminergic neurotoxin MPTP. Life Sci. 46:379–390.

Barker S., Harrison R.E.W., Monti J., Brown G.B., and Christian S.T. (1981) Identification and quantification of 1,2,3,4-tetrahydro-β-carboline, 2-methyl-1,2,3,4-tetrahydro-β-carboline, and 6-methoxy-1,2,3,4-tetrahydro-β-carboline as *in vivo* constituents of rat brain and adrenal gland. Biochem. Pharmacol. 30:9–17.

Beck O., Faull K., and Repke, D. (1986) Rapid hydroxylation of methtryptoline (1-methyl-tetrahydro-β-carboline) in rat: identification of metabolites by chiral gas chromatography-mass spectrometry. Arch. Pharmacol. 333:307–312.

Bosin T.R., and Jarvis C.A. (1985) Derivatization in aqueous solution, isolation and separation of tetrahydro-β-carbolines and their precursors by liquid chromatography. J. Chromatog. 341:287–293.

Bosin T.R., Krogh S., and Mais D. (1986) Identification and quantitation of 1,2,3,4-tetrahydro-β-carboline-3-carboxylic acid and 1-methyl-1,2,3,4-tetrahydro-β-carboline-3-carboxylic acid in beer and wine. J. Agric. Food Chem. 34:843–847.

Braestrup C., and Nielsen M. (1993) Discovery of β-carboline ligands for benzodiazepine receptors. Psychopharm. Ser. 11:1–6.

Breyer-Pfaff U., Wiatr G., Stevens I., Gaertner H.J., Mundle G., and Mann K. (1996) Elevated norharman plasma levels in alcoholic patients and control resulting from tobacco smoking. Life Sci. 58:1425–1432.

Bringmann G., Feineis D., Friedrich H., and Hille A. (1991) Endogenous alkaloids in man—synthesis, analytics. Planta Med. 57 [Suppl.]:73–84.

Bringmann G., God R., Feineis D., Wesemann W., Riederer P., Rausch W.-D., Reichmann H., and Sontag K.-H. (1995) The TaClo concept: 1-trichloromethyl-1,2,3,4-tetrahydro-β-carboline, a new toxin for dopaminergic neurons. J. Neural Transm. [Suppl.] 46: 235–244.

Bringmann G., Feineis D., God R., Fahr S., Wesemann W., Clement H.-W., Grote C., Kolasiewicz W., Sontag K.-H., Heim C., Sontag T., Reichmann H., Janetzkey B., Rausch W.-D., Abdel-Mohsen M., Koutsilieri E., Gotz M., Gsell W., Zielke B., and Riederer P. (1996) Neurotoxic effects on the dopaminergic system induced by TaClo (1-trichloromethyl-1,2,3,4-tetrahydro-β-carboline), a potential mammalian alkaloid: in vivo and in vitro studies. Biogen. Amines 12:83–102.

Buckholtz N.S. (1980) Neurobiology of tetrahydro-β-carbolines. Life Sci. 27:893–903.

Buckholtz N.S., and Boggan W.O. (1977) Monoamine oxidase inhibition in brain and liver produced by β-carbolines: structure-activity relationships substrate specificity. Biochem. Pharmacol. 26:1991–1996.

Burns R., Chiueh C., Markey S., Ebert M., Jacobowitz D., and Kopin I. (1983) A primate model of parkinsonism: selective destruction of dopaminergic neurons in the pars compacta of the substantia nigra by N-methyl-4-phenyl-1,2,3,6-tetrahydropyridine. Proc. Natl. Acad. Sci. USA 80:4546–4550.

Cheeke P.R. (1995) Endogenous toxins and mycotoxins in forage grasses and their effects on livestock. J. Anim. Sci. 73:909–915.

Cleeter M., Cooper J.M., and Schapira A.H.V. (1992) Irreversible inhibition of mitochondrial complex I by MPP$^+$: evidence for the free radical involvement. Biochem. Biophys. Res. Commun. 105:1368–1373.

Cobuzzi R. Jr., Neafsey E.J., and Collins M.A. (1994) Differential cytotoxicities of N-methyl-β-carbolinium analogues of MPP$^+$ in PC12 cells: insights into potential neurotoxicants in Parkinson's disease. J. Neurochem. 62:1503–1510.

Collins M.A., and Neafsey E.J. (1985) β-Carboline analogs of N-methyl-4-phenyl-1,2,3,6-tetrahydropyridine (MPTP): endogenous factors underlying idiopathic parkinsonism? Neurosci. Lett. 55:179–184.

Collins M.A., Neafsey E.J., Cheng B.Y., Hurley-Gius K., Ung-Chhun N.A., Pronger D.A., Christiansen M.A., and Hurley-Gius D. (1986) Endogenous analogs of MPTP: Indoleamine-derived tetrahydro-β-carbolines as potential causative factors in Parkinson's disease. Adv. Neurol. 45:179–182.

Collins M.A., Neafsey E.J., Matsubara K., Cobuzzi R., and Rollema H. (1992) Indole-N-methylated β-carbolinium ions as potential brain-bioactivated neurotoxins. Brain Res. 570:154–160.

Collins M.A., Slobodnik L., and Neafsey E.J. (1995) Inhibitors of NO synthase and poly (ADP-ribose) synthase (PARS) do not block toxic actions of β-carbolinium cations or MPP⁺ in mesencephalic cultures. Abst. Soc. Neurosci. 21:1259.

Collins M.A., Neafsey E.J., and Matsubara K. (1996) β-Carbolines: metabolism and neurotoxicity. Biogen. Amines 12:171–180.

Crooks P.A., Godin C.S., Nwosu C., Ansher S., and Jacoby W.B (1986) Reevaluation of the products of tryptamine catalyzed by rabbit liver N-methyltransferases. Biochem. Pharmacol. 35:1600–1603.

Dillon J., Spector A., and Nakanishi K. (1976) Identification of β-carbolines from fluorescent human lens proteins. Nature 259:422–423.

Drucker G., Raikoff K., Neafsey E.J., and Collins M.A. (1989) Dopamine uptake inhibitory capacities of β-carboline and 3,4-dihydro-β-carboline analogs of MPTP oxidation products. Brain Res. 509:125–133.

Eatough V.M., Kempster P.A., Stem G.M., and Lees A.J. (1990) Premorbid personality and idiopathic Parkinson's disease. Adv. Neurol. 53:335–337.

Fekkes D., Schouten M., Pepplinkhuizen L., Bruinvels J., Lauwers W., and Brinkman U. (1992) Norharman, a normal body constituent. Lancet 339:506.

Felton J.S., and Knize M.G. (1990) Heterocyclic-amine mutagens/carcinogens in foods. Hdbk. Exp. Pharmacol. 94:471–501.

Fields J.Z., Albores R., Neafsey E.J., and Collins M.A. (1992) Inhibition of mitochondrial succinate oxidation—similarities and differences between N-methylated β-carbolines and MPP⁺. Arch. Biochem. Biophys. 294:539–543.

Fukushima S., Matsubara K., Akane A., and Shiono H. (1991) 1-Methyl-tetrahydro-β-carboline-3-carboxylic acid is present in rat brain and is not increased after acute ethanol injection with cyanamide treatment. Alc. 9:31–35.

Gearhart D.A., Collins M.A., and Neafsey E.J. (1995) Preliminary characterization of β-carboline 2-N-methyltransferase from mammalian brain. Abst. Soc. Neurosci. 21:1252.

Gearhart D.A., Neafsey E.J., and Collins M.A. (1996) β-Carboline-N-methyltransferase activity in human brain tissue from control and Parkinson's disease subjects. Soc. Neurosci. Abst. 22:217.

Gearhart D.A., Collins M.A., and Neafsey E.J. (1997) Characterization of brain β-carboline 2-N-methyltransferase, an enzyme that may play a role in idiopathic Parkinson's disease. Neurochem. Res. 22:113–121.

Gearhart D.A. (1997) N-Methylation of β-carbolines as a potential bioactivation route in Parkinson's disease. Ph.D. Thesis, Loyola University Chicago.

Godin C.S., Crooks P.A., and Damani L. (1986) N-Methylation o phenylpyridines and bipyridyls as a potential toxication route. Tissue distribution of azaheterocycle N-methyltransferase activity. Toxicol. Lett. 34:217–222.

Godin C.S., and Crooks P.A. (1989) N-Methylation as a toxication route for xenobiotics. II. *In vivo* formation of the N,N'-dimethyl-4,4'-bipyridyl ion (Paraquat) from 4,4'-bipyridyl in the guinea pig. Drug Metab. Dispos. 17:180–185.

Grote C., Clement H.-W., Wesemann W., Bringmann G., Feineis D., Riederer P., and Sontag K.-H. (1995) Biochemical lesions of the nigrostriatal system by TaClo (1-trichloromethyl-1,2,3,4-tetrahydro-β-carboline) and derivatives. J. Neural Transm. [Suppl.] 46:275–281.

Harrison R.E.W. (1982) Stress elevation of brain and adrenal levels of non-polar tryptophan metabolites. Ph.D. Thesis, University of Alabama, Birmingham, AL.

Hasegawa S., Matsubara K., Takahashi A., Naoi M., and Nagatsu T. (1995) Inhibition of type A monoamine oxidase by N-methyl β-carbolinium ions. Biogen. Amines 11:295–303.

Hayashi T., Todoriki H., and Iida Y. (1990) Highly sensitive method for the determination of 1-methyl-1,2,3,4-tetrahydro-β-carboline using combined capillary gas chromatography and negative-ion chemical ionization mass spectrometry. J. Chromatog. 528:1–8.

Heikkila R.E., Sieber B.A., Manzino L., and Sonsalla P. (1989) Some features of the nigrostriatal dopaminergic neurotoxin MPTP in the mouse. Mol. Cell. Neuropathol. 10: 171–185.

Herraiz T., Huang Z., and Ough S. (1993) 1,2,3,4-Tetrahydro-β-carboline-3-carboxylic acid and 1-methyl-1,2,3,4-tetrahydro-β-carboline-3-carboxylic acid in wines. J. Agric. Food Chem. 41:455–459.

Higashimoto M., Yamamoto T., Kinouchi T., Matsumoto H., and Ohnishi Y. (1996) Mutagenicity of 1-methyl-1,2,3,4-tetrahydro-β-carboline-3-carboxylic acid treated with nitrite in the presence of alcohols. Mutat. Res. 367:43–49.

Holman R.B., Elliott G.R., Faull K., and Barchas J.D. (1980) Tryptolines: the role of indoleamine-aldehyde condensation products in the effects of alcohol. In: Psychopharmacology of Alcohol (Sandler M., ed.), pp. 155–169, Raven Press, New York.

Hoppel C.L., Greenblatt D., Kwok H.-C., Arora P.K., Singh M.P., and Sayre L.M. (1987) Inhibition of mitochondrial respiration by analogs of 4-phenylpyridine and MPP$^+$, the neurotoxic metabolite of MPTP. Biochem. Biophys. Res. Commun. 148:684–693.

Hung H.C., Tao P.L., and Lee E.H. (1995) MPP$^+$ uptake does not explain the differential toxicity of MPP$^+$ in the nigrostriatal and mesolimbic pathways. Neurosci. Left. 196:93–96.

Janetzky B., God R., Bringmann G., and Reichmann H. (1995) 1-Trichloromethyl-1,2,3,4-tetrahydro-β-carboline, a new inhibitor of Complex I. J. Neural Transm. [Suppl.] 46: 265–273.

Javitch J.A., D'Amato R.J., Strittmatter S.M., and Snyder S.H. (1985) Parkinsonism-inducing neurotoxin, MPTP: Uptake of metabolite MPP$^+$ by dopamine neurons explains selective toxicity. Proc. Natl. Acad. Sci. USA 82:2173–2177.

Jenner P., Schapira A.H.V., and Marsden C.D. (1992) New insight into the cause of Parkinson's disease. Neurol. 42:2241–2250.

Johnson J.V., Yost R.A., Beck O., and Faull K.F. (1985) The use of tandem mass spectrometry for the identification and quantitation of tryptolines (tetrahydro-β-carbolines) in tissue extracts. In: Aldehyde Adducts in Alcoholism (Collins, M.A., ed.) pp. 161–177, A.R. Liss, Inc., New York.

Kim H., Sablin S.O., and Ramsay R.R. (1997) Inhibition of monoamine oxidase A by β-carboline derivatives. Arch. Biochem. Biophys. 337: 137–142.

Krueger M.J., Tan A.K., Ackrell B.A., and Singer T.P. (1993) Is Complex II involved in the inhibition of mitochondrial respiration by MPP$^+$ and N-methyl-β-carbolines? Biochem. J. 291:673–676.

Kuhn W., Muller Th., Grobe H., Dierks T., and Rommelspacher H. (1995) Plasma levels of the β-carbolines, harman and norharman, in Parkinson's disease. Acta Neurol. Scand. 92:451–454.

Langston J.W., Tetrud J.W., and Irwin I. (1983) Chronic parkinsonism in humans due to a product of meperidine-analog synthesis. Sci. 219:979–980.

Manabe S., Yuan J., Takahashi T., and Urban R.C. Jr (1996) Age-related accumulation of 1-methyl-1,2,3,4-tetrahydro-β-carboline-3-carboxylic acid in human lens. Exp. Eye Res. 63:179–186.

Matsubara K. (1996) Occurrence of neurotoxic β-carbolinium cations in mammalian central nervous system. Biogen. Amines 12:161–169.

Matsubara K., Collins M.A., and Neafsey E.J. (1992a) Mono-N-methylation of 1,2,3,4-

tetrahydro-β-carbolines in brain cytosol: absence of indole methylation. J. Neurochem. 59:505–510.

Matsubara K., Neafsey E.J., and Collins M.A. (1992b) Novel S-adenosylmethionine-dependent indole-N-methylation of β-carbolines in brain particulate fractions. J. Neurochem. 59:511–518.

Matsubara K., Collins M.A., Akane A., Ikebuchi J., Neafsey E.J., Kagawa M., and Shiono H. (1993) Potential bioactivated neurotoxicants, N-methylated β-carbolinium ions, are present in human brain. Brain Res. 610:90–96.

Matsubara K., Kobayashi S., Kobayashi Y., Yamashita K., Koide H., Hatta M., Iwamoto K., Tanaka O., and Kimura K. (1995) β-Carbolinium cations, endogenous MPP$^+$ analogs, in the lumbar cerebrospinal fluid of patients with Parkinson's disease. Neurol. 45: 2240–2245.

McIsaac W. M. (1961) Formation of 1-methyl-6-methoxy-1,2,3,4-tetrahydro-2-carboline under physiological conditions. Biochim. Biophys. Acta 52:607–609.

Melchior C.M., and Collins M.A. (1982) The routes and significance of endogenous synthesis of alkaloids in animals. CRC Crit. Rev. Toxicol. 10:313–356.

Myers R.D., and Melchior C. (1977) Differential action on voluntary alcohol intake of tetrahydroisoquinolines or a β-carboline infused chronically in the ventricle of the rat. Pharmacol. Biochem. Behav. 7:381–386.

Neafsey E.J., Drucker G., Raikoff K., and Collins M.A. (1989) Striatal dopaminergic toxicity following intranigral injection in rats of 2-methyl-norharman, a β-carbolinium analog of N-methyl-4-phenylpyridinium ion. Neurosci. Lett. 105:344–349.

Neafsey E.J., Albores R., Gearhart D., Kindel G., Raikoff K., Tamayo F., and Collins M.A. (1995) Methyl-β-carbolinium analogs of MPP$^+$ cause nigrostriatal toxicity after substantia nigra injections in rats. Brain Res. 675:279–288.

Neef G., Eder U., Petzoldt K., Seeger A., and Wieglepp H. (1982) Microbial hydroxylations of β-carboline derivatives. J. Chem. Soc. Chem Commun. 366–367.

Naoi M., Matsuura S., Takahashi T., and Nagatsu T. (1989) A methyltransferase in human brain catalyzes N-methylation of 1,2,3,4-tetrahydroisoquinoline into N-methyl-1,2, 3,4-tetrahydroisoquinoline, a precursor of a dopaminergic neurotoxin, N-methylisoquinolinium ion. Biochem. Biophys. Res. Commun. 161:1213–1219.

Nicklas W., Vyas I., and Heikkila R. (1985) Inhibition of NADH-linked oxidation in brain mitochondria by 1-methyl-4-phenylpyridine, a metabolite of the neurotoxin, 1-methyl-4-phenyl-1,2,3,6-tetrahydropyridine. Life Sci. 36:2503–2508.

Ohkubo S., Toshihiko H., and Oka K. (1985) Methyltetrahydro-β-carbolines and Parkinson's disease. Lancet 1:1272–1273.

Papavergou E.J., and Clifford M.N. (1992) Tetrahydro-β-carboline-3-carboxylic acids in smoked foods. Food Additiv. Contamin. 9:83–95.

Perry T.L., Yong V.W., Wall R.A., and Jones K. (1986) Paraquat and two endogenous analogs of the neurotoxic substance MPTP do not damage dopaminergic nigrostriatal neurons in the mouse. Neurosci. Lett. 69:285–289.

Popl M., Fahnrich J., and Tatar V. (1990) Chromatographic Analysis of Alkaloids, Vol. 53, Chromatographic Science Series, Marcel Dekker, Inc., New York.

Przedborski S., Jackson-Lewis V., Yokoyama R., Shibata T., Dawson V.L., and Dawson T.M. (1996) Role of neuronal nitric oxide in MPTP-induced dopaminergic neurotoxicity. Proc. Natl. Acad. Sci. USA 93:4565–4571.

Raha A., Wagner C., MacDonald R., and Bresnick E. (1994) Rat liver cytosolic 4S polycyclic aromatic hydrocarbon-binding protein is glycine-N-methyltransferase. J. Biol. Chem. 269:5750–5756.

Ramsden D.B., and William A.C. (1985) Production in nature of compounds resembling MPTP, a possible cause of Parkinson's disease. Lancet 1:215–216.

Robinson T. (1981) The Biochemistry of Alkaloids. pp. 113–126, Springer-Verlag, New York.

Rollema H., Booth R., and Castagnoli N.J. (1988) *In vivo* dopaminergic neurotoxicity of the 2-β-methylcarbolinium ion, a potential endogenous MPP$^+$ analog. Eur. J. Pharmacol. 153:131–134.

Rommelspacher H., May T., and Susilo R. (1991) β-Carbolines and tetrahydroisoquinolines: Detection and function in mammals. Planta Med. 57:S85–92.

Rommelspacher H., and Schmidt L. (1995) Tetrahydroisoquinolines and β-carbolines: putative natural substances in plants and mammals. Prog. Drug Res. 415–459.

Saavedra J.M., Coyle J.T., and Axelrod J. (1973) The distribution and properties of the nonspecific N-methyltransferase in brain. J. Neurochem. 20:743–752.

Saxton J.E. (1960) The indole alkaloids. In: The Alkaloids, Chemistry and Physiology (Vol. VII) (Manske R.H.F., ed.) pp. 4–199, Academic Press, New York.

Sayre L.M, Wang F., Arora P.K., Riachi N.J., Harik S.I., and Hoppel C.L. (1991) Dopaminergic neurotoxicity in vivo and inhibition of mitochondrial respiration in vitro by possible endogenous pyridinium-like substances. J. Neurochem. 57:2106–2115.

Schultes R.E. (1982) The beta-carboline hallucinogens of South America. J. Psychoact. Drugs 14:205–214.

Schulz J.B., Matthews R.T., Muqit M., Browne SE., and Beal M.F. (1995) Inhibition of neuronal nitric oxide synthase by 7-nitroindazole protects against MPTP-induced neurotoxicity in mice. J. Neurochem. 64:936–939.

Segonzac A., Schoemaker H., Tateishi T., and Langer S.Z. (1985) 5-Methoxytryptoline, a competitive endocoid acting at [3H]imipramine recognition sites in human platelets. J. Neurochem. 45:249–256.

Sen N.P., Seaman S.W., Lau B., Weber D., and Lewis D. (1995) Determination and occurrence of various tetrahydro-β-carboline-3-carboxylic acids and the corresponding N-nitroso compounds in foods and alcoholic beverages. Food Chem. 54:327–337.

Sontag K.-H., Heim C., Sontag T., God R., Reichmann H., Wesemann W., Rausch W., Riederer P., and Bringmann G. (1995) Long-term behavioral effects of TaClo (1-trichloromethyl-1,2,3,4-tetrahydro-β-carboline) after subchronic treatment in rats. J. Neural Transm. [Suppl.] 46:283–289.

Spies C.D., Rommelspacher H., Schnapper C., Muller C., Marks C., Berger G., Conrad C., Blum S., Specht M., Hannemann L., Striebel H., and Schaffartzik W. (1995) β-Carbolines in chronic alcoholics undergoing elective resection. Alc. Clin. Exp. Res. 19:969–976.

Sugimura T., and Nagao M. (1979) Mutagenic factors in cooked foods, CRC Crit. Rev. Toxicol. 6:189–209.

Tanner C.M., and Langston (1990) Do environmental toxins cause Parkinson's disease? A critical review. Neurol. 40:17–30.

Testa B., Naylor R., Costall B., Jenner P., and Marsden C.D. (1985) Does an endogenous methylpyridinium analogue cause Parkinson's disease? J. Pharm. Pharmacol. 37:679–680.

Tipton K.F., and Singer T.P. (1993) Advances in our understanding of the mechanism of the neurotoxicity of MPTP and related compounds. J. Neurochem. 61:1191–1202.

Tsuchiya H., Todoriki H., and Hayashi T. (1995a) Metabolic hydroxylation of 1-methyl-1,2,3,4-tetrahydro-β-carboline in humans. Pharmacol. Biochem. Behav. 52:677–682.

Tsuchiya, H., Yamada, K., Ohtani, S., Takagi, N., Todoriki, H., and Hayashi, T. (1995b) Determination of tetrahydro-β-carbolines in rat brain by gas chromatography-negative ion chemical ionization mass spectrometry without interference from artifactual formation. J. Neurosci. Meth. 62:37–41.

Tsuchiya, H., Yamada, K., Tajima, K., and Hayashi, T. (1996) Urinary excretion of tetrahydro-β-carbolines relating to ingestion of alcoholic beverages. Alc. Alcohol. 31:197–203.

Turner, B.B., Katz, R.J., Roth, K.A., and Carroll, B.J. (1978) Central elevation of phenylethanolamine-N-methyltransferase following stress. Brain Res. 153:419–422.

Ushiyama, H., Oguri, A., Totsuka, Y., Itoh, H., Sugimura, T., and Wakabayashi, K. (1995) Norharman and harman in human urine. Proc. Jpn. Acad. 71B:57–60.

Wakabayashi, K., Ochiai, M., Saito, H., Tsuda, M., Suwa, Y., Nagao, M., and Sugimura, T. (1983) Presence of 1-methyl-1,2,3,4-tetrahydro-β-carboline-3-carboxylic acid, a precursor of mutagenic nitroso compound, in soy sauce. Proc. Natl. Acad. Sci. USA 80:2912–2916.

Whaley, W.M., and Govindachari, T.R. (1951a) The Pictet-Spengler synthesis of tetrahydroisoquinolines and related compounds. Org. React. VI:151–190.

Whaley, W.M., and Govindachari, T.R. (1951b) The preparation of 3,4-dihydroisoquinolines and related compounds by the Bischler-Napieralski reaction. Org. React. VI:74–150.

Williams, A.C., Pall, H.S., Steventon, G.B., Green, S., Buttrum, S., Molloy, H., and Waring, R.H. (1993) N-Methylation of pyridines and Parkinson's disease. Adv. Neurol. 60:194–196.

Chapter 6

Highly Halogenated Tetrahydro-β-Carbolines as a New Class of Dopaminergic Neurotoxins

Gerhard Bringmann, Doris Feineis, Christoph Grote, Ralf God, Hans-Willi Clement, Karl-Heinz Sontag, Bernd Janetzky, Heinz Reichmann, Wolf-Dieter Rausch, Peter Riederer and Wolfgang Wesemann

Contents in Brief

1. Introduction

The Pictet-Spengler condensation of 2-arylethylamines with aldehydes or α-keto acids (Callaway et al., 1994) is not only the most efficient pathway for the chemical synthesis of tetrahydro-β-carbolines (THβCs), but has also been found to play a role in human organisms, leading to endogenous "mammalian alkaloids" (Bringmann, 1979; Buckholtz, 1980; Airaksinen and Kari, 1981a; Airaksinen and Kari, 1981b; Collins, 1986a; Rommelspacher and Susilo, 1985; Brossi, 1993). During the last three decades, the biological potential of the simple, formaldehyde- and acetaldehyde-derived THβCs tryptoline (1) and eleagnine (2) (see Fig. 1) has been investigated thoroughly because these compounds and related derivatives were regarded as causative links between alcoholism and opioid mania (Davis and Walsh, 1970; Rommelspacher et al., 1984; Myers, 1989). Furthermore, since the merely synthetic neurotoxin MPTP (1-methyl-4-phenyl-1,2,3,6-tetrahydropyridine) was found to induce parkinsonism in humans, monkeys, and mice (Burns et al., 1983; Singer et al., 1993), special attention has been focused on the potential role of THβCs as inducers of parkinsonism, closely related in structure, yet occurring in Nature. Indeed, for several β-

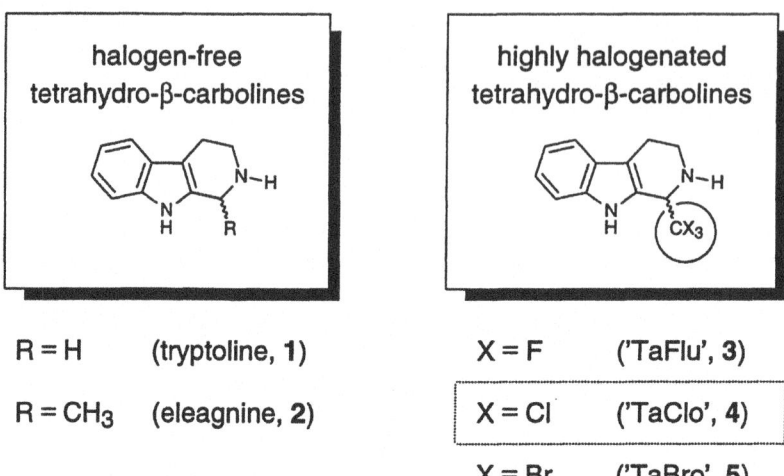

R = H   (tryptoline, **1**)   X = F   ('TaFlu', **3**)

R = CH₃   (eleagnine, **2**)   X = Cl   ('TaClo', **4**)

                                                           X = Br   ('TaBro', **5**)

Fig. 1   The halogen-free THβCs tryptoline (1) and eleagnine (2) are well-established mammalian alkaloids, which were detected in mammalian body fluids after alcohol consumption (Rommelspacher et al., 1980; Bosin et al., 1989). The highly chlorinated THβC 'TaClo' (4), presumably formed endogenously after intake of the drug, chloral hydrate, is a novel neurotoxic lead. Also shown are the closely related highly halogenated THβCs, are 'TaFlu' (3) and 'TaBro' (5), which are formally derived from the aldehydes, fluoral and bromal.

carbolines toxic behavior towards dopaminergic neurons was demonstrated (Collins et al., 1986b; Albores et al., 1990; Sayre et al., 1991).

In this chapter, we report highly halogenated THβCs as a novel class of neurotoxic agents. Our special interest is focused on the chloral-derived heterocycle 'TaClo' (1-trichloromethyl-1,2,3,4-tetrahydro-β-carboline, 4) (see Figs. 1 and 2) (Bringmann and Hille, 1990; Bringmann et al., 1992; Bringmann et al., 1995a; Bringmann et al., 1996a), which is readily formed *in vitro* under quasi-physiological conditions (buffered water, pH = 7.4, 37°C) from the biogenic amine tryptamine ('Ta', 6) and the synthetic trichloroacetaldehyde ('Clo', 7) (see Fig. 2).

This observation prompted us to postulate (Bringmann et al., 1995a; Bringmann et al., 1996a) that a spontaneous *in vivo* formation of TaClo (4) in the mammalian organism has to be taken into account under special conditions, i.e. after intake of the hypnotic drug, chloral hydrate, or after exposure to the frequently used industrial solvent, trichloroethylene (see Fig. 2). Thus, a neuropharmacological investigation of 4 seemed rewarding, since TaClo (4) might possibly be a "natural" inducer of parkinsonian-type neurodegenerative processes.

By contrast, 'TaFlu' (1-trifluoromethyl-1,2,3,4-tetrahydro-β-carboline, 3) and 'TaBro' (1-tribromomethyl-1,2,3,4-tetrahydro-β-carboline, 5) certainly are compounds of exclusively synthetic origin. These TaClo analogs are of special importance for a comparison of the influence of the halogen (i.e., chlorine vs. fluorine resp. bromine) on the neurotoxic potential of highly halogenated THβCs.

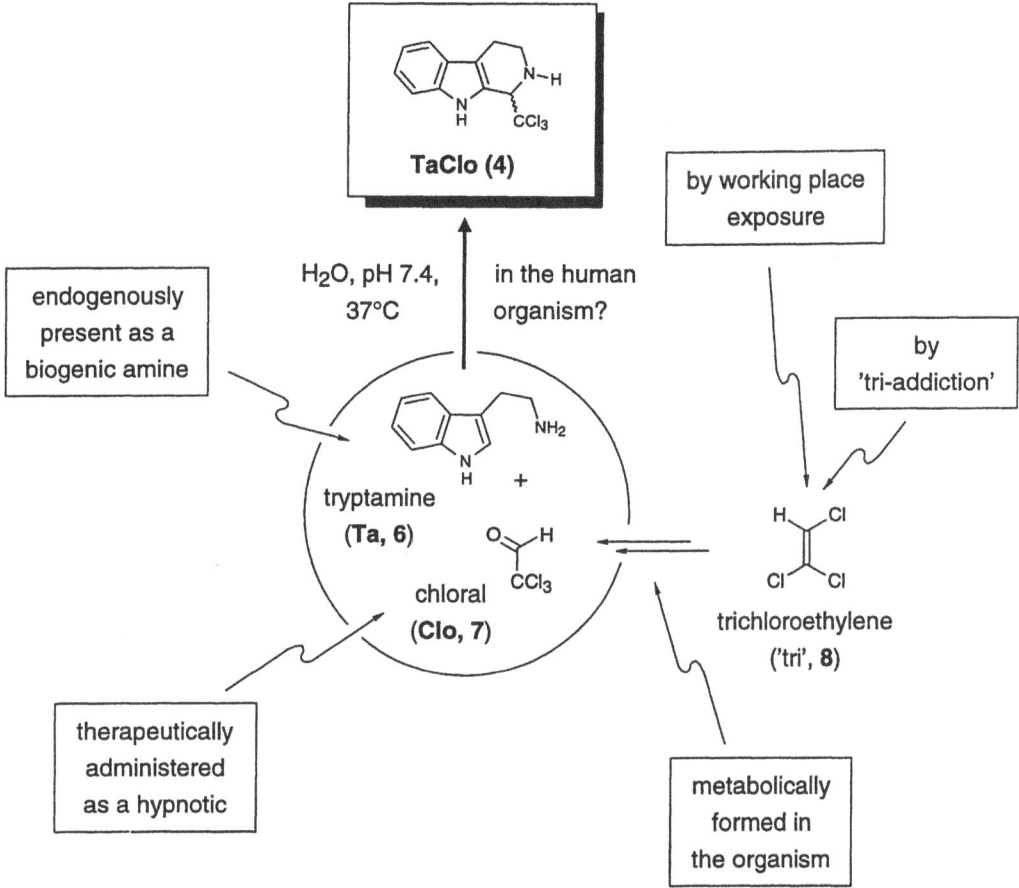

Fig. 2 Possible *in vivo* formation of the highly chlorinated and lipophilic tetrahydro-β-carboline 'TaClo' (4) from the endogenously present tryptamine ('Ta', 6) and chloral ('Clo', 7) by a Pictet-Spengler type cyclization.

2. Chloral-derived THβCs as Potential Mammalian Alkaloids with Expected Neurotoxic Properties

Chloral (7) in a form of its hydrate is usually administered on a gram scale even to children (Rall, 1990). The reactivity of 7, for example towards the biogenic amine tryptamine (6) or the amino acid tryptophan is of special interest, due to the fact that this oldest synthetic narcotic is today undergoing a comeback as a soporific, since it does not shorten or suppress the REM- and the non-REM-type sleep (Kuschinsky and Lüllmann, 1978; Mutschler, 1986). Furthermore, 7 can be formed endogenously as a metabolite of trichloroethylene ('tri', 8) (Bruckner et al., 1989). Thus, in the course of "tri-intoxication" or "tri-addiction", an enhanced concentration of this synthetic, highly reactive aldehyde 7 might induce the formation of hitherto unprecedented trichloromethyl-containing "mammalian alkaloids," such as TaClo (4) (see Fig. 2).

We postulated 4 to induce neurodegenerative processes in the central nervous system (CNS) due to the structural analogy of its β-carboline framework to the dopaminergic neurotoxin MPTP (9) (Bringmann et al., 1995a). Furthermore, in comparison to other psychotropically active β-carbolines, e.g. eleagnine (2) (see Buckholtz, 1980), TaClo (4) exhibits an additional structural peculiarity, namely the huge trichloromethyl group that dominates the molecule. The well-known insecticide DDT (p,p′-dichlorodiphenyl trichloroethane, 10), which exerts chronic toxic effects on the CNS after having accumulated during long-term exposure (Deichmann, 1981), is also characterized by a CCl_3-unit. The lipophilic character of the CCl_3 group should also favor a storage of TaClo (4) in fat-containing tissues, as already demonstrated for 10. Furthermore, compared with the halogen-free THβCs 1 and 2, the enhanced lipophilicity of 4 gives rise to the assumption that the ability of TaClo (4) to penetrate membranes, especially of crossing the blood-brain barrier, could also be increased, leading to an accumulation in neuronal tissue (Bringmann et al., 1995a, 1996a). In addition, similar to other highly halogenated compounds (Henschler, 1987), radical-inducing processes triggering a severe damage of neuronal cell membranes might also be caused by the trichloromethyl group.

In view of our hypothesis about the chloral-derived THβC TaClo (4) - the "TaClo concept" (see Fig. 3)—we aim at an intensive investigation of the scope and mechanism of the neurotoxicity of TaClo and its actual role in the pathogenesis of neurodegenerative processes in man.

2.1. Synthetic route for the preparation of TaClo

To thoroughly investigate the neurotoxic potential of TaClo (4), and also for the preparation of structurally modified analogs, an efficient synthetic pathway leading to 4 was established with a good yield and high purity (Bringmann et al., 1995b). Although 4 may be prepared, according to its presumably *in vivo* formation, via a direct condensation reaction of tryptamine (8) and chloral (9) in aqueous solution, or, more rationally, in toluene (Bringmann and Hille, 1990), it is advisable to proceed via the corresponding formamide, *N*-formyl-TaClo (11). This useful intermediate can easily be prepared by running the reaction in formic acid as a solvent, with simultaneous *N*-formylation. Due to its much higher stability and crystallization properties, 11 can be handled and purified far more easily, allowing virtually unlimited storage. By a simple deformylation reaction, TaClo itself can easily be set free at any time, to give the toxin 4 in a crystalline and extremely pure form. By this efficient procedure, 4 can be obtained on a 100 g scale.

2.2. TaClo as a chiral compound: elucidation of the absolute configuration

TaClo (4) as a chiral substance has as yet been prepared and analyzed only as a racemic mixture of its two enantiomeric forms, named (*R*)-TaClo [(*R*)-4] and (*S*)-TaClo [(*S*)-4]. Given the sometimes extremely different biological activities of enantiomers [c.f. the teratogenic versus sedative properties of the antipodes of thalidomide (contergan®) (see Büch and Büch, 1987)] and the increasing importance of TaClo, the investigation of the stereo-

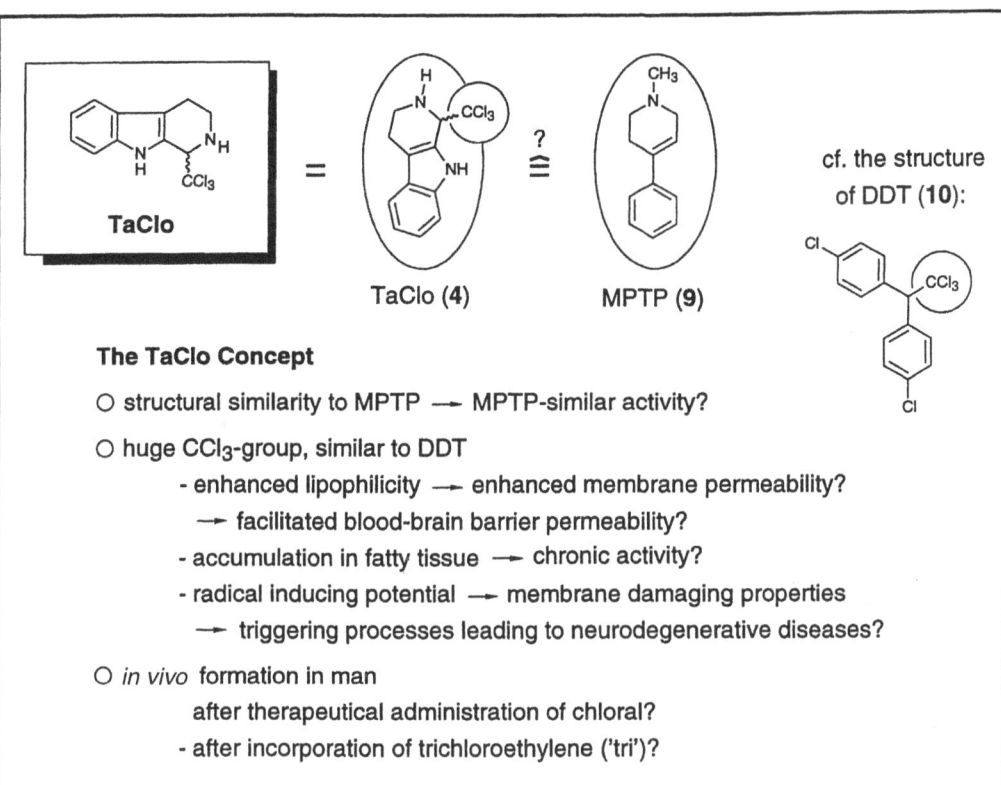

Fig. 3 The TaClo concept (Bringmann et al., 1995a): Due to its structural analogy to the well-known neurotoxin MPTP (9) and the insecticide DDT (10), TaClo (4) was expected to exhibit a distinct neurotoxicity. Furthermore, a *de novo* formation of 4 in man under special conditions was postulated.

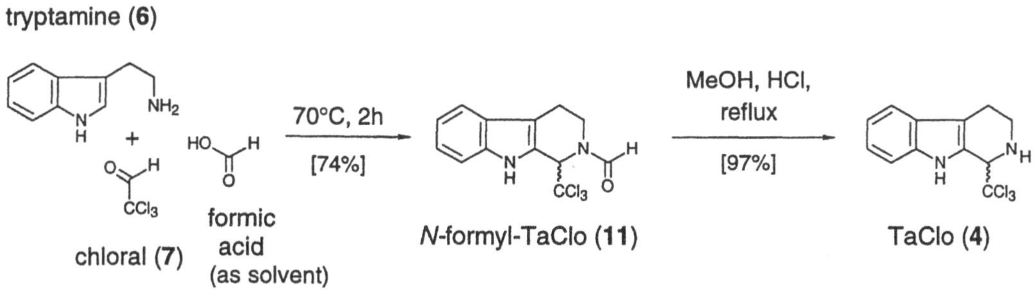

tryptamine (6)

Fig. 4 Synthetic route to obtain highly pure TaClo (4) via *N*-formyl-TaClo (11) as an intermediate by performing the condensation reaction of tryptamine (6) and chloral (7) in formic acid as a solvent; subsequent treatment with methanolic hydrochloric acid to yield the target molecule 4.

chemical aspects of this toxin seemed rewarding, including the resolution, structure elucidation, and separate testing of (*R*)-4 and (*S*)-4.

The discovery that racemic *N*-formyl-TaClo (11) could be partially precipitated as
enantiomerically pure crystals, which were suitable for an X-ray structure analysis, was an
important milestone in the elucidation of the absolute configuration of the two TaClo enantiomers, (*R*)-4 and (*S*)-4 (Bringmann et al., 1995b). The mirror-image structures of the isomers (*R*)-11 (with the CCl₃-group above the graphical plane) and (*S*)-11 (with the CCl₃-
group below the graphical plane), as established by X-ray crystallography, are shown in
Fig. 5. Based on chromatography in a chiral HPLC phase, we elaborated an efficient analytical device suited for a rapid assignment of the stereochemical homogeneity of the crystalline material of 11 (Bringmann et al., 1995b). The enantiomers of TaClo, (*R*)-4 and (*S*)-
4, can be separately obtained by deformylation reaction (see the above section) without
racemization at C-1.

To attribute which of the two series of enantiomerically pure TaClo crystals thus

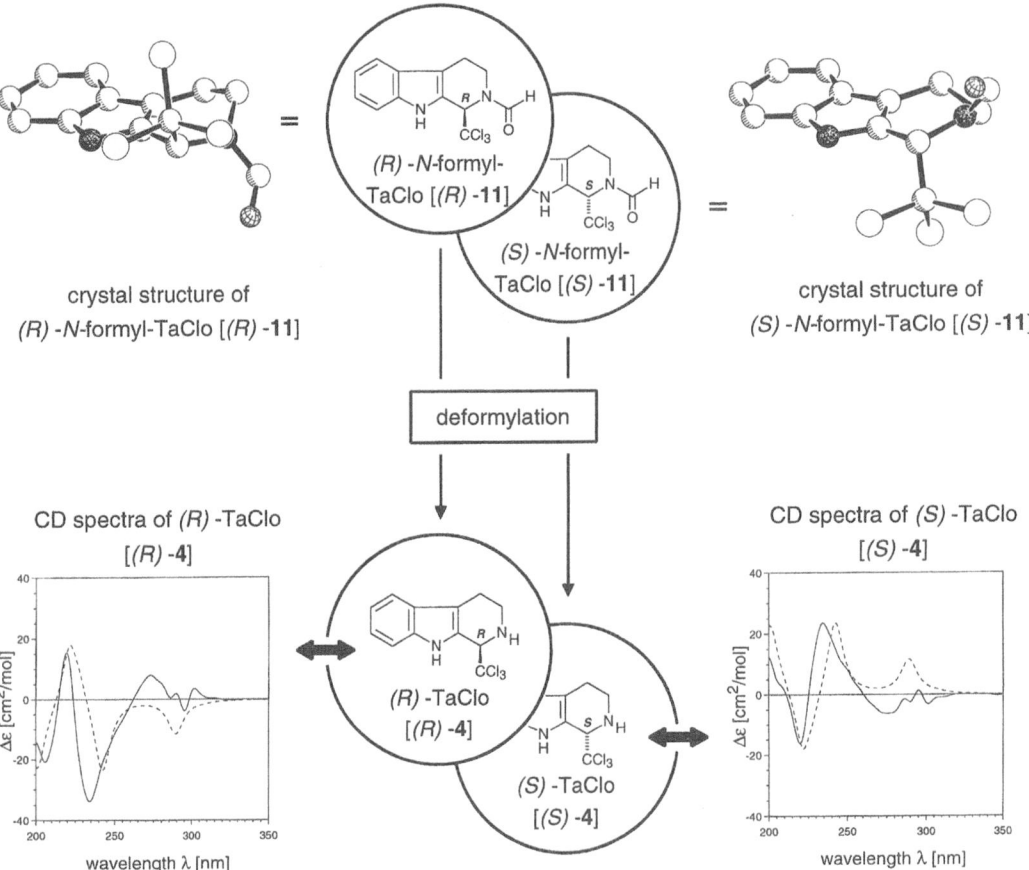

Fig. 5 Elucidation of the absolute configuration of the two TaClo antipodes (*R*)-4 and (*S*)-4 by
X-ray crystallography of enantiomerically pure crystals of *N*-formyl-TaClo (11), and by
comparison of experimental (——— = shown as full lines) and theoretically predicted CD
spectra (- - - - = shown as dotted lines) of the enantiomers (*R*)-4 and (*S*)-4.

obtained consisted of (*R*)-4 and which contained the (*S*)-antipode, we used circular dichroism spectroscopy (CD). That the two separated compounds indeed were enantiomeric substances was to be seen from the fact that their measured CD spectra (shown as full lines, see Fig. 5, left and right) exhibited exactly opposite curves. Although TaClo represents a new structural type of chiral compounds, and its absolute configuration thus cannot be deduced empirically (by comparison with substances with known configuration), we succeeded in an unequivocal assignment of the stereostructure by theoretically predicting CD spectra. This methodology, which we have previously used mainly for the structural elucidation of a broad variety of axially chiral natural products (Bringmann et al., 1993, 1994, 1995c) was now applied for the first time to centro-chiral β-carbolines. The procedure is based upon the comparison of experimentally measured CD spectra with the ones obtained by theoretical calculation. These theoretical CD spectra are calculated for a whole series of different conformations, and then the single CD spectra thus obtained are added up according to the Boltzmann statistics (i.e., according to the energies of these conformations), to give an averaged overall CD spectrum. Due to the excellent agreement (see Fig. 5) of the measured (full lines) and the calculated (dotted lines) CD curves, it was possible to stereochemically attribute the enantiomers of TaClo. This assignment was furthermore confirmed by an X-ray crystallographic determination of the absolute configuration of (*S*)-*N*-formyl-TaClo [(*S*)-11] (Bringmann et al., 1995b).

2.3. Ability of TaClo to cross the blood-brain barrier

Since TaClo (4) was expected to occur only in small amounts in the mammalian organisms, we first elaborated a sensitive and reliable analytical device using gas chromatography after derivatization of 4 with perfluorinated anhydrides (Bringmann et al., 1996b). On the base of this method, we started to study the pharmacokinetics of 4. After peripheral administration of TaClo (4) in relatively high amounts (dose applied: 40 mg/kg, i.p.), only the traces were recovered in various body fluids (e.g., urine, feces, blood, bile) as well as in organ tissues (e.g., liver, heart, lung, kidneys), indicating a rapid metabolic turnover of the compound (Bringmann et al., 1996b). Interestingly, after separation of whole blood samples obtained from TaClo-treated rats into plasma- and an erythrocytes-containing fraction, gas chromatography/mass spectrometry (GC-MS) investigations indicated that the nonpolar TaClo molecule is capable of penetrating membranes. The compound was determined mainly in the fraction of the lysed erythrocytes (Bringmann et al., 1996b).

For the evaluation of the relevance of highly halogenated THβC to induce neurodegenerative processes, it was of great interest whether this permeability could be attributed to other membranes, in particular to the blood-brain barrier (BBB). And indeed, the ability of 4 to cross the BBB was proven by its identification in various brain regions obtained from rats (*n* = 7) systematically treated with TaClo (daily dose: 4 mg/kg, applied for six days) (Bringmann et al., 1995a, 1996b).

After selective sample workup based on solid-phase extraction on C_{18} cartridges, the brain samples were derivatized with heptafluorobutyric anhydride (HFBA) and subsequently submitted to GC-MS analysis in selected-ion monitoring (SIM) mode. The identification of the THβC 4 was achieved on registration of characteristic molecular fragments of its HFB derivative 12, as indicated in Fig. 6. Apart from the *cerebellum,* with ca. 30 ng TaClo/g wet tissue, the detected average TaClo content in the brain material was calculated to be ca. 80 ng/g wet tissue (see Fig. 6).

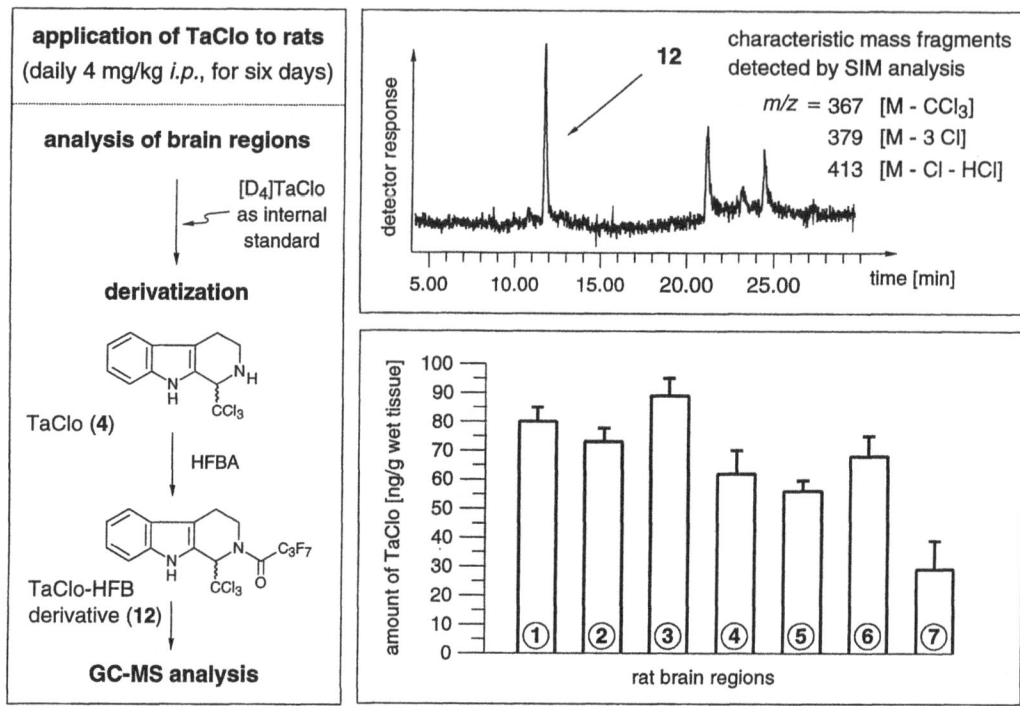

Fig. 6. Detection of TaClo (4) in various brain regions by GC-MS. After derivatization with heptafluorobutyric anhydride (HFBA), characteristic ion fragments of the resulting TaClo-HFB
derivative (12) were detected in selected-ion monitoring (SIM) mode. By spiking the brain
samples with four-fold deuterated TaClo ([D$_4$]-TaClo) as the internal standard prior to
workup, quantification of the amounts of 4 detected in *cortex frontalis* (①), *cortex pari-
etalis* (②), *cortex occipitalis* (③), *telencephalon* and *diencephalon* (④), *mesencephalon
and metencephalon* (⑤), *medulla* (⑥), and *cerebellum* (⑦) was accomplished indicating a
nearly equal distribution of 4 (see inset bar graph).

2.4. *De novo* formation of TaClo in rats treated with its putative precursors

The particular importance of TaClo is based upon the assumption that the condensation
reaction of tryptamine (6) and chloral (7) may also occur in man. This hypothesis was supported by the finding that TaClo (4) was formed in rats after administration of its putative
precursors (doses applied: 5 mg/kg i.p. of 6, 10 mg/kg i.p. of 7, for 21 d, five times per
week) (Bringmann et al., 1995a, 1996a). In whole blood samples taken on the last day of
rat treatment and separated into serum and clot, TaClo was identified unambiguously by
GC/MS analysis according to the procedure described as follows and indicated in Fig. 7.

After separation of interfering compounds and derivatization with trifluoroacetic anhydride (TFAA), the molecular ion peak of the resulting TaClo-TFA derivative 13 was monitored in SIM mode. Due to the natural distribution of the chlorine isotopes ^{35}Cl and ^{37}Cl,
the [M]$^{+\cdot}$ peak of 13 is accompanied by three peaks according to the characteristic isotopic
pattern of three chlorine atoms in the TaClo molecule. As demonstrated in Fig. 7, the
expected statistic intensity distribution of 100:96:31:3 of the four chlorine isotopic peaks at

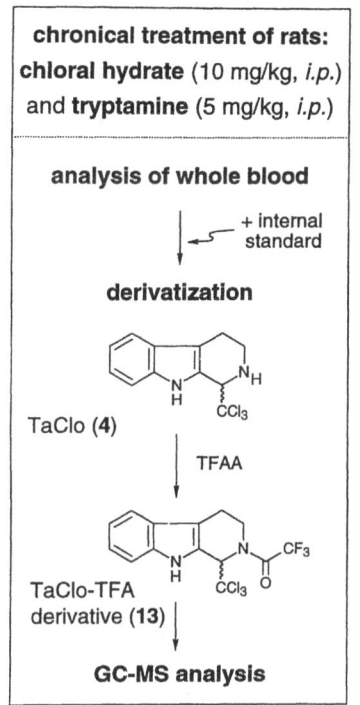

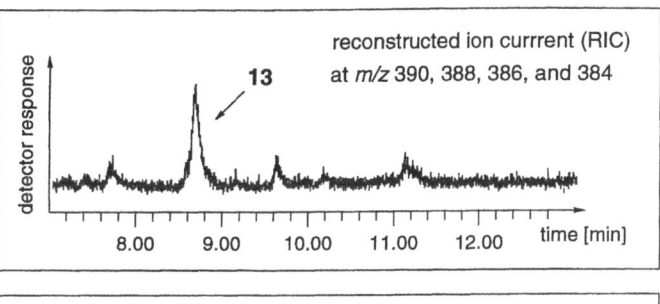

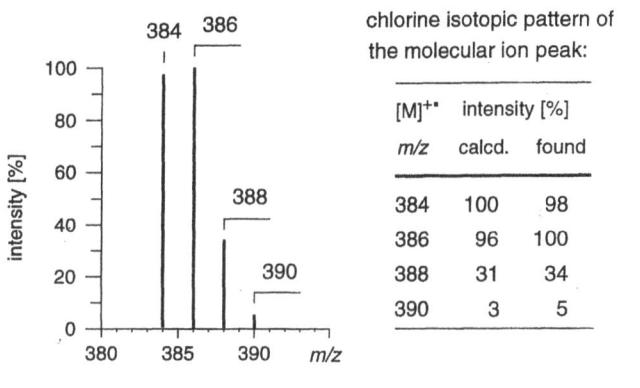

Fig. 7 *De novo* formation of TaClo (4) in rats after application of its putative precursors tryptamine and chloral hydrate. After derivatization with trifluoroacetic anhydride (TFAA), the characteristic chlorine isotopic pattern of the molecule ion from the resulting TaClo-TFA derivative (13) was detected by GC/MS in SIM mode by registration of the ion traces at *m/z* 390, 388, 386, and 384.

m/z 384, 386, 388, and 390 was clearly found in three of the 10 rat blood samples investigated. Hence, from these findings, it becomes evident that, in accordance to our hypothesis, TaClo (4) has indeed to be considered as a potential mammalian alkaloid, the traces of which may also occur in man, under special conditions.

3. Lesion Studies

For investigations of the neurotoxicological potential of TaClo (4) and related analogs, the effects on the dopaminergic system were examined by *in vitro* and *in vivo* methods. Behavioral and biochemical studies were performed to evaluate the mode of action of 4 on the nigrostriatal system.

3.1. Effects of TaClo in cell culture on cell integrity and dopamine metabolism

The effects of TaClo on mesencephalic primary cell cultures were studied by observation of the morphological changes in the cells and by biochemical measurement of tyrosine-3-hydroxylase (E.C. 1.14.16.2.) activity, dopamine (DA) content, and the DA uptake.

For the preparation of the neuronal cell cultures, dopaminergic neurons were obtained from the ventral *mesencephalon* of embryonic brains (C57BL/6 mice, gestation day 14–15) (Rausch et al., 1995). The cultures were grown for 10 days and exposed to 10, 25, 50, and 100 µM of TaClo for 24 h. The immunohistochemistry analysis was carried out by incubation of the cell cultures with anti-tyrosine hydroxylase (TH) antibody (Rausch et al., 1995). The positively stained cells were counted, and a computerized video system was used for morphometric analysis. The impairment of the DA metabolism was determined by measurement of the ^{3}H-DA uptake (Rausch et al., 1995) and of the DA concentration in the culture medium by high-pressure liquid chromatography (HPLC) (Sofic, 1986).

The effects of different concentrations of TaClo (4) on dopaminergic parameters in the cell culture are demonstrated in Table 1. The number of tyrosine-3-hydroxylase immunoreactive (TH-IR) neurons was reduced, dose-dependently, with a significant reduction obtained at a concentration of 100 µM. The metabolism of DA was also impaired and the DA concentration in the culture decreased significantly. Furthermore, when 4 was applied at a dose of 100 µM, it reduced the uptake of ^{3}H-DA.

The histochemical assays in cell culture as described above indicate the neurotoxicity of TaClo (4) for dopaminergic cells. As described previously (Rausch et al., 1995; Bringmann et al., 1996a), morphological changes such as swelling of axons and dendrites following the exposure of TaClo were observed. The degenerative effects caused by the THβC 4 were similar to the toxic processes induced by MPTP respectively MPP⁺ (1-methyl-4-phenyl-pyridinium ion) (Koutsilieri et al., 1993), even though a 10- to 100-fold higher dose had to be used. In contrast to MPTP, the survival of astrocytes in cell cultures was also impaired by TaClo (4) (Rausch et al., 1995).

3.2. Inhibition of the mitochondrial respiration

One of the possible pathogenic factors for Parkinson's disease is a decrease in the activity of complex I of the respiratory chain in dopaminergic neurons of the *substantia nigra* (Mizuno et al., 1989; Janetzky et al., 1994). In addition to the bioactivated product of MPTP, MPP⁺ (Heikkila et al., 1985), β-carbolines are also under investigation because of their analogy (Fields et al., 1992; Bringmann et al., 1995b; Janetzky et al., 1995). All these compounds are characterized by their ability to inhibit complex I of the mitochondrial res-

Table 1. Degenerative effects on tyrosine hydroxylase immunoreactive (TH-IR) neurons in primary cell cultures induced by TaClo (4). Ten wells were analyzed for each measurement (n = 3–5, ±S.D.; *p < 0.05, **p < 0.01, Student's *t*-test).

TaClo (µM)	TH-IR cells/well	DA content pmoles/well	^{3}H-DA uptake pmoles/well
0	186 ± 74	0.8 ± 0.3	0.06 ± 0.01
10	172 ± 69	0.7 ± 0.2	0.05 ± 0.01
25	164 ± 67	0.6 ± 0.2	0.05 ± 0.01
50	128 ± 47	0.4 ± 0.2*	0.05 ± 0.01
100	83 ± 46*	0.3 ± 0.1*	0.04 ± 0.01**

piratory chain highly selectively. To evaluate the mechanism of the toxicity of highly halogenated THβC, such as TaClo (4), the inhibitory potential of these compounds on the mitochondrial respiration was determined *in vitro* in rat brain homogenates as well as in submitochondrial particles (SMP).

Rat brain homogenates and intact mitochondria or SMP, from rat liver were prepared according to Janetzky et al. (1995). Activities of enzymes such as complex I (NADH-ubiquinone 1-reductase and NADH-dehydrogenase), complex II (succinate dehydrogenase), complex II/III (succinate-cytochrome c-reductase), complex I/III (NADH-cytochrome c-reductase) and complex IV (cytochrome c-oxidase) were measured using a Gilford Response spectrophotometer. The mitochondrial respiration of intact mitochondria and SMP were assayed polarographically using a Clark-type oxygen electrode (Janetzky et al., 1995).

The activity of NADH-ubiquinone 1-reductase (complex I) was totally inhibited by 800 µM of TaClo (4); the inhibition activity on the other enzyme complexes had a smaller extent (see Table 2). No significant differences were found using either brain homogenate or SMP.

In addition to TaClo (4), its presumable metabolite *N*-methyl-TaClo (14) and its brominated analog TaBro (5) were also tested in comparison to MPTP (9) and MPP+. Although, as indicated in Table 3, the concentrations of TaClo respectively TaBro needed for total inhibition of complex I (IC_{100}) were less than one-tenth that of MPP+, it should be mentioned that the high neurotoxic potential of MPP+ for dopaminergic neurons is the result of at least two effects, the inhibition of the respiratory chain and the interaction with the active transport system into mitochondria (Ramsay et al., 1986). Apparently, *N*-methyl-TaClo (14) exhibits an even higher toxic potential compared to TaClo itself, since, already at a concentration of 250 µM, a total inhibition of complex I was obtained.

Noteworthy, as compared to TaClo (4), *N*-methyl-TaClo (14) showed a distinctly higher inhibitory potential on complex I, presumably due to its still close structural similarity to MPTP and MPP+. In addition, the activity of complex II of the respiratory chain is also totally inhibited by 14 at a concentration of 250 µM (Janetzky et al., 1995).

Furthermore, in a comparative *in vitro* study testing the halogen-free THβCs tryptoline (1) and eleagnine (2), it had been clearly demonstrated that highly lipophilic trichloro- and tribromomethyl groups exert a significant influence, since within this series of examined heterocycles, the highly halogenated THβCs 4, 5, and 14 are by far the most active compounds.

Table 2. Inhibition of enzymes of the energy metabolism induced by 800 µM of TaClo (4) in rat brain homogenate. The enzyme activity is given as nmol/min/mg total protein.

Enzymes	Enzyme activity control	Enzyme activity TaClo	Inhibition (%)
complex I (NUR)	10.9	<0.1	100
complex II	29.6	30.1	0
complex I/III	24.6	9.8	60
complex II/III	11.9	8.6	27
complex IV	45.8	38.9	20

NUR = NADH-ubiquinone 1-reductase

Table 3.   Extent of the inhibitory activity of TaClo (4), TaBro (5), and *N*-methyl-TaClo (14) on complexes I and II of the mitochondrial respiratory chain.

compound	X	R	complex I IC_{100} NUR	complex II extent of inhibition SDH/SCCR
TaClo (4)	Cl	H	700 µM	30% (at 1 mM)
N-methyl-TaClo (14)	Cl	CH_3	250 µM	100% (at 250 µM)
TaBro (5)	Br	H	650 µM	n.d.
tryptoline (1)			$IC_{25} = 1000$ µM	n.d.
eleagnine (2)			$IC_{50} = 1200$ µM	n.d.
MPTP			n.d.	n.d.
MPP$^+$			≥ 8 mM	n.d.

NADH-ubiquinone 1-reductase (NUR); succinate-dehydrogenase (SDH); succinate-cytochrome c-reductase (SCCR); not detectable (n.d.)

3.3.   Behavioral studies on rats after intraperitoneal application of TaClo

In order to substantiate the neurodegenerative action of TaClo (4) by *in vivo* experiments, rats were treated systematically with low doses of TaClo for up to 7 weeks (subchronical application). The effects on behavior, especially on motor function, were followed by long-term observations for up to 9 months (Sontag et al., 1995).

Adult, female Wistar rats (aged 3–4 months) were used. They had free access to food and water and were kept on a 12/12 h light-dark cycle at a room temperature of 21°C and at 55% of humidity. The animals were injected intraperitoneally with TaClo at a dose of 0.2 mg/kg in 0.9 % NaCl daily for 7 weeks. The behavioral studies were carried out between the 4th and 9th day, and 9 months after the end of the injection period in a computerized open-field system. The apomorphine-induced (0.4 mg/kg subcutaneously) locomotor behavior, expressed as percentage of time spent running and distance traveled, was observed for 60 min. Analysis of variance for unequal groups (ANOVA) was used for testing statistical significance.

Four to nine days after the injection period there was no difference in the apomorphine-induced locomotor activity expressed as percent of time spent running or distance traveled, respectively, either of TaClo- or NaCl-treated rats. However, it was remarkable to observe a greater stimulation of both parameters by apomorphine in the TaClo-treated group (** $p < 0.01$ vs. NaCl, ANOVA) when the animals were tested 9 months after the end of the subchronic treatment (see Fig. 8).

The results obtained from the studies of locomotor behavior point to a progressive neurotoxic effect of TaClo (4) with hypersensitive postsynaptic receptors revealed by systemic application of apomorphine nine months after a subchronic treatment with TaClo. These results suggest that 4 might cause a very slowly progressing degeneration of dopaminergic neurons resulting in a hypersensitivity of dopaminergic receptors within the mesolimbic system. Further studies are necessary to show whether this progressive degeneration will finally result in a severe impairment of the nigrostriatal system.

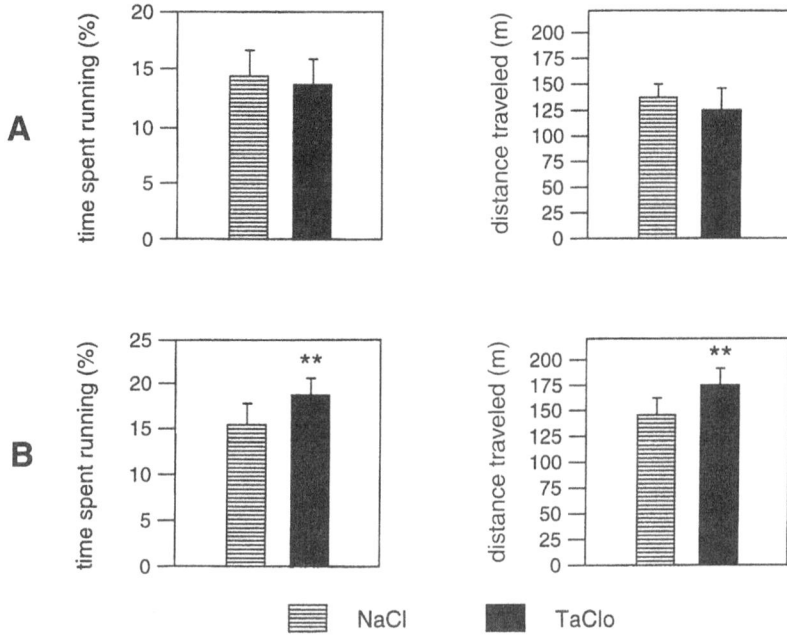

Fig. 8 Apomorphine-induced locomotor activity plotted as % of time spent running (left), and distance traveled (right) measured over 60 min in a computerized actimeter 4–9 days (A) or 9 months (B) after the end of a 7-week period of daily injection (five times a week) of either NaCl or 0.2 mg/kg of TaClo, respectively. Apomorphine was injected subcutaneously in a dose of 0.4 mg/kg. Values are means ± S.E.M.; ** $p < 0.01$ or *** $p < 0.001$ vs. NaCl, ANOVA.

3.4. Striatal dopamine metabolism in the rat after intranigral injection of TaClo

Rats, subjected to a unilateral intracerebral injection of neurotoxins, such as 6-OHDA (6-hydroxydopamine) or MPTP, had been used as a model for Parkinson's disease (Ungerstedt et al., 1971; Wesemann et al., 1993). The effect of a TaClo-induced impairment of the dopaminergic activity in the *striatum* was measured by *in vivo* pulse voltammetry after a single unilateral intranigral injection of TaClo (4) or *N*-methyl-TaClo (14). With regard to the neurotransmitter DA, voltammetric analysis of the extracellular concentration of the DA metabolite DOPAC (3,4-dihydroxyphenylacetic acid) is a reliable indicator for DA metabolism.

Male Han-Wistar rats, 3–4 months old (250–300 g body weight), were anesthetized with a solution of chloral hydrate (400 mg/kg i.p.) and used for measurement by *in vivo* voltammetry with carbon fiber electrodes (Gonon et al., 1980). The working electrodes were implanted in the *striata* of both hemispheres using stereotactic coordinates according to Paxinos and Watson (1982). Forty min after beginning the voltammetric measurement, the DA precursor L-DOPA (L-3,4-dihydroxyphenylalanine) was intraperitoneally injected to test the restitution capacity of the nigrostriatal system. The THβCs 4 and 14 were stereotactically injected (10 μg/2 μl) in the right *substantia nigra pars compacta* (SN$_C$) 1 week before analysis of striatal DA metabolism. The changes of the extracellular DOPAC con-

centration in the *striatum* were obtained by measurement of the height of the catechol peak
at 80 mV. The toxic effect of 4 and 14 on dopaminergic neurons was determined by comparison of the DA metabolism of the ipsilateral *striatum* with the contralateral side. The
data were expressed as means ± S.E.M. The paired Student's *t*-test was used to compare the
means of the extracellular DOPAC contents of the lesioned and the intact side of the *striatum*.

One week after the unilateral injection of TaClo (4) and *N*-methyl-TaClo (14), respectively, the dopaminergic metabolism was reduced in the ipsilateral *striatum*. The two compounds showed a different neurotoxic potential. As compared to the contralateral side,
TaClo (4) decreased the DOPAC signal to about 45% (see Fig. 9 left), whereas *N*-methyl-
TaClo (14) reduced the signal to about 10% of the contralateral side (see Fig. 9 right). After
systemic injection of L-dopa (100 mg/kg) the signal was restored.

The results of the voltammetric analysis of the nigrostriatal dopaminergic activity after
the intranigral injection of TaClo (4) or *N*-methyl-TaClo (14) demonstrate the neurotoxicity of these substances. The impairment of the dopaminergic metabolism caused by 4 was
enhanced by an application of the *N*-methylated derivative 14. In a quantitative sense, the
neurotoxic potency of 14 against dopaminergic neurons is comparable with that of MPP$^+$
(Wesemann et al., 1993). This *in vivo* finding agrees well with the observation mentioned
before that 14 is a more potent inhibitor of the respiratory chain than 4 itself. Since
N-methylation is a well-known biotransformation, further investigations will have to show
whether TaClo (4) is bioactivated to *N*-methyl-TaClo (14), which means that neurotoxicity
is increased by metabolism. As already mentioned above, *N*-methyl-TaClo (14) has by far

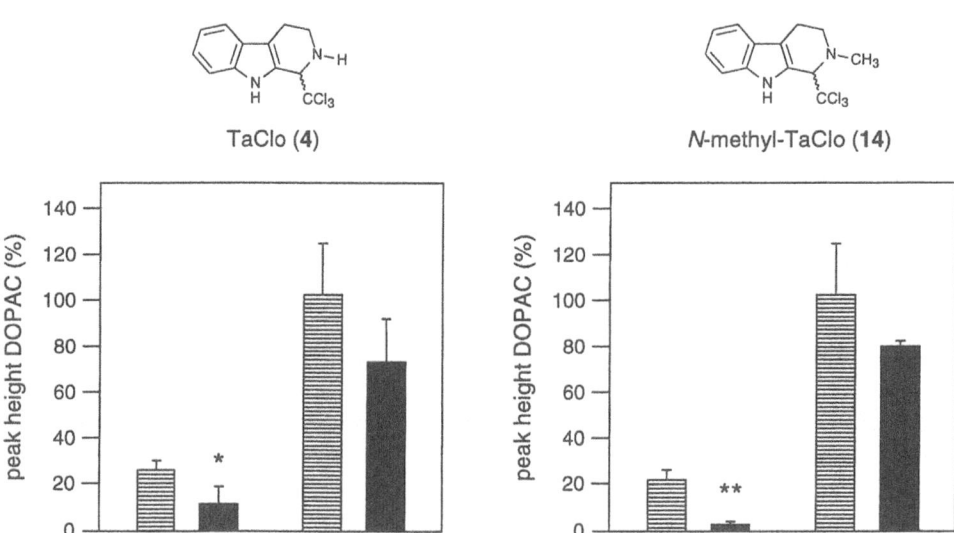

Fig. 9   Effect of an injection of TaClo (10 µg/2 µl) (left column) respectively *N*-methyl-TaClo
(10 µg/2 µl) (right column) in the right substantia nigra pars compacta of the rat after 1
week on the extraneuronal DOPAC concentration in the striatum measured by *in vivo* pulse
voltammetry. L-dopa was applied intraperitoneally at a dose of 100 mg/kg. Concentrations
are shown as percentage of intact (contralateral) side after L-dopa ($n = 5$, ± S.E.M.; * p <
0.05, ** p < 0.01 ipsilateral-lesioned side *vs.* contralateral side, paired Student's *t*-test).

the most distinct structural similarity to the parkinsonism-inducing model toxin MPTP (Langston et al., 1983). Furthermore, several other *N*-methyl-β-carbolines have already been described as neurotoxins, severely affecting the energy metabolism (Collins and Neafsey, 1985; Sayre et al., 1991). *N*-methyl-β-carbolinium analogs of MPP$^+$ are known to reduce the catecholamine levels in the *striatum* of rats after an intranigral injection (Neafsey et al., 1989; Neafsey et al., 1995). These effects are described to be similar to the ones observed after application of MPP$^+$ (Sayre et al., 1991).

4. Outlook

In conclusion, these *in vitro* and *in vivo* studies on rats concerning the ability of TaClo (4) to induce neurodegeneration have revealed a distinct toxic potential of 4 for the dopaminergic system. This is of special interest due to the observation that TaClo (4) may indeed be formed endogenously in man under particular conditions. Recently, by GC/MS investigations, TaClo (4) has been identified unambiguously in whole blood samples obtained from patients treated with chloral hydrate (Bringmann et al., 1997). Current research is now focusing on the elucidation of the metabolic turnover of 4 after administration of [^{14}C]radiolabeled TaClo to rats. This work is in progress.

Acknowledgments

This work was supported by the Bundesministerium für Bildung, Wissenschaft, Forschung und Technologie (BMBF-Schwerpunkt "Morbus Parkinson und andere Basalganglienerkrankungen", Förderkennzeichen 01 KL 9405, 01 KL 9101/0, 01 KL 9191/0 and 01 KL 9013) and by the Fonds der Chemischen Industrie. Our special thanks are due to Dr. K. Peters (Max-Planck-Institut für Festkörperforschung, Stuttgart), Prof. Dr. H. Burzlaff, and Dr. J. Lange (Institut für Angewandte Physik, Erlangen) for preparing X-ray structure analyses.

References

Airaksinen M.M., and Kari I. (1981a) β-Carbolines, psychoactive compounds in the mammalian body. Part II: Effects Med. Biol. 59:190–211.

Airaksinen M.M., and Kari I. (1981b) β-Carbolines, psychoactive compounds in the mammalian body. Part I: Occurrence, origin and metabolism. Med. Biol. 59:21–34.

Albores R., Neafsey E.J., Drucker G., Fields J.Z., and Collins M.A. (1990) Mitochondrial respiratory inhibition by *N*-methylated β-carboline derivatives structurally resembling *N*-methyl-4-phenylpyridine. Proc. Natl. Acad. Sci. USA 87:9368–9372.

Bosin T.R., Borg S., and Faull K.F. (1989) Harman in rat brain, lung and human CSF: effect of alcohol consumption. Alcohol 5:505–511.

Bringmann G. (1979) Chemische Mechanismen der Alkohol-Wirkung. Naturwissenschaften 66:22–27.

Bringmann G., and Hille A. (1990) 1-Trichloromethyl-1,2,3,4-tetrahydro-β-carboline—a potential chloral-derived indole alkaloid in man. Arch. Pharm. 323:567–569.

Bringmann G., Friedrich H., and Feineis D. (1992) Trichloroharmanes as potential endogenously formed inducers of Morbus Parkinson: synthesis, analytics, and first *in vivo*
investigations. J. Neural Transm. [Suppl.] 38:15–26.

Bringmann G., Gulden K.P., Busse H., Fleischhauer J., Kramer B., and Zobel E. (1993) Circular dichroism of naphthyltetrahydroisoquinoline alkaloids: calculation of CD spectra by semiempirical methods. Tetrahedron 49:3305–3312.

Bringmann G., Gulden K.-P., Hallock Y.F., Manfredi K.P., Cardellina II J.H., Boyd M.R.,
Kramer B., and Fleischhauer J. (1994) Circular dichroism of michellamines: independent assignment of axial chirality by calculated and experimental CD spectra. Tetrahedron 50:7807–7814.

Bringmann G., God R., Feineis D., Wesemann W., Riederer P., Rausch W.-D., Reichmann
H., and Sontag K.-H. (1995a) The TaClo concept: 1-trichloromethyl-1,2,3,4-tetrahy-
dro-β-carboline (TaClo), a new toxin for dopaminergic neurons. J. Neural Transm.
[Suppl.] 46:235–244.

Bringmann G., God R., Feineis D., Janetzky B., and Reichmann H. (1995b) TaClo as a neurotoxic lead: improved synthesis, stereochemical analysis, and inhibition of the mitochondrial respiratory chain. J. Neural Transm. [Suppl.] 46:245–254.

Bringmann G., Ledermann A., Stahl M., and Gulden K.-P. (1995c) Bismurrayaquinone A:
synthesis, chromatographic enantiomer resolution, and stereoanalysis by computa-
tional and experimental CD investigations. Tetrahedron 51:9353–9360.

Bringmann G., Feineis D., God R., Fähr S., Wesemann W., Clement H.-W., Grote C.,
Kolasiewicz W., Sontag K.-H., Heim C., Sontag T.A., Reichmann H., Janetzky B.,
Rausch W.-D., Abdelmohsen M., Koutsilieri E., Götz M.E., Gsell W., Zielke B., and
Riederer P. (1996a) Neurotoxic effects on the dopaminergic system induced by TaClo
(1-trichloromethyl-1,2,3,4-tetrahydro-β-carboline), a potential mammalian alkaloid:
in vivo and *in vitro* studies. Biogenic Amines 12:83–102.

Bringmann G., Friedrich H., Birner G., Koob M., Sontag K.-H., Heim C., Kolasiewicz W.,
Fähr S., Stäblein M., God R., and Feineis D. (1996b) Determination of the dopaminergic neurotoxin 1-trichloromethyl-1,2,3,4-tetrahydro-β-carboline (TaClo) in biological samples using gas chromatography with selected ion monitoring. J. Chromatogr. B
687:337–348.

Bringmann G., God R., Feineis D., Fornadi K., and Fornadi F. (1997) First identification of
the dopaminergic neurotoxin TaClo (1-trichloromethyl-1,2,3,4-tetrahydro-β-carbo-
line) in chloral-treated patients. In preparation.

Brossi A. (1993) Mammalian Alkaloids II. In: The Alkaloids (Cordell G.A., ed.), Vol. 43,
pp. 119–183, Academic Press, New York.

Bruckner J.V., Davis B.D., and Blancato J.N. (1989) Metabolism, toxicity, and carcino-
genicity of trichloroethylene. Crit. Rev. Toxicol. 20:31–50.

Büch H.P., and Büch U. (1987) Hypnotika - Pharmakotherapie bei Schlafstörungen und
Erregungszuständen. In: Allgemeine und spezielle Pharmakologie und Toxikologie 5th
edn., (Forth, W., Henschler, D. and Rummel, W., eds). pp. 501–504, Wissenschaftsverlag, Mannheim.

Buckholtz N.S. (1980) Neurobiology of tetrahydro-β-carbolines. Life Sci. 27:893–903.

Burns R.S., Chiueh C.C., Markey S.P., Ebert M.H., Jacobowitz D.M., and Kopin I.J. (1983)
A primate model of parkinsonism: selective destruction of dopaminergic neurons in
the *pars compacta* of the *substantia nigra* by *N*-methyl-4-phenyl-1,2,3,6-tetrahy-
dropyridine. Proc. Natl. Acad. Sci. USA 80:4546–4550.

Callaway J.C., Gynther J., Poso A., Vepsäläinen J., and Airaksinen M.M. (1994) The Pictet-Spengler reaction and biogenic tryptamines: formation of tetrahydro-β-carbolines at physiological pH. J. Heterocyclic Chem. 31: 431–435.

Collins M.A., and Neafsey E.J. (1985) β-Carboline analogues of *N*-methyl-4-phenyl-1,2,5,6-tetrahydropyridine (MPTP): endogenous factors underlying idiopathic parkinsonism? Neurosci. Lett. 55:179–184.

Collins M.A. (1986a) Mammalian Alkaloids. In: The Alkaloids, (Brossi, A., ed.). Vol. 27, pp. 323–358, Academic Press, New York.

Collins M.A., Neafsey E.J., Cheng B.Y., Hurley-Gius K., Ung-Chhun N.A., Pronger D.A., Christensen M.A., and Hurley-Gius D. (1986b) Endogenous analogs of *N*-methyl-4-phenyl-1,2,3,6-tetrahydropyridine: indoleamine derived tetrahydro-β-carbolines as potential causative factors in Parkinson's disease. Adv. Neurol. 45:179–182.

Davis V.E., and Walsh M.J. (1970) Alcohol, amines, and alkaloids: A possible biochemical basis for alcohol addiction. Science 167:1005–1007.

Deichmann W.B. (1981) Halogenated cyclic hydrocarbons. In: Patty's Industrial Hygiene and Toxicology, 3rd edn., (Clayton G. D., Clayton F. E., eds.), Vol. 2B, pp. 3687–3701, Wiley and Sons, New York, Chichester, Brisbane, Toronto, Singapore.

Fields J.Z., Albores R.R., Neafsey E.J., and Collins M.A. (1992) Inhibition of mitochondrial succinate oxidation - similarities and differences between *N*-methylated β-carbolines and MPP+. Arch. Biochem. Biophys. 294:539–543.

Gonon F., Buda M., Cespuglio R., Jouvet M., and Pujol J.F. (1980) *In vivo* electrochemical detection of catechols in the *neostriatum* of anaesthetized rats: dopamine or DOPAC? Nature 286:902–904.

Grote C., Clement H.-W., Wesemann W., Bringmann G., Feineis D., Riederer P., and Sontag K.-H. (1995) Biochemical lesions of the nigrostriatal system by TaClo (1-trichloromethyl-1,2,3,4-tetrahydro-β-carboline) and derivatives. J. Neural Transm. [Suppl.] 46:275–281.

Heikkila R.E., Nicklas W.J., and Duvoisin D.C. (1985) Dopaminergic toxicity of rotenone and the 1-methyl-4-phenylpyridinium ion after their stereotactic administration to rats: implications for the mechanism of 1-methyl-4-phenyl-1,2,3,6-tetrahydropyridine toxicity. Neurosci. Lett. 62:389–394.

Henschler D. (1987) Wichtige Gifte und Vergiftungen. In: Allgemeine und spezielle Pharmakologie und Toxikologie, 5th edn., (Forth W., Henschler D. and Rummel W., eds.), pp. 800–801, Wissenschaftsverlag, Mannheim.

Janetzky B., Hauck S., Youdim M.B., Riederer P., Jellinger K., Pantucek F., Zöchling R., Boissl K.W., and Reichmann H. (1994) Unaltered aconitase activity, but decreased complex I activity in *substantia nigra pars compacta* of patients with Parkinson's disease. Neurosci. Lett. 169:126–128.

Janetzky B., God R., Bringmann G., and Reichmann H. (1995) 1-Trichloromethyl-1,2,3,4-tetrahydro-β-carboline, a new inhibitor of complex I. J. Neural Transm. [Suppl.] 46: 265–273.

Koutsilieri E., Chan W.W., Reinitzer D., and Rausch W.D. (1993) Functional changes in cocultures of *mesencephalon* and striatal neurons from embryonic C57BL/6 mice due to low concentrations of 1-methyl-4-phenylpyridinium (MPP+). J. Neural Transm. 94: 189–197.

Kuschinsky G., and Lüllmann H. (1978) Kurzes Lehrbuch der Pharmakologie und Toxikologie. 8th ed., p. 210, Thieme Verlag, Stuttgart.

Langston J.W., Ballard P.A., Tetrud J.W., and Irwin I. (1983) Chronic parkinsonism in humans due to a product of meperidine-analog synthesis. Science 219:979–980.

Mizuno Y., Ohta S., Tanaka M., Takamiya S., Suzuki K., Sato T., Oya H., Ozawa T., and Kagawa Y. (1989) Deficiencies in complex I subunits of the respiratory chain in Parkinson's disease. Biochem. Biophys. Res. Commun. 163:1450–1455.

Mutschler E. (1986) Arzneimittelwirkungen, 5th edn., p. 160, Wissenschaftliche Verlagsgesellschaft, Stuttgart.

Myers R.D. (1989) Isoquinolines, beta-carbolines and alcohol drinking: involvement of opioid and dopaminergic mechanisms. Experientia 45:436–443.

Neafsey E.J., Drucker G., Raikoff K., and Collins M.A. (1989) Striatal dopaminergic toxicity following intranigral injection in rats of 2-methyl-norharman, a β-carbolinium analog of N-methyl-4-phenylpyridinium ion (MPP$^+$). Neurosci. Lett. 105:344–349.

Neafsey E.J., Albores R., Gearhart D., Kindel G., Raikoff K., Tamayo F., and Collins M.A. (1995) Methyl-β-carbolinium analogs of MPP$^+$ cause nigrostriatal toxicity after *substantia nigra* injections in rats. Brain Res. 675:279–288.

Paxinos A., and Watson C. (1982) The Rat Brain in Stereotaxic Coordinates. Academic Press, Sydney.

Rall T.W. (1990) Hypnotics and sedatives; ethanol. In: Goodman Gilman's The Pharmacological Basis of Therapeutics, 8th edn., (Goodman Gilman A., Rall T.W., Nies A.S., Taylor P., eds.), pp. 357, 464–365, Pergamon Press, New York, Oxford, Beijing, Frankfurt, São Paulo, Sydney, Tokyo, Toronto.

Ramsay R.R., Dadgar J., Trevor A., and Singer T.P. (1986) Energy-driven uptake of N-methyl-4-phenylpyridine by brain mitochondria mediates the neurotoxicity of MPTP. Life Sci. 39: 581–588.

Rausch W.-D., Abdel-mohsen M., Koutsilieri E., Chan W.W., and Bringmann G. (1995) Studies of the potentially endogenous toxin TaClo (1-trichloromethyl-1,2,3,4-tetrahydro-β-carboline) in neuronal and glial cell cultures. J. Neural Transm. [Suppl.] 46: 255–263.

Rommelspacher H., Strauβ S., and Lindemann J. (1980) Excretion of tetrahydroharmane and harmane into the urine of man and rat after load with ethanol. FEBS Lett. 109: 209–212.

Rommelspacher H., Damm H., Strauβ S., and Schmidt G. (1984) Ethanol induces an increase of harman in the brain and urine of rats. Naunyn-Schmiedeberg's Arch. Pharmacol. 327:107–113.

Rommelspacher H., and Susilo R. (1985) Tetrahydroisoquinolines and β-carbolines: putative natural substances in plants and mammals. Prog. Drug Res. 29:415–459.

Sayre L.M., Wang F., Arora P.K., Riachi N.J., Harik S.I., and Hoppel C.L. (1991) Dopaminergic neurotoxicity *in vivo* and inhibition of mitochondrial respiration *in vitro* by possible endogenous pyridinium-like substances. J. Neurochem. 57:2106–2115.

Singer T.P., Ramsay R.R., Sonsalla P.K., Nicklas W.J.k., and Heikkila R.E. (1993) Biochemical mechanism underlying MPTP-induced and idiopathic parkinsonism. Adv. Neurol. 60:300–305.

Sofic E. (1986) Untersuchung von biogenen Aminen, Metaboliten, Ascorbinsäure und Glutathion mittels HPLC-ECD und deren Verhalten in ausgewählten Lebensmitteln und im Organismus von Tier und Mensch. Thesis, Technical University of Vienna.

Sontag K.-H., Heim C., Sontag T.A., God R., Reichmann H., Wesemann W., Rausch W.-D., Riederer P., and Bringmann G. (1995) Long-term behavioural effects of TaClo

(1-trichloromethyl-1,2,3,4-tetrahydro-β-carboline) after subchronic treatment in rats. J. Neural Transm. [Suppl.] 46:283–289.

Ungerstedt U. (1971) Postsynaptic supersensitivity after 6-hydroxy-dopamine-induced degeneration of nigrostriatal dopamine system. Acta Physiol. Scand. [Suppl.] 367: 69–93.

Wesemann W., Grote C., Clement H.-W., Block F., and Sontag K.-H. (1993) Functional studies on monoaminergic transmitter release in parkinsonism. Prog. Neuro-Psychopharmacol. & Biol. Psychiat. 17:487–499.

pros-*Methylimidazoleacetic Acid: A Potential Neurotoxin in Brain?*

George D. Prell

Contents in Brief

1. Introduction

pros-Methylimidazoleacetic acid (p-MIAA; N^{π}-methylimidazoleacetic acid; 1-methylimidazole-5-acetic acid) (Fig. 1) is routinely measured (Khandelwal et al., 1982; Green and Khandelwal, 1985; Prell et al., 1996b) in our studies of its isomer *tele*-methylimidazoleacetic acid (t-MIAA; N^{τ}-methylimidazoleacetic acid; 1-methylimidazole-4-acetic acid) (Fig. 1). The latter is a metabolite of histamine (Schayer and Cooper, 1956; Tham et al., 1966a; Kelvin, 1970; Green et al., 1987); p-MIAA is not (Prell et al. 1989a). In our studies of the histaminergic system in brain, we generally measure levels of both *tele*-methylhistamine (t-MH), histamine's primary metabolite in brain, and levels of its metabolite, t-MIAA. Levels of t-MH and t-MIAA are indices of brain histaminergic activity (Prell and Green, 1994). Comparative measurements of p-MIAA (e.g. Prell et al., 1988a, 1991a) have helped us in evaluating the distinctiveness of findings obtained about t-MIAA.

Little is known about p-MIAA. Interest about p-MIAA's actions in brain was stimulated by the adventitious discovery (Prell et al., 1991b) that concentrations of p-MIAA in cerebrospinal fluid (CSF) from patients with Parkinson's disease were strongly positively

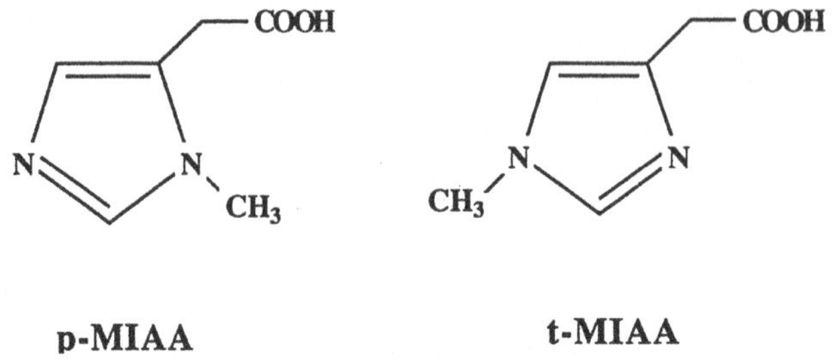

Fig. 1   Structures of (left) *pros*-methylimidazoleacetic acid (p-MIAA; N^{π}-methylimidazoleacetic acid) and (right) *tele*-methylimidazoleacetic acid (t-MIAA; N^{τ}-methylimidazoleacetic acid). t-MIAA is a metabolite of histamine; p-MIAA is not (see text).

correlated with the severity of patients' symptoms. This suggested that p-MIAA might have neurotoxic effects, which prompted us to examine (Prell et al., 1991b) effects of 1-methyl-4-phenyl-1,2,3,6-tetrahydropyridine (MPTP) on striatal levels of p-MIAA in mice. MPTP is toxic to the dopaminergic system of mice (Hallman et al., 1984; Pileblad et al., 1985; Sonsalla and Heikkila, 1986; Radke et al., 1987; Date et al., 1990; Bernardini et al., 1990; Sundström et al., 1990) and produces a Parkinson-like syndrome in man and other primates (Davis et al., 1979; Langston et al., 1983; Burns et al., 1983, 1985; German et al. 1988). In an effort to account for the association between nigro-striatal damage and p-MIAA, we also examined (Blandina et al., 1995) p-MIAA's influence on the release of the excitatory neurotoxins, glutamate and aspartate.

2. Biochemical Origin of p-MIAA

The precise biochemical origin(s) of p-MIAA is unknown. It was once claimed that $[^{14}C]$p-MIAA was recovered in urine of mice injected with $[^{14}C]$histamine (Karjala and Turnquest, 1955). However, numerous studies of metabolism of histamine (exogenous or endogenous) failed to confirm that p-MIAA was a metabolite (see Green et al., 1987). Although loading rats with L-histidine stimulated formation of histamine in brains of rats, it did not affect levels of p-MIAA (Prell et al., 1989a, 1996a). Inhibition of the histamine synthetic enzyme, L-histidine decarboxylase (Green, 1994), by acute or chronic administration of its irreversible inhibitor, α-fluoromethylhistidine (Kollonitsch et al., 1978), depleted levels of histamine, t-MH and t-MIAA. But levels of p-MIAA were not affected (Prell et al., 1989a, 1996b). Lastly, among regions of rat brain, there is no correlation between the distribution of p-MIAA levels and distributions of histidine, histamine, t-MH, t-MIAA, the activity of histidine decarboxylase or rates of histamine turnover (Prell et al., 1989a). The latter are all mutually correlated (Prell and Green, 1994).

   Other observations support the conclusion that p-MIAA and t-MIAA arise from different sources. Samples of monkey ventricular CSF, collected continuously throughout 12 h lights on/12 h lights off cycles, showed different diurnal fluctuations in levels of t-MIAA and p-MIAA (Prell et al., 1989b). Peak levels of t-MIAA occurred during periods of illumination and lagged 2 h behind peak and trough levels of t-MH, whereas p-MIAA levels peaked in the middle of the dark period. In CSF of monkey (Prell et al., 1988a) and man (Prell et al., 1989c), t-MIAA (and t-MH) showed large rostral-caudal concentration gradients, but no gradient was observed for p-MIAA. In mice, inhibition of monoamine oxidase (MAO) depleted urinary content of t-MIAA, but not that of p-MIAA (Kelvin, 1970). In brains of rats, inhibition of MAO reduced endogenous levels of t-MIAA (Khandelwal et al., 1984), but those of p-MIAA were unchanged (Prell et al., 1989a). In clinical studies of effects of age on brain histaminergic activity, CSF levels of t-MH and t-MIAA increased with age, while p-MIAA did not (Prell et al., 1988b, 1991a). Levels of t-MH and t-MIAA were each higher in females; p-MIAA levels were higher in CSF of males (Prell et al., 1991a).

In the periphery, it has been repeatedly observed that *pros*-methylhistidine (p-MeHis; 1-methylhistidine) is a (the?) physiological precursor of p-MIAA (Tham et al., 1966a, b, c; Granerus, 1968) (see below). In rats administered *pros*-methylhistidine (p-MeHis; 1000 mg/kg, i.p.), brain levels of *pros*-methylhistamine (p-MH) and p-MIAA, each measured by gas chromatography/mass spectrometry (GC/MS), increased dramatically (Prell et al., 1989a). This is analogous to studies in rats in which L-histidine (given intracerebroventricularly) was decarboxylated to form histamine, which was then converted to t-MH, then t-MIAA (Schwartz et al., 1971). Thus p-MIAA in brain may also rise from p-MeHis. The enzyme(s) that decarboxylates p-MeHis has yet to be identified. Although p-MeHis is the only certain precursor for p-MIAA, the physiological significance of this pathway *in brain* remains unclear. p-MH levels in brain are generally below limits of detection (Prell et al., 1989a) although recent preliminary (unpublished) studies detected trace amounts. Furthermore, p-MH was not detected in brain samples from rats given the irreversible MAO inhibitor, pargyline (Hough et al., 1984), whereas levels of t-MH invariably increase. Alternatively, if p-MH was shown to be a normal constituent of brain that exhibited high turnover, then one might anticipate its levels to be evanescent and difficult measure.

p-MeHis is present in the human diet (see below). p-MeHis can also be formed endogenously in the brains of mammals. p-MeHis can be produced by methylation of histidine (Brown et al., 1960; Tocci and Bessman, 1967) or methylation of carnosine by carnosine methyltransferase, present in mammalian brain (McManus, 1962), to produce anserine (β-alanyl-*pros*-methylhistidine; *pros*-methylcarnosine). Endogenous methylation could account for the persistent excretion of p-MeHis by subjects starved as long as 20 days (Young et al., 1973) or excretion of either p-MeHis or anserine in those whose diets were devoid of any p-MeHis (free or conjugated) (Block et al., 1965). Homoanserine (γ-aminobutyryl-*pros*-methylhistidine) could be yet another source of p-MeHis (Crush, 1970) (and thus p-MIAA). As a constituent of myosin light chain kinase, p-MeHis is almost certainly formed by post-translational methylation of histidine residues in protein (Meyer and Mayr, 1987). p-MeHis, anserine, homoanserine and myosin light chain kinase are all present in mammalian brain (Hosein and Smart, 1960; Nakajima et al., 1967). Human CSF contains both free and conjugated p-MeHis (Lakke and Teelken, 1976; Ferraro and Hare, 1985).

p-MeHis can derive from hydrolysis of anserine (Lenny et al., 1985; Lenny, 1985) by carnosinase, present in both CSF (Murphy et al., 1973) and brain (Kish et al., 1979; Lenny et al., 1985; Lenny, 1985). Brain has the highest carnosinase activity of all human organs or tissues examined (Lenny, 1985); human basal ganglia has particularly high carnosinase activity (Kish et al., 1979). Conversely, reduced carnosine synthetase activity would retard incorporation of p-MeHis into p-MeHis-containing dipeptides. It has been speculated (Prell and Green, 1991) that the fall in carnosine synthetase activity that occurs in Parkinson's disease could lead to greater availability of p-MeHis which could augment production of p-MIAA. CSF levels of p-MIAA correlated with severity of Parkinson patients' symptoms (Prell et al., 1991b; see below). Interestingly, levels of iron are elevated in the substantia nigra of Parkinson patients (Drayer et al., 1986; Riederer et al., 1989; Dexter et al., 1989;

Youdim and Riederer, 1993). Iron and aluminum salts generate free radicals (Riederer et al., 1989; Dexter et al., 1989) that can catalyze transamination of p-MeHis to form the α-keto-acid, *pros*-methylimidazolepyruvic acid (Doctor and Oro, 1967). One free radical, the superoxide anion, decarboxylates α-keto-acids. Thus, heavy metals in brains of Parkinson patients might promote formation of *pros*-methylimidazolepyruvic acid and thus p-MIAA.

3. Presence of p-MIAA in Nature

There are no data to suggest that p-MIAA exists in water. In contrast, it is likely that at least some p-MIAA is ingested with meals since p-MIAA is present in tissues (and plasma and urine) of animals consumed by humans as food. However, it is doubtful that significant quantities of p-MIAA are passively absorbed because nearly all p-MIAA would be charged at ambient pH within the lumen of the intestines. Although p-MIAA may not be obtained from the diet, there is little question that its precursor, p-MeHis, is present in food and is absorbed. The content of p-MeHis differs greatly among foods and has been tabulated (Crush, 1970; Sjölin et al., 1987; Suzuki et al., 1987). A general ranking by species of p-MeHis content in muscle suggests that chicken and deer > beef and sheep > pig. Among fish, cod and tuna have high content. Little or no p-MeHis is present in milk, eggs and vegetables. Experiments with laboratory personnel (unpublished) showed that p-MIAA levels in urine increased markedly within hours of consumption of chicken or yogurt. In humans, variations in urinary levels of p-MeHis (Sjölin et al., 1989) and p-MIAA (Tham, 1966a; Sharpless et al., 1975; Khandelwal et al., 1982) are probably attributable, at least in part, to variations of p-MeHis in the diet (Datta and Harris, 1951; Block et al., 1965; Butt and Fleshler, 1965; Tham, 1966a; Crush, 1970; Kelvin, 1970; Young et al., 1973; Sjölin et al., 1987; Suzuki et al., 1987).

4. Methods of Measurement of p-MIAA

p-MIAA in brain and CSF were measured exclusively by GC/MS using either electron impact ionization (EI) (Khandelwal et al., 1982; Green and Khandelwal, 1985) or methane positive chemical ionization (PCI) (Prell et al., 1989a, 1996b). The latter mode is more sensitive and is used for routine analyses. A method for determination of p-MIAA, histamine and its metabolites (including t-MIAA) in the same biological samples has been described (Prell et al., 1997). p-MIAA is synthesized from p-MeHis (modification of Prell, 1991).

For determination of p-MIAA levels in tissue, brains were homogenized in ice-cold water (5 or 10 vol); homogenates (300 μl) were mixed with 1.7 ml of 0.118 M HCl. Tubes that contained samples were placed in boiling water (20 min), then cooled and sealed before being stored at −80°C. At the time of analysis, constant amounts of internal standard, d_3-*tele*-methylimidazoleacetic acid (d_3-t-MIAA), were added to authentic standards (0.03–300 ng in 10 mM HCl) and thawed biological samples. All were mixed by vortex at room temperature for ≥30 min. Samples were centrifuged (50,000 g; 20 min at 4°C); supernatants were retained. d_3-t-MIAA was also used as internal standard for analysis of t-MIAA. Samples and standards were processed in parallel. Blanks contained only 10 mM HCl.

CSF from human subjects (who gave informed consent for participation in our studies) was collected as described elsewhere (Prell et al., 1991a, 1991b). Briefly, subjects were maintained on the same diet (low in monoamines, free of tyramine and caffeine) for at least 5 days before collection, fasted and were recumbent from midnight until 09.00 h when lumbar punctures (L_3–L_4 level) were performed. Aliquots between the 14th–17th milliliter were retained for measurement of p-MIAA and t-MIAA. Samples were collected into coded vials without preservative, immediately frozen on dry ice and stored at –70°C. When analyzed, samples were acidified with an equal volume of 0.2 M HCl, before addition of internal standards. After analytes were measured, the coded information was appraised.

Samples and standards were mixed by vortex with 4 ml of *n*-butanol-chloroform (1:1), 100 μl of 50 mM TRIS-acetate buffer (pH 9), and 100 μl of 10 M NaOH, then centrifuged (2000 g, 5 min). Aqueous layers were retained, re-extracted with *n*-butanol-chloroform, then applied to an anion exchange column (Bio-Rad AG1 X-4 100–200 mesh, acetate form). Contents were washed with water, then eluted with 4 ml of 0.5 M acetic acid into a silanized vial containing 100 μl 10 mM HCl, then dried overnight in a vacuum centrifuge. The residue was esterified with 100 μl of boron trifluoride-butanol (14%) at 90°C for 90 min then mixed with 400 μl toluene and 300 μl saturated TRIS. After centrifugation, the lower aqueous layer was discarded. The mixture was washed with 200 μl of water; the aqueous phase was again discarded. The organic phase was mixed with 100 μl of 0.1 M HCl and centrifuged. The upper organic phase was aspirated away. Chloroform (50 μl) and saturated TRIS (50 μl) were added to the remaining aqueous phase, then mixed and centrifuged. The upper aqueous phase was carefully removed. The remaining organic material was dried with anhydrous crystalline sodium sulfate, then transferred to vials for injection onto a fused-silica capillary column (DB-WAX, polyethylene glycol phase with 0.25 μm phase film thickness; 15 m × 0.25 mm id; J&W Scientific).

Samples were analyzed on a combined Hewlett-Packard gas chromatograph (HP-5890)-mass spectrometer (HP5988A) with a dual EI/PCI source, interfaced with a HP-59970B workstation. Samples were chromatographed in the splitless mode with helium (32 ml/min; 15 psi head pressure) as carrier gas. Methane pressure was 1 mm Hg in the ionization source. Both methane and helium were of ultra high purity. Oven temperature, initially equilibrated at 45°C, was ramped at 30°C/min after sample injection, to 250°C. Injection port, GC/MS transfer line and ion source were maintained at 175°, 250° and 200°C, respectively. Derivatized p-MIAA or t-MIAA and d_3-t-MIAA were routinely analyzed by methane PCI-selected ion monitoring (SIM) at *m/z* 197 and *m/z* 200, respectively (and *m/z* 95 and *m/z* 98 in EI-SIM). Ratios of their area counts were linearly related to standards of both p-MIAA and t-MIAA. Under conditions of our assay, the derivative of p-MIAA was retained on GC columns about 0.6–1.5 min longer than the derivative of t-MIAA.

5. Localization of p-MIAA in Brain

In a large study of rats (N = 34) (Prell et al., 1989a), levels of p-MIAA in whole brain ranged from (approx.) 40 to 200 pmol/g of wet tissue weight (94 ± 7 pmol/g, mean ± SEM). Distribution of p-MIAA among regions of rat brain was hypothalamus> corpus striatum> hippocampus> olfactory cortex> frontal cortex> thalamus> midbrain> cerebellum> medulla/pons, with only a 3.5-fold difference between regions of highest and lowest concentrations (Fig. 2). The variance of p-MIAA levels among regions was such that levels of many regions (e.g. hypothalamus, corpus striatum, hippocampus, olfactory cortex and frontal cortex) did not differ significantly (p > 0.05). The statistically significant, albeit minor, heterogeneity in concentrations of p-MIAA among regions suggests that p-MIAA is not simply an ultrafiltrate of plasma. Nearly all p-MIAA is charged at physiological pH; thus it is unlikely that p-MIAA diffuses across the blood-brain barrier. Even though plasma concentrations of p-MIAA exceed those of CSF (see Prell et al., 1988a), its concentrations

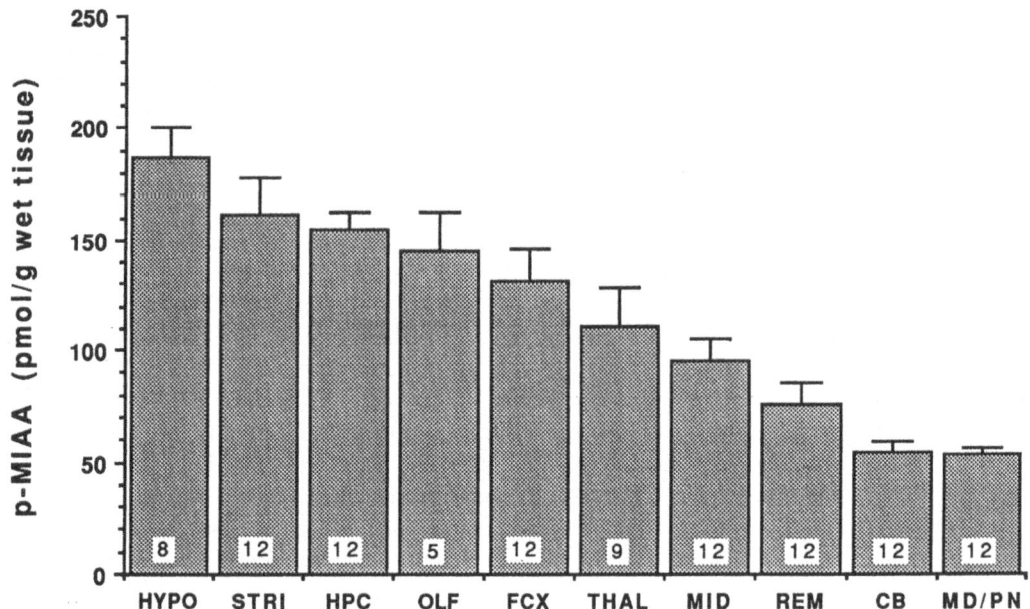

Fig. 2   Concentrations (mean ± SEM, pmol/g) of *pros*-methylimidazoleacetic acid (p-MIAA) in regions of rat brain. p-MIAA was measured in hypothalamus (HYPO), corpus striatum (STRI), hippocampus (HPC), olfactory cortex (OLF), frontal cortex (FCX) (i.e. cerebral cortex rostral to the optic chiasma), thalamus (THAL), midbrain (MID), cerebellum (CB), the medulla-pons together (MD/PN) and the remainder of the brain (REM). Numbers of replicates for each region are shown in each bar. Note that there was no significant difference (p > 0.05; Newman-Keuls test) among levels of p-MIAA in the hypothalamus, corpus striatum, hippocampus, olfactory cortex and frontal cortex. Additional information about the regional distribution of p-MIAA is described elsewhere (Prell et al., 1989a).

in whole brain (mean of 94 nmolal-see above) are higher than levels in plasma (Prell et al., 1988a). Therefore, it is most likely that p-MIAA is synthesized (or otherwise enriched) within the brain.

Probenecid did not affect levels of p-MIAA in rat brain (Prell et al., 1989a). Thus, like t-MIAA, whose levels in brain are also probenecid-insensitive (Khandelwal et al., 1984), p-MIAA may be eliminated from brain by another acid transport system(s), e.g. those related to transport of 3,4-dihydroxyphenylacetic acid (Wilk et al., 1975) or lactate or pyruvate (Miller and Oldendorf, 1986).

6. p-MIAA in CSF of Patients with Parkinson's Disease

As mentioned above, interest in p-MIAA as a possible neurotoxin arose adventitiously from results of a study to evaluate if changes in the histaminergic system occur in Parkinson's disease. p-MIAA levels were measured in CSF of 13 patients with Parkinsonism (Prell et al., 1991b). All patients (5F, 8M) had symptoms of bradykinesia, resting tremor and rigidity. Their mean (±SD) age was 57.9 ± 9.3 years (range 40–69). One male patient (age 69) had Parkinson's disease for 10 years; duration of illness of the others ranged from 1–5 years (3.2 ± 1.3 SD). At the time of the study none of the patients was taking medications, including drugs for Parkinson's disease. Two to 3 days before collection of CSF, disease severity was rated using the Columbia University Rating Scale (CURS) (Yahr et al., 1969) following explicit criteria (Duvoisin, 1971; Hunter and Shaw, 1975). One rater graded all patients. Nine volunteers (4F, 5M) in good health and not taking any medication served as controls. Their mean (±SD) age was 63.3 ± 4.0 years (range 60–72).

Severity of disease (scores on the CURS) correlated positively with concentrations of p-MIAA in CSF (Spearman's $\rho = 0.75$, $p < 0.005$; Fig. 3) (Prell et al., 1991b). p-MIAA levels ranged from 10.5-89.6 pmol/ml. Although rating scores are ordinal values, CURS scores and p-MIAA levels were normally distributed; this corresponded to a Pearson correlation of $r = +0.81$, $p = 0.0007$ (Fig. 3). CURS scores correlated with levels of p-MIAA in both males (N = 8; $\rho = +0.77$, $p < 0.05$) and females (N = 5; $\rho = +1.0$, $p < 0.05$). The mean (±SEM) level of p-MIAA (pmol/ml) of males (61.0 ± 8.8) *tended* ($p = 0.06$) to be higher than the mean of females (33.9 ± 8.6). Neither the CURS scores ($p > 0.8$) nor p-MIAA levels ($p > 0.2$) correlated with age, and neither measurement correlated with duration of illness ($p > 0.4$). The only patient to have received Sinemet (L-dopa plus carbidopa) within the previous 6 months had a p-MIAA level of 71.5 pmol/ml which was not remarkable.

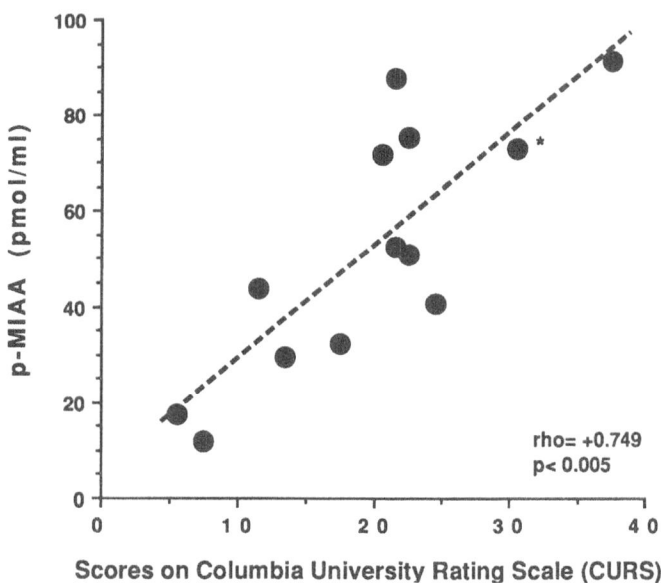

Fig. 3 Correlation between patients' scores on the Columbia University Rating Scale (CURS), which rates severity of symptoms of Parkinson's disease, and concentrations of p-MIAA in cerebrospinal fluid of these patients. At the times of ratings and collection of CSF, all but one (marked *) of the patients either had never taken Sinemet or had been withdrawn > 6 months. All subjects consumed the same diet. Scores correlated positively (Spearman's $\rho = +0.749$, $p < 0.005$) with levels of p-MIAA. Values of both parameters were normally distributed; the Pearson product-moment method yielded a correlation coefficient of $r = +0.814$ ($p = 0.0007$). (Data adapted from Prell et al., 1991b).

Despite the strong correlation between disease severity and p-MIAA levels in CSF of patients (Fig. 3), the mean (±SEM) level (pmol/ml) of the latter (50.6 ± 7.2) did not differ significantly (p > 0.1) from the mean p-MIAA level of controls (61.1 ± 10.9). Among the latter, a single outlier skewed the mean and standard error; its deletion yielded a mean for controls (N = 8; 52.8 ± 8.0 pmol/ml) that was nearly identical to the mean of the patients. Levels of the histamine metabolite, t-MIAA, were not correlated with CURS scores (p > 0.3) or with levels of p-MIAA (p > 0.6). Similar to p-MIAA, levels of t-MIAA in CSF of patients (6.5 ± 0.6) did not differ significantly (p > 0.4) from those of controls (7.3 ± 1.0). When males and females were analyzed separately, p-MIAA levels of controls and patients likewise did not differ significantly.

7. p-MIAA and Studies with Mice Given MPTP

Relationships observed with p-MIAA in CSF of patients with Parkinson's disease suggested that p-MIAA may also be affected in brains of mice given MPTP (Prell et al., 1991b). Male C57BL/6 mice (≈25 g) were injected with MPTP (80 mg/kg, i.p.) in four equally divided doses (each separated by 60 min) following the method of Sonsalla and Heikkila (1986). Control mice were given saline at the same intervals. Seven days after injections, mice were killed by cervical dislocation. *Striata* and frontal cortices were retained and processed (outlined above). p-MIAA and t-MIAA were measured by GC/MS (Green and Khandelwal, 1985; Prell et al., 1989a, 1997; see above). Dopamine (DA), homovanillic acid (HVA), 3,4-dihydroxyphenylacetic acid (DOPAC) and norepinephrine (NE) were measured by high pressure liquid chromatography with electrochemical detection (Blandina et al., 1989).

In *corpus striatum,* mean levels of DA, DOPAC and NE were each significantly lower, and levels of HVA *tended* (p = 0.054) to be lower, in MPTP-treated mice than in controls. In cortex, levels of DA, HVA and NE were each significantly lower in MPTP-treated mice than in controls (Prell et al., 1991b). However, *only in the corpus striatum of MPTP-treated mice* did p-MIAA levels correlate negatively with levels of DA (r = –0.85, p < 0.008), HVA (r = –0.79, p < 0.03), DOPAC (r = –0.84, p < 0.01) and NE (r = –0.91, p < 0.003). In the frontal cortex of these same mice, or in either corpus striatum or cortex of control mice, p-MIAA levels showed no significant correlation (p > 0.2) with any of these analytes. Levels of t-MIAA did not correlate with p-MIAA or any of the other analytes in either brain region of controls or treated mice (Prell et al., 1991b). Interestingly, mean levels of p-MIAA in either *corpus striatum* or cortex of MPTP-treated mice did not differ significantly (p > 0.25) from respective levels of p-MIAA in either *corpus striatum* or cortex of controls (Prell et al., 1991b). Likewise, levels of t-MIAA in either brain region did not differ (p > 0.8) between controls and treated mice. These latter findings are consonant with concentration gradient studies of CSF from monkeys, some of which had been given MPTP (Prell et al., 1988a), in that CSF levels of p-MIAA and t-MIAA of treated monkeys did not differ from controls.

Results of experiments on mice given MPTP offered a parallel to those observed with the Parkinson patients. The mean level of p-MIAA in corpus striatum of MPTP-treated mice did not differ from controls, just as the mean level of p-MIAA in CSF of patients with Parkinson's disease did not differ from controls. Yet p-MIAA levels in MPTP-treated mice were inversely correlated with the fall in levels of DA, HVA and DOPAC, recalling the correlation of p-MIAA levels in CSF with severity of Parkinson's disease. In contrast, in cortex of MPTP-treated mice and in corpus striatum and cortex of controls, p-MIAA levels did not correlate with levels of any other analyte. Therefore, p-MIAA concentrations in human patients and mice appeared to reflect the degree of disease severity even though levels of p-MIAA were not pathognomonic of Parkinson's disease, i.e. they did not distinguish patients from volunteers.

The striking correlations between p-MIAA levels and severity of Parkinson's disease ($r = +0.81$) and depletion of DA and its metabolites in corpus striatum of MPTP-treated mice (each $r \geq -0.79$) provoke speculation that a causal relationship may exist between p-MIAA and indices of striatal dopaminergic function. The simplest hypothesis to account for these correlations (concomitant with no difference in mean levels of p-MIAA of controls) is that accumulation of p-MIAA (or a process that regulates its accumulation) is a factor that influences disease severity. Thus, even though levels of p-MIAA remain within "the normal range," subjects with higher levels of p-MIAA would show greater disease severity than subjects with lower levels. The injured or compromised nigrostriatum may be sensitive to p-MIAA or a process that regulates it. Perhaps relevant is the report (Coughlin et al., 1992) that showed a correlation between deaths due to Parkinson's disease in 17 nations and each country's per capita consumption of meat; the latter is a source of p-MeHis (see above).

8. p-MIAA and the Release of the Excitoneurotoxin Glutamate

One possibility to account for our findings is that p-MIAA influences the release of glutamate or aspartate, which are excitoneurotoxins (Dingledine and McBain, 1994; Plaitakis and Shashidharan, 1995). In Parkinson patients, CSF concentrations of aspartate correlated negatively with clinical outcome (Araki et al., 1986). Conversely, antagonists of glutamate ameliorate or act in synergy with L-3,4-dihydroxyphenylalanine (*L-dopa*) in alleviating Parkinson-like effects produced by MPTP (Carlsson and Carlsson, 1989; Greenamyre, 1993). p-MIAA's effects on amino acid release were studied in rats subjected to transcerebral microdialysis. Details of this study have been published (Blandina et al. 1995).

Briefly, microdialysis tubing was implanted into the corpus striatum, hippocampus and cortex of anesthetized rats. The following day, with animals freely moving, tubing was perfused with dialysis fluid (2 µl/min). After an equilibration period (60 min), fractions (each 20 µl) were collected at 10-min intervals. Spontaneous release of glutamate or aspartate in each region was determined from collections of five (each 10 min) dialysis samples. Thereafter, tissues were exposed for 20 min to dialysis fluid containing p-MIAA or t-MIAA. Data from animals were accepted only if (a) veratridine (250 µM), added at the end of each experiment, elicited >two-fold increase in glutamate and aspartate release over basal levels, and (b) gross visualization of coronal sections postmortem indicated proper placement of dialysis probes. Glutamate and aspartate were measured using high pressure liquid chromatography with fluorometric detection by a method described elsewhere (Blandina et al.,1995).

In the corpus striatum, release of glutamate was stimulated by p-MIAA (500 µM). After its removal, glutamate release reverted to spontaneous basal levels. The extent of glutamate release by p-MIAA (225–300%) was slightly higher than amounts of glutamate released by 250 µM veratridine (200–250%) (Blandina et al., 1995). A concentration-response curve, obtained by averaging striatal glutamate release produced by increasing concentrations of p-MIAA (each rat receiving a single dose, 3–6 experiments per concentration), indicated that the EC_{50} for p-MIAA was 24 ± 4 µM (Blandina et al., 1995). Results were not due to inhibition of glutamate uptake; high-affinity uptake carriers for glutamate exist on both neuronal and glial cells (Kanner and Schuldiner, 1987; Kanai and Hediger, 1992) and keep glutamate concentrations below neurotoxic levels (Fonnum, 1984; Nicholls and Attwell, 1990). p-MIAA (either at 100 μM or 1 mM) incubated with rat striatal slices did not alter uptake of L-[^{14}C]glutamic acid (Blandina et al., 1995).

p-MIAA's effect appeared to be somewhat specific for the corpus striatum since p-MIAA (up to concentrations of 1 mM) did not affect glutamate release in the hippocampus or cortex. Furthermore, p-MIAA's effects appeared to be specific for glutamate because in the same dialysis collections in which glutamate was measured, concentrations of aspartate were not significantly altered in any brain region examined. t-MIAA did not affect release of either glutamate or aspartate in any brain region.

9. p-MIAA Measured in CSF of Patients with Chronic Schizophrenia

Our limited data about effects of p-MIAA (Prell et al., 1991b; Blandina et al., 1995) suggested that its accumulation was associated with neurotoxicity or exacerbation of neurodegenerative processes. However, recent findings about p-MIAA in patients with schizophrenia (Prell et al., 1996c) suggest that p-MIAA may be associated with other actions in the central nervous system. p-MIAA was measured in CSF of 30 inpatients (8F, 22M) who met Research Diagnostic Criteria and DSM-III criteria for chronic schizophrenia and were refractory to antipsychotic medications at the time of the study. Their mean (± SD) age and duration of illness were 31 ± 7 (range 21–45) and 11 ± 6 (range 3–26) years, respectively. Patients were maintained for 6 weeks on their admission medications. To allow a drug-free CSF collection, all but six patients were then withdrawn from medications for up to 6 weeks (average ± SD period was 30 ± 8 days). CSF was collected and processed as outlined in the Parkinson study (Prell et al., 1991b) described above.

Patients were rated with the Psychiatric Symptom Assessment Scale (PSAS) (Bigelow and Berthot, 1989). Cluster scores were used to rate positive (e.g. hallucinations, grandiosity) and negative (e.g. emotional withdrawal, blunted affect) symptoms (Bigelow and Berthot, 1989). Ventricular brain ratios (VBR), i.e. ratio of the lateral ventricles to brain areas measured on computed tomographic brain scans, were also measured (Weinberger et al., 1979).

Among all patients, levels of p-MIAA showed a negative correlation with mean positive cluster scores of the PSAS (r = –0.48, p < 0.02). Among patients withdrawn from neuroleptics (N = 24), this correlation was maintained (p < 0.05) (Prell et al., 1996c). No correlation was observed with negative cluster scores (p > 0.6). Levels of p-MIAA also correlated negatively with VBR values (r = –0.48, p < 0.03). Among those withdrawn from medications, this relationship was maintained (p < 0.02). Based on VBR values <8.4% used to define abnormal ventricular enlargement (Weinberger et al., 1979), patients with enlarged ventricles had markedly lower (p < 0.03) levels (pmol/ml; mean ± SEM) of p-MIAA (14.8 ± 3.0) than patients with normal ventricular size (42.7 ± 5.9) (Prell et al., 1996c).

The inverse correlations between p-MIAA levels in CSF and both positive scores and ventricular brain ratios may suggest that processes that *reduce* accumulation of p-MIAA in brain may be associated with increased severity of symptoms among patients with schizophrenia. This conclusion stands in sharp contrast to observations made in Parkinson's disease, in mice given MPTP and with p-MIAA-induced release of glutamate in rat corpus striatum, which suggested an association between accumulation of p-MIAA and stimulation or exacerbation of neurodegenerative processes. Interestingly, despite these correlations between p-MIAA levels in CSF and indices of severity of schizophrenia, p-MIAA levels in CSF of chronic schizophrenic patients did not differ significantly from levels in controls (see Prell et al., 1995). Thus, our current information about p-MIAA suggests that p-MIAA or processes that affect its levels even within the "normal range" may influence or reflect severity of neurological and psychiatric disorders associated with the brain dopaminergic system.

10. Lack of Change in p-MIAA Levels with Drugs that Affect the Dopaminergic System

Even though our data on p-MIAA appears to show correlations with indices of altered dopaminergic activity, i.e. in patients with Parkinson's disease, chronic schizophrenia or in mice given MPTP (see above), other manipulations (unpublished) of the dopaminergic system did not affect p-MIAA levels in brains of rats. For example, compared to control rats injected with saline, p-MIAA levels were not significantly changed in either the corpus striatum or cerebral cortex of rats given (i.p.) reserpine (5 then 2.5 mg/kg, 48 h and 24 h, respectively before decapitation) or carbidopa (200 mg/kg) and L-dopa (200 mg/kg), 3 h and 2 h respectively before decapitation. These results were consonant with those of a concentration gradient study of CSF of monkeys, some of which had been given MPTP (Prell et al., 1988a). p-MIAA levels in CSF of MPTP-treated monkeys given Sinemet [100 mg L-dopa, 10 mg carbidopa] were similar to levels of controls. Likewise, in male rats, p-MIAA levels in corpus striatum and cortex were unaffected 3 h after administration (i.p.) of either haloperidol (0.6 mg/kg) or thioridazine (100 mg/kg). Therefore, if there are interactions between the dopaminergic system and p-MIAA in brain, they may not be direct. Furthermore, changes in one system may not necessarily cause changes in the other.

11. Summary and Conclusions

Presently, we know very little about the activity of p-MIAA in mammalian brain. Although p-MIAA concentrations correlated with the intensity of neurological and/or psychiatric disorders, it has been difficult to envision a mechanism(s) by which p-MIAA acts in the brain because its levels in CSF of patients (or in brains of mice given MPTP) did not differ significantly from those of healthy controls. Therefore, one major possibility to account for present observations is that processes (presently unknown) that regulate p-MIAA's presence in brain and/or CSF (e.g. synthetic enzymes, membrane transporters) may have more direct or important roles in disorders such as Parkinson's disease and schizophrenia.

Further research about the neurochemistry of p-MIAA in brain may clarify its role, if any, in normal brain function or in pathophysiology of the central nervous system. For example, if p-MIAA forms a metabolite, levels of the latter might be a better index of endogenous p-MIAA turnover or p-MIAA activity, than levels of p-MIAA alone. This might be analogous to quinolinic acid whose levels in brain and CSF of patients with Huntington's disease do not differ from controls (Schwartz et al., 1988a; Reynolds et al. 1988). Yet, turnover of quinolinic acid was increased in Huntington's disease (Schwartz et al.,

1988b) and quinolinic acid produced in rat brains the neurochemical and neurodegenerative changes observed in this disorder (Ellison et al., 1987; Schwartz et al., 1989).

Acknowledgment

The author thanks Drs. Jack Peter Green and Patrizio Blandina for their enormous contributions to research done on p-MIAA. The author sincerely thanks Dr. Green for his scholarly comments about this manuscript and those that preceeded it. The work of Albert Morrishow and Erwin Douyon, who assisted with many of the tissue preparations and performed analyses by GC/MS, is gratefully acknowledged. Findings about p-MIAA arose from research supported by grants (to Dr. Blandina) from M.U.R.S.T.-Universitá di Firenze and 93.04025.04 from C.N.R. (Italy), (to Dr. Green) from the National Institute of Mental Health (MH-31805) (USA) and (to Dr. Prell) from the National Institute of Neurological Diseases and Stroke (NS-28012) of the National Institutes of Health (USA).

References

Araki K., Takino T., Ida S., and Kuriyama K. (1986) Alteration of amino acids in cerebrospinal fluid from patients with Parkinson's disease and spinocerebellar degeneration. Acta Neurol. Scand. 73:105–110.

Bernardini G.L., Specialte S.G., and German D.C. (1990) Increased midbrain dopaminergic cell activity following $2'CH_3$-MPTP-induced dopaminergic cell loss: an *in vitro* electrophysiological study. Brain Res. 527:123–129.

Bigelow L., and Berthot B. (1989) The psychiatric symptom assessment scale (PSAS). Psychopharmacol. Bull. 25:168–179.

Blandina P., Knott P. J., Leung L.K.H., and Green J.P. (1989) Stimulation of histamine H_2 receptor in rat hypothalamus releases endogenous norepinephrine. J. Pharmacol. Exp. Ther. 249:44–51.

Blandina P., Cherici G., Moroni F., Prell G.D., and Green J.P. (1995) Release of glutamate from striatum of freely moving rats by *pros*-methylimidazoleacetic acid. J. Neurochem. 64:788–793.

Block W.D., Hubbard R.W., and Steele B.F. (1965) Excretion of histidine and histidine derivatives of human subjects ingesting protein from different sources. J. Nutr. 85: 419–425.

Brown D.D., Silva O.M, McDonald P.B., Snyder S.H., and Kies M.W. (1960) The mammalian metabolism of L-histidine. III. The urinary metabolites of L-histidine-C^{14} in the monkey, human and rat. J. Biol. Chem. 235:154–159.

Burns R.S, Chiueh C.C., Markey S.P., Ebert M.H., Jacobowitz D.M., and Kopin I.J. (1983) A primate model of Parkinsonism: selective destruction of dopaminergic neurons in the pars compacta of the substantia nigra by N-methyl-4-phenyl-1,2,3,6-tetrahydropyridine. Proc. Natl. Acad. Sci. USA 80:4546–4550.

Burns R.S., LeWitt P.A., Ebert M.H., Pakkenberg H., and Kopin I.J. (1985) The clinical syndrome of striatal dopamine deficiency. Parkinsonism induced by 1-methyl-4-phenyl-1,2,3,6-tetrahydropyridine (MPTP). New Engl. J. Med. 312:1418–1421.

Butt J.H., and Fleshler B. (1965) Anserine, a source of 1-methylhistidine in urine of man. Proc. Soc. Exp. Biol. Med. 118:722–725.

Carlsson M., and Carlsson A. (1989) The NMDA antagonist MK-801 causes marked loco-motor stimulation in monoamine-depleted mice. J. Neural Transm. 75:221–226.

Coughlin S.S., Pincus J.H., and Karstaedt P. (1992) An international comparison of dietary protein consumption and mortality from Parkinson's disease. J. Neurol. 239:236–237.

Crush K.G. (1970) Carnosine and related substances in animal tissues. Comp. Biochem. Physiol. 34:3–30.

Date J., Felten D.L., and Felton S.Y. (1990) Long-term effect of MPTP in the mouse brain in relation to aging: neurochemical and immunocytochemical analysis. Brain Res. 519: 266–276.

Datta S.P., and Harris H. (1951) Dietary origin of urinary methylhistidine. Nature 168: 296–297.

Davis G.C., Williams A.C., Markey S.P, Ebert M.H., Caine E.D., Reichert C.M., and Kopin I.J. (1979) Chronic parkinsonism secondary to intravenous injection of meperidine analogues. Psychiatry Res. 1:249–254.

Dexter D.T., Wells F.R., Lees A.J., Agid F., Agid Y., Jenner P., and Marsden C.D. (1989) Increased nigral content and alterations in other metal ions occuring in brain in Parkinson's disease. J. Neurochem. 52:1830–1836.

Dingledine R., and McBain C.J. (1994) Excitatory amino acid transmitters. In: Basic Neurochemistry (G.J. Siegel, B.W. Agranoff, R.W. Albers and P.B. Molinoff, eds.), pp. 367–387. Raven Press, New York.

Doctor V.M., and Oro I. (1967) Non-enzymatic transamination of histidine with α-keto acids. Naturwissenschaften 54:1–3.

Drayer B.P., Olanow W., Burger P., Johnson G.A., Herfkens R., and Riederer S. (1986) Parkinson plus syndrome: diagnosis using high field MR imaging of brain iron. Radiology 159:493–498.

Duvoisin R.C. (1971) The evaluation of extrapyramidal disease. In: Monoamines Noyaux Gris Centraux et Syndrome de Parkinson (de Ajuriaguerra J., Gautheir G., eds.), pp. 313–325. Masson, Paris.

Ellison D.W., Beal M.F., Mazurek M.F., Malloy J.R., Bird E.D., and Martin J.B. (1987) Amino acid neurotransmitter abnormalities in Huntington's disease and the quinolinic acid animal model of Huntington's disease. Brain 10:1657–1673.

Ferraro T.N., and Hare T.A. (1985) Free and conjugated amino acids in human CSF: influence of age and sex. Brain Res. 338:53–60.

Fonnum F. (1984) Glutamate: a neurotransmitter in mammalian brain. J. Neurochem. 42: 1–11.

German D.C., Dubach M., Askari S., Speciale S.G., and Bowden D.M. (1988) 1-Methyl-4-phenyl-1,2,3,6-tetrahydropyridine-induced Parkinsonian syndrome in *Macaca fascicularis:* which midbrain dopaminergic neurons are lost? Neuroscience 24:161–174.

Granerus G. (1968) Urinary excretion of histamine, methylhistamine and methylimidazoleacetic acids in man under standardized dietary conditions. Scand. J. Clin. Lab. Invest. 22 (Suppl. 104):59–68.

Green J.P. (1994) Histamine. In: Basic Neurochemistry (Siegel G.J., Agranoff B.W., Albers R.W., Molinoff P.B., eds.), pp. 309–319. Raven Press, New York.

Green J.P., and Khandelwal J.K. (1985) Histamine turnover in regions of rat brain. Adv. Biosci. 51:185–195.

Green J.P., Prell G.D., Khandelwal J.K., and Blandina P. (1987) Aspects of histamine metabolism. Agents Actions 22:1–15.

Greenamyre J.T. (1993) Glutamate-dopamine interactions in the basal ganglia: relationship to Parkinson's disease. J. Neural Transm. [Gen. Sect.] 91:255–269.

Hallman H., Olson L., and Jonsson G. (1984) Neurotoxicity of the meperidine analogue N-methyl-4-phenyl-1,2,3,6-tetrahydropyridine on brain catecholamine neurons in the mouse. Eur. J. Pharmacol. 97:133–136.

Hosein E.A., and Smart M. (1960) The presence of anserine and carnosine in brain tissue. Can. J. Biochem. Physiol. 38:569–573.

Hough L.B, Khandelwal J.K., and Green J.P. (1984) Histamine turnover in regions of rat brain. Brain Res. 291:103–109.

Hunter K.R., and Shaw K.M. (1975) Therapeutic effects. In: The Clinical Uses of Levodopa, (Stern G., ed.), pp. 41–71. University Park Press, Baltimore.

Kanai Y., and Hediger M.A. (1992) Primary structure and functional characterization of a high-affinity glutamate transporter. Nature 360:467–471.

Kanner B.I., and Schuldiner S. (1987) Mechanism of transport and storage of neurotransmitters. CRC Crit. Rev. Biochem. 22:1–38.

Karjala S.A., and Turnquest B.W. (1955) The characterization of two methylimidazoleacetic acids as radioactive histamine metabolites. J. Amer. Chem. Soc. 77: 6358–6359.

Kelvin A.S. (1970) Evidence that 1-methylimidazole-5-acetic acid is not a metabolite of histamine. Brit. J. Pharmacol. 38:437p–438p.

Khandelwal J.K., Hough L.B., Pazhenchevsky B., Morrishow A. M., and Green J. P. (1982) Presence and measurement of methylimidazoleacetic acids in brain and body fluids. J. Biol. Chem. 257:12815–12819.

Khandelwal J.K., Hough L.B., and Green J.P. (1984) Regional distribution of the histamine metabolite, *tele*-methylimidazoleacetic acid, in rat brain: effects of pargyline and probenecid. J. Neurochem. 42:519–522.

Kish S.J., Perry T.L., and Hansen S. (1979) Regional distribution of homocarnosine, homocarnosine-carnosine synthetase and homocarnosinase in human brain. J. Neurochem. 32:1629–1636.

Kollonitsch J., Patchett A.A., Marburg S., Maycock A.L., Perkins L.M., Doldouras G.A., Duggan D. E., and Aster S.D. (1978) Selective inhibitors of biosynthesis of aminergic neurotransmitters. Nature 274:906–908.

Lakke J.P.W.F., and Teelken A.W. (1976) Amino acid abnormalities in cerebrospinal fluid of patients with Parkinsonism and extrapyramidal disorders. Neurology 26:489–493.

Langston J.W., Ballard P., Petrud J.W., and Irwin J. (1983) Chronic Parkinsonism in humans due to a product of meperidine analogue synthetics. Science 219:979–980.

Lenney J.F. (1985) Carnosinase and homocarnosinosis. J. Oslo City Hosp. 35:27–40.

Lenney J.F., Peppers S.C., Kucera-Orallo C.M., and George R.P. (1985) Characterization of human tissue carnosinase. Biochem. J. 228:653–660.

McManus I.R. (1962) Enzymatic synthesis of anserine in skeletal muscle by N-methylation of carnosine. J. Biol. Chem. 237:1207–1211.

Meyer H.E., and Mayr G.W. (1987) N^{π}-Methylhistidine in myosin-light-chain kinase. Biol. Chem. Hoppe-Seyler 368:160–1161.

Miller L.P., and Oldendorf W.H. (1986) Regional kinetic constants for blood-brain barrier pyruvic acid transport in conscious rats by a monocarboxylic acid cycle. J. Neurochem. 46:1412–1416.

Murphy W.H., Lindmark D.G., Patchen L.I., Housler M.E., Harrod E.K., and Mosovich L. (1973) Serum carnosinase deficiency concomitant with mental retardation. Pediatr. Res. 7:601–606.

Nakajima T., Wolfgram F., and Clark W.G. (1967) The isolation of homoanserine from bovine brain. J. Neurochem. 14:1107–1112.

Nicholls D., and Attwell D. (1990) The release and uptake of excitatory amino acids. Trends Pharmacol. Sci. 11:462–468.

Pileblad E., Fornstedt B., Clark D., and Carlsson A. (1985) Acute effects of 1-methyl-4-phenyl-1,2,3,6-tetrahydropyridine on dopamine metabolism in mouse and rat striatum. J. Pharmacol. 37:707–711.

Plaitakis A., and Shashidharan P. (1995) Amyotrophic lateral sclerosis, glutamate, and oxidative stress. In: Psychopharmacology: The Fourth Generation of Progress (Bloom F.E., Kupfer, D.J., eds.), pp. 1531–1543. Raven Press, New York.

Prell G.D. (1991) Synthesis of ^{15}N-imidazoleacetic acid. J. Label. Comp. Radiopharmaceut. 29:111–115.

Prell G.D., and Green J.P. (1991) Histamine metabolites and *pros*-methylimidazoleacetic acid in human cerebrospinal fluid. Agents Actions (Suppl.) 33:343–363.

Prell G.D., and Green J.P. (1994) Measurement of histamine metabolites in brain and cerebrospinal fluid provides insights into histaminergic activity. Agents Actions 41: C5–C8.

Prell G.D., Khandelwal J.K., Burns R.S., and Green J.P. (1988a) Histamine metabolites in cerebrospinal fluid of the rhesus monkey (*Macaca mulatta*): cisternal-lumbar concentration gradients. J. Neurochem. 50:1194–1199.

Prell G.D, Khandelwal J.K., Burns R.S., LeWitt P.A., and Green J.P. (1988b) Elevated levels of histamine metabolites in cerebrospinal fluid of aging, healthy humans. Comp. Gerontol. A. (Clin. Sci.) 2:114–119.

Prell G.D., Khandelwal J.K., Hough L.B., and Green J.P. (1989a) *pros*-Methylimidazoleacetic acid in rat brain: its regional distribution and relationship to metabolic pathways of histamine. J. Neurochem. 52:561–567.

Prell G.D., Khandelwal J.K., Burns R.S., and Green J.P. (1989b) Diurnal fluctuations in levels of histamine metabolites in cerebrospinal fluid of rhesus monkey. Agents Actions 26:279–286.

Prell G.D., Khandelwal J.K., LeWitt P.A., and Green J.P. (1989c) Rostral-caudal concentration gradients of histamine metabolites in human cerebrospinal fluid. Agents Actions 26:267–272.

Prell G.D., Khandelwal J.K., Burns R.S., LeWitt P.A., and Green J.P. (1991a) Influence of age and sex on the levels of histamine metabolites and *pros*-methylimidazoleacetic acid in lumbar cerebrospinal fluid from healthy controls and neurological subjects. Arch. Gerontol. Geriatr. 12:1–12 and 71.

Prell G.D., Khandelwal J.K., Burns R.S., Blandina P., Morrishow A.M., and Green J.P. (1991b) Levels of *pros*-methylimidazoleacetic acid: correlation with severity of Parkinson's disease in CSF of patients and with depletion of striatal dopamine and its metabolites in MPTP-treated mice. J. Neural Transm. [P-D Sect] 3:109–125.

Prell G.D., Green J.P., Kaufmann C.A., Khandelwal J.K., Morrishow A.M., Kirch D.G., Linnoila M., and Wyatt R.J. (1995) Histamine metabolites in cerebrospinal fluid of patients with chronic schizophrenia: their relationships to levels of other aminergic transmitters and ratings of symptoms. Schiz. Res. 14:93–104, 268.

Prell G.D., Hough L.B., Khandelwal J.K., and Green J.P. (1996a) Lack of precursor-product relationship between histamine and its metabolites in brain after histidine loading. J. Neurochem. 67:1938–1944.

Prell G.D., Douyon E., Sawyer W.F., and Morrishow A.M. (1996b) Disposition of histamine, its metabolites, and pros-methylimidazoleacetic acid in brain regions of rats chronically infused with α-fluoromethylhistidine. J. Neurochem. 66:2153–2159.

Prell G.D., Green J.P., Khandelwal J.K., Wyatt R.J., Lawson W.B., Jaeger A.C., Kaufmann

C.A., and Kirch D.G. (1996c) *pros*-Methylimidazoleacetic acid in cerebrospinal fluid of patients with chronic schizophrenia: relationships to ratings of symptoms, ventricular brain ratios, and rates of urine excretion. Clin. Neuropharmacol. 19:415–419.

Prell G.D., Morrishow A.M., Douyon E., and Lee W.S. (1997) Inhibitors of histamine methylation in brain promote formation of imidazoleacetic acid, which interacts with GABA receptors. J. Neurochem. 68:142–151.

Radke J.M., Cummings P., and Vincent S.R. (1987) Effects of MPTP poisoning on central somatostatin and substance P levels in the mouse. Eur. J. Pharmacol. 134: 105–108.

Reynolds G.P., Pearson S.J., Halket J., and Sandler M. (1988) Brain quinolinic acid in Huntington's disease. J. Neurochem. 50:1959–1960.

Riederer P., Sofic E., Rausch W.-D., Schmidt B., Reynolds G.P., Jellinger K., and Youdim M.B.H. (1989) Transition metals, ferritin, glutathione, and ascorbic acid in Parkinsonian brains. J. Neurochem. 52:515–520.

Schayer R.W., and Cooper J.A.D. (1956) Metabolism of ^{14}C-histamine in man. J. Appl. Physiol. 9:481–483.

Schwartz J.-C., Pollard H., Bischoff S., Rehault M.C., and Verdière-Sahuque M. (1971) Catabolism of ^{3}H-histamine in the rat brain after intracisternal administration. Eur. J. Pharmacol. 16:326–335.

Schwartz R., Tamminga C.A., Kurlan R., and Shoulson I. (1988a) Cerebral spinal fluid levels of quinolinic acid in Huntington's disease and schizophrenia. Ann. Neurol. 24: 580–582.

Schwartz R., Okuno E., White R.J., Bird E.D., and Whetselli W.O. (1988b) 3-Hydroxyanthranilate oxygenase activity is increased in the brains of Huntington's disease victims. Proc. Natl. Acad. Sci. USA 85:4079–4081.

Schwartz R., Okuno E., and White R.J. (1989) Brain ganglia lesions in the rat: effects on quinolinic acid metabolism. Brain Res. 490:103–109.

Sharpless N.S., Muenter M.D., and Tyce G.M. (1975) Effects of L-DOPA on endogenous histamine metabolism. Med. Biol. 53:85–92.

Sjölin J., Hjört G., Friman G., and Hambraeus L. (1987) Urinary excretion of 1-methylhistidine: A qualitative indicator of exogenous 3-methylhistidine and intake of meats from various sources. Metabolism 36:1175–1184.

Sjölin J., Stjernström H., Henneberg S., Hambraeus L., and Friman G (1989) Evaluation of urinary 3-methylhistidine excretion in infection by measurements of 1-methylhistidine and the creatinine ratios. Amer. J. Clin. Nutr. 49:62–70.

Sonsalla P.K., and Heikkila R.E. (1986) The influence of dose and dosing interval on MPTP-induced dopaminergic neurotoxicity in mice. Eur. J. Pharmacol. 129:339–345.

Sundström E., Fredriksson A., and Archer T. (1990) Chronic neurochemical and behavioral changes in MPTP-lesioned C57BL/6 mice: a model for Parkinson's disease. Brain Res. 528:181–188.

Suzuki T., Hirano T., and Suyama M. (1987) Free imidazole compounds in white and dark muscles of migratory marine fish. Comp. Biochem. Physiol. 87B:615–619.

Tham R. (1966a) Gas chromatographic analysis of histamine metabolites in urine. Excretion of labelled material in dogs. J. Chromatogr. 22:245–250.

Tham R. (1966b) Gas chromatographic analysis of histamine metabolites in urine. Quantitative determination of ring methylated imidazoleacetic acids in healthy man. J. Chromatogr. 23:207–216.

Tham R. (1966c) Liberation of histamine in man. Gas chromatography of ring methylated imidazoleacetic acids in urine. Scand. J. Clin. Lab. Invest. 18:603–616.

Tocci P.M., and Bessman S.P. (1967) Histidine peptiduria. In: Amino Acid Metabolism and Genetic Variation (Nyhan W. L., ed.), pp. 161–168. McGraw-Hill, New York.

Weinberger D., Torrey E., Neophytides A., and Wyatt R. (1979) Lateral cerebral ventricular enlargement in chronic schizophrenia. Arch. Gen. Psychiatr. 36:735–739.

Wilk S., Watson E., and Travis B. (1975) Evaluation of dopamine metabolism in rat striatum by a gas chromatographic technique. Eur. J. Pharmacol. 30:238–243.

Yahr M.D., Duvoisin R.C., Schear M.J., Barret R.E., and Hoehn M.M. (1969) Treatment of Parkinsonism with levodopa. Arch. Neurol. 21: 343–354.

Youdim M.B.H., and Riederer P. (1993) The role of iron in senescence of dopaminergic neurons in Parkinson's disease. J. Neural Transm. (Suppl.) 40:57–67.

Young V.R., Haverberg L.N., Bilmazes C., and Munro H.N. (1973) Potential use of 3-methylhistidine excretion as an index of progressive reduction in muscle protein catabolism during starvation. Metabolism 22:1429–1436.

Part B

Metabolism

Bioactivation of Azaheterocyclic Amines via S-Adenosyl-L-Methionine-Dependent N-Methyltransferases

Kazuo Matsubara

Contents in Brief

In this chapter, I focus on the N-methyltransferases capable of catalyzing S-adenosyl-L-methionine (SAM)-dependent methylation of azaheterocyclic amines, and on their substrates underlying neurodegenerative disease. Epidemiological studies indicate that idiopathic Parkinson's disease is associated with certain environmental factors, such as early exposure to rural life (Rajput et al., 1987; Koller et al., 1990; Morano et al., 1994), drinking water from rural wells (Rajput et al., 1987; Morano et al., 1994), and exposure to certain pesticides (Semchuk et al., 1993; Fleming et al., 1994; Seidler et al., 1996), wood preservatives (Seidler et al., 1996) and industrial toxicants (Tanner and Langston, 1990). The discovery of 1-methyl-4-phenyl-1,2,3,6-tetrahydropyridine (MPTP) opened the possibility that Parkinson's disease may be initiated or precipitated by environmental or endogenous toxins with a structure similar to MPTP, acting in genetically-predisposed individuals. Since several N-methylated azaheterocyclic amines are known to be toxic, the question is whether azaheterocyclics can be bioactivated by N-methyltransferases *in vivo* and *in vitro*. In particular, indoleamine-related β-carbolines (βCs), catecholamine-derived tetrahydroisoquinolines (6,7-DHTIQs) and phenethylamine-derived tetrahydroisoquinolines (TIQs) are of interest as endogenous MPTP-like toxins or protoxins. These substances are

N-methylated directly or following oxidation to quaternary amines, structurally related to 1-methyl-4-phenylpyridinium (MPP$^+$).

1. N-Methyltransferase

Among a number of N-methyltransferases found in plants and animal tissues, several enzymes could be involved in N-methylation of azaheterocyclic amines to form neurotoxic products in mammals. The enzymes require SAM as a methyl donor, and most of them have selective specificity to substrates. All these SAM-dependent methyltransferase are potently inhibited by the methyltransferase-reaction product, S-adenosyl-L-homocysteine (SAH). Possible enzymes which could methylate azaheterocyclics and their substrates are summarized in the following sections.

1.1 Nicotinamide N-methyltransferase (NNMT, EC 2.1.1.1)

NNMT is a monomer peptide and catalyzes the N-methylation of nicotinamide and other pyridines to directly form pyridinium ions. This enzyme belongs to a family of NNMT, phenylethanolamine N-methyltransferase (EC 2.1.1.28) and thioether S-methyltransferase (EC 2.1.1.96). The entire human nicotinamide N-methyltransferase cDNA has been cloned recently (Aksoy et al., 1995), and is located on chromosome 11. The enzyme molecular size is 27000 daltons (Alston and Abeles, 1988). N^1-Methylnicotinamide potently decreases the enzyme activity to 6% of control value at a concentration of 1 mM, but Ca^{2+} does not affect the enzyme activity (Rini et al., 1990). The enzyme activity is predominantly in the liver, and lower expression is seen in the kidney, lung, skeletal muscle, placenta and heart. The activity in the brain is extremely low or negative (Seifert et al., 1984; Sano et al., 1992). Activities are generally high in mammalian omnivores and carnivores (human, pig, dog, cat, rat, mouse) while absent, or nearly so, in many herbivores (ox, cow, horse, sheep, rabbit). The activities in various tissues in rats are higher than those in mice (Seifert et al., 1984). Human hepatic NNMT is a cytoplasmic enzyme with a pH optimum of approximately 7.4. Specific substrates for NNMT are nicotinamide and its derivatives. Apparent K_m values of the enzyme for the substrate, nicotinamide, and SAM are 347 and 1.76 µM, respectively. As with other methyl group acceptors, isoquinolines and tetrahydroisoquinolines are also N-methylated, but are poorer substrates for this enzyme than niconatimide, however (Alston and Abeles, 1988).

Human liver NNMT activity varies five-fold among individuals, with a bimodal frequency distribution (Rini et al., 1990). Approximately 26% of the population is in a subgroup with high NNMT activity. Thus, it is possible that individual differences in NNMT activity might be related to variations in the N-methylation of pyridine and related compounds similar to nicotinamide, as well as to individual differences in their toxicity. The N-methylation activity is proposed to be aberrant in parkinsonian patients. After the ingestion of nicotinamide, the urinary excretion of N^1-methylnicotinamide was significantly elevated in Parkinson's patients with decreased excretion of N^1-methyl-2-pyridone-5-carboxyamide as compared with control subjects (Green et al., 1991). Okada and Matsubara (unpublished data) re-examined the N^1-methylnicotinamide excretion in parkinsonians after a nicotinamide loading with the use of an improved chromatographic procedure; N^1-Methylnicotinamide excretion was several times higher in parkinsonians than in patients with cerebral infarction, without any changes in the excretion of N^1-methyl-2-pyridone-5-carboxyamide

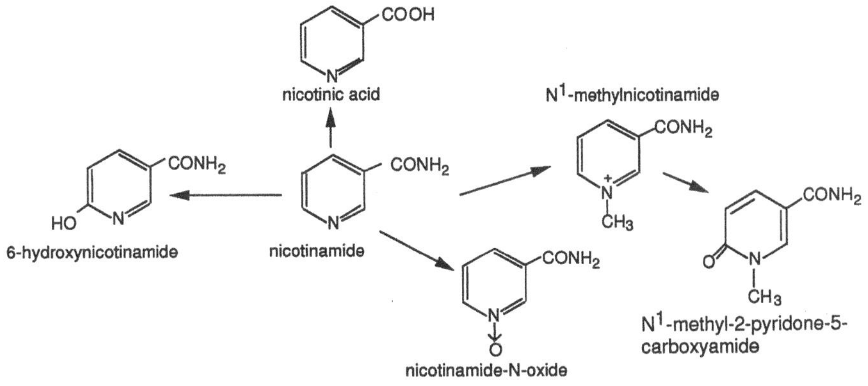

Fig. 1 Nicotinamide metabolic pathway.

or other nicotinamide metabolites. The metabolic pathway of nicotinamide is shown in Fig. 1. N^1-Methylnicotinamide itself is toxic to mitochondria respiration enzyme *in vitro* and is proposed as one of the candidates involved in idiopathic Parkinson's disease (Fukushima et al., 1995). However, its specific accumulation steps into the dopaminergic neurons and mitochondria need to be clarified.

Nicotinate N-methyltransferase (EC 2.1.1.7) catalyzes N-methylation of nicotinic acid to N-methylnicotinic acid and is different from NNMT. The enzyme-catalyzed nicotinic acid N-methylation exists in plants, but is unknown in mammals.

1.2   Histamine N-methyltransferase (HNMT, EC 2.1.1.8)

HNMT is the major enzyme involved in histamine metabolism. Histamine is methylated by HNMT on the *tele*-nitrogen to form *tele*-methylhistamine, but not on the other two nitrogens in its structure. HNMT gene maps on chromosome 2 (Aksoy et al., 1996) and the enzyme activity is localized in postsynaptic sites in neurons, glia and cerebrospinal fluid, and is also found in kidney, the intestine and lung. The guinea pig enzyme shows optima at pH 7.5 and 9, whereas the bovine enzyme shows no clear pH optimum (Gitomer and Tipton, 1986). The bovine enzyme has a different molecular mass of 34000 daltons from that of guinea pig, rat or mouse (29000 daltons) (Gitomer and Tipton, 1986). The substrate selectivity of this enzyme has been known to be highly specific for histamine and structurally related compounds. However, many biogenic amines, including tyramine, tryptamine and their hydroxy derivatives, are strong inhibitors of HNMT activity (Fuhr and Kownatzki, 1986). Quinoline and βC analogs also are inhibitors of HNMT, but do not act as methyl acceptors with this enzyme (Cumming and Vincent, 1992). Interestingly, nicotine is also a significant inhibitor of HNMT, and *R*-(+)-nicotine is methylated by this enzyme to nicotinium ion (Gairola et al., 1988). Thus, HNMT might methylate some species of heterocyclic amines.

1.3   Phenylethanolamine N-methyltransferase (PNMT, EC 2.1.1.28)

PNMT catalyzes the synthesis of epinephrine from norepinephrine, the last step of catecholamine biosynthesis. Human PNMT has 282 amino acid residues with a predicted molecular weight of 30853 (Kaneda et al., 1988). The human PNMT gene localized on chromosome 17 is a candidate gene for hypertension (Koike et al., 1995). The enzyme can methylate a variety of phenylethanolamines, i.e., norepinephrine, epinephrine, norephedrine, and p-hydroxynoroephedrine, but not phenylethylamines. Thus a β-hydroxy group is essential in the substrate. Maximal enzyme activity occurs between pH 7.5 and 8.2 in 0.05 M phosphate buffer, and between 8.0 and 9.0 in 0.1 M Tris buffer. The K_m for the N-methylation of norepinephrine is 10 μM. PNMT exists in the soluble fraction of adrenal gland, heart and brain (Beart et al., 1979). Enzyme activity is almost completely inhibited with p-chloromercuribenzoate, and the stimulation of PNMT is blocked by inhibitors of protein synthesis. 4,6,7-Trihydroxy-TIQ, a condensation product from norepinephrine, is in a class of 4-hydroxylated TIQs, and could be methylated by this enzyme.

A similar enzyme is tyramine N-methyltransferase (EC 2.1.1.27) which is involved in tyrosine metabolism and has some activity on phenylethylamine analogs. However, the biological importance of this enzyme is not clear in mammals.

1.4   Amine N-methyltransferase (ANMT, EC 2.1.1.49)

Alternative names of this enzyme are nicotine N-methyltransferase, tryptamine N-methyltransferase, arylamine N-methyltransferase and azaheterocyclic N-methyltransferase. Originally, two groups independently found this enzyme. Jakoby and co-workers (Ansher and Jakoby, 1986b) have isolated two forms of nonspecific ANMT (designated A and B, distinct but overlapping specificity), having a molecular mass of 30000 daltons, that act on a variety of alkyamines and aryl amines from rabbit liver. Crooks and co-worker (Godin et al., 1986) also obtained a similar enzyme catalyzing nicotine N-methylation, namely azaheterocyclic N-methyltransferase, from guinea pig tissues. Pyridine and related compounds are good substrate for this enzyme, but nicotinamide does not serve as a detectable substrate. These observations distinguish this enzyme from NNMT. However, other physical properties between NNMT and ANMT are similar.

ANMT is located in the cytosolic fraction of lung, liver and spleen in the brain of guinea-pig and rabbit. However, the enzyme activity in the brain is low; it is necessary to concentrate the brain extract more than four-fold with Amicon PM10 membrane (Ansher et al., 1986). In the tissue preparations, there are some low molecular inhibitors for the enzyme activities; thus, the dialyzed sample gives high activities compared with the undialyzed sample. ANMT activities in the brain of rats decrease gradually between 3 and 14 weeks of age without any differences between males and females (Sano et al., 1993). A wide range of primary, secondary and tertiary amines can act as methyl acceptors via this enzyme, including tryptamine, aniline, nicotine and variety of drugs and other xenobiotics. Thus, this enzyme could primarily be involved in the *in vivo* methylation of TIQs, 6,7-DHIQs, tetrahydro-βCs (THβCs) and other MPTP analogs. Because of the broad substrate specificity of ANMT, it could play an important role in the methylation of xenobiotics *in vivo*. The fact that N-methylation of nicotine and other pyridines to pyridiniums appears dominantly in the lung may contribute to the observed pulmonary toxicity in tobacco users (Godin et al., 1986). Maximal enzyme activity occurs between pH 7.0 and 9.0, depending on the substrate used.

Interestingly, the transmethylation hypothesis of schizophrenia had been introduced in the 1970s. The hypothesis was that endogenously formed N-methylated indoleamines might play roles in the pathogenesis of schizophrenia (Nestoros et al., 1977; Luchins et al., 1978 and references cited therein). Indeed, N-methylated indoleamines can be produced *in vivo* and do have significant psychophotomimetic effects; however, there is little evidence for a specific increase in the methylation of indoleamines in schizophrenic patients. Recent studies on this issue that might relate to ANMT activity have not been published.

1.5   Others

There are two interesting N-methylation enzymes found in plants. (*R,S*)-Tetrahydrobenzylisoquinoline N-methyltransferase (EC 2.1.1.115) has broad specificity for (*R,S*)-tetrahydrobenzylisoquinolines, such as norreticline, tetrahydropapaverine, and participates in the pathway leading to morphinan alkaloid synthesis in plants (Fig. 2). (*S*)-Tetrahydroprotoberberine N-methyltransferase (EC 2.1.1.122) methylates tetrahydroprotoberberine and involves in the synthesis of isoquinoline alkaloids. If these enzymes exist in the human tissues, they would methylate especially 1-benzyl-TIQs and 1-phenyl-TIQs as summarized in the later section.

Other uncharacterized N-methyltransferases are possibly present in human brain, such as "β-carboline N-methyltransferase," which is reviewed later in a separate section. This enzyme(s) has a unique characteristic in the cell localization, nuclear and cytosol fractions, that is clearly different from other novel N-methyltransferases, NNMT, HNMT, PNMT, and ANMT.

2.   Assay Procedures

In general, the radiochemical method using [³H-methyl]- or [¹⁴C-methyl]-SAM as a methyl donor has been utilized. After the incubation with substrate in either the whole homogenate or subfraction of tissues, a radioactive product is detected by HPLC/radiochemical detection. This method is highly sensitive and can be utilized for most substrate and inhibitor studies. Also, other chromatographic methods using non-radiolabeled SAM, i.e., GC/MS, HPLC/ECD and HPLC/fluorescence detection, are applicable, although a specific analytical method for each product has to be employed. Sano et al. (1992) reported the simple and

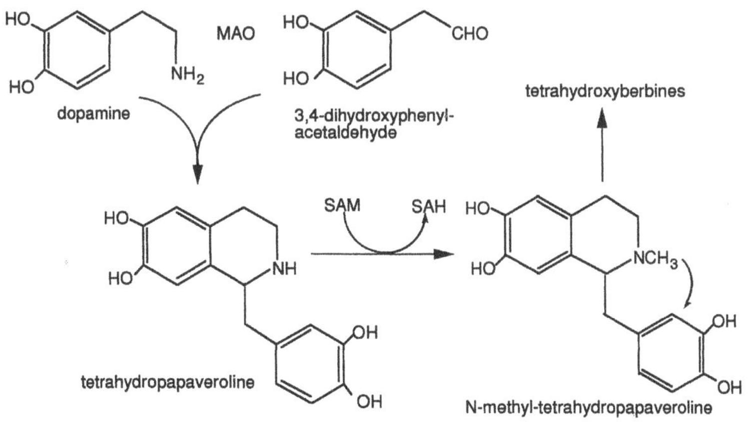

Fig. 2   Reaction sequence for the formation of tetrahydroxyberbines from the 1-benzyl-TIQ derivative, tetrahydropapaveroline (THP), via SAM-dependent N-methylation.

sensitive method for the determination of activities of NNMT and ANMT in the crude cytosolic fractions of tissues. The N-methylated products are determined fluorometrically by their reaction with acetophenone or 4-methoxybenzaldehyde to form fluorescent 2,7-naphthyridine derivatives, and the lower limits of the determination were 8–30 pmol/100 µl. Activities of NNMT can be determined using 5-methylnicotinamide, which is a selective substrate for NNMT but not a methyl acceptor of ANMT. Although 4-methylnicotinamide serves as a methyl acceptor for both NNMT and ANMT, it can be used as a selective substrate for brain ANMT because of the absence of NNMT activity in this organ. However, this method is difficult to employ in studies of substrate specificity.

3. Methyl Donor, SAM

The methyl transfer pathway is important in many areas of metabolism in the central nervous system. It is the sole pathway that provides methyl groups to modify proteins, nucleic acids, fatty acids, phospholipids and polysaccharides. It is also necessary for the inactivation of catecholamines and other biogenic amines, and it provides precursors of polyamine, purine and pyrimidine synthesis. SAM is best known as a methyl donor in these methyl transfer pathways. SAH is formed when the methyl group of SAM has been transferred.

The enzyme methionine adenosyltransferase (MAT, EC 2.5.1.6) catalyzes the formation of SAM from methionine and ATP. Two isoforms of MAT (I and III) have been identified in human liver (Cabrero et al, 1988). Type III is less active than type I (Kunz et al., 1980) and is activated by the addition of DMSO in the *in vitro* assay. Genetic deficiencies in human MAT isoforms have been reported (Gahl et al., 1987). The activity in the liver of a genetically deficient individual was reported to be 28% of normal subjects. The activities of MAT in the nucleus caudate and putamen are higher than those in other regions of human brain (Trolin et al., 1994). Also, there is a significant correlation between age and the activity of MAT in the frontal cortex, but not in the other brain regions. Slightly lower SAM and higher SAH levels are observed in the corpus striatum of the rat (Yu, 1978; Trolin et al., 1994), possibly resulting from an enhanced SAM utilization in the basal nuclei (Stramentinoli and Maffei, 1978). Age-related changes in adult human brain SAM content have not been observed, although a rapid decrease in SAM has been detected during the first year of life (Surtees and Hyland, 1990). There are conflicting reports with regard to the influence of age on SAH level in the brain; however, a recent study by Trolin et al. (1994) showed increased SAH levels in various regions of older rat brains. The biochemical nature of SAM and MAT are reviewed in detail by Hoffman (1994).

Disturbances of the methyltransfer pathway have been implicated in neurological symptoms, the etiology of depression, and reduced cognition in normal aging (Baldessarini, 1987). Interestingly, marked impairment of motor function in mice and rats following the intracerebroventricular administration of SAM has been reported (Charlton and Crowell, 1992; Crowell et al., 1993; Charlton and Mack, 1994). The dominant effects of SAM are Parkinson's-like symptoms that include hypokinesia, tremor, rigidity and abnormal posture. These symptoms are blocked by L-dopa administration (Crowell et al., 1993). The investigators postulate that aberrant methylation in the brain would be involved in the etiology of Parkinson's disease. The molecular mechanism in SAM's adverse effects is not clear; however, exogenous SAM may decrease dopamine levels in the synaptic cleft through the activation of catechol-*O*-methyltransferase (COMT, EC 2.1.16), or increase the N-methylation of heterocyclic amines. SAM is a methyl donor utilized by COMT to catalyze the transfer of methyl groups, principally to the *m*-hydroxyl position of catecholamines. Concentrations of COMT are substantial within the brain, and the levels of SAM have been shown to be lower in the striatum of adult rats (Yu, 1978; Gharib et al., 1982). Based on the high demand for SAM and its instability, SAM is likely to be the limiting factor in methylation reactions in the brain that possibly underlies the activation of heterocyclic amines.

In experimental rats, SAM improves energy metabolism and reduces brain edema. SAM dose-dependently prevents the delayed death of hippocampal CA1 neurons in rats subjected to transient and brief forebrain ischemia, and its effect is suppressed by the administration of SAH (Matsui et al., 1987; Sato et al., 1988).

4. Substrate for N-methyltransferase, a Possible Neurotoxin Precursor

Several classes of heterocyclic molecules, structurally related to MPTP, have been advanced as possible neurotoxin precursors underlying the nigrostriatal degeneration in Parkinson's disease. While a number of compounds have been shown to be methylated, the responsible N-methyltransferase enzyme in each case has not been well identified. In this section, N-methylation of MPTP derivatives, βCs and TIQs is summarized. The compounds having an aromatic substitution at position 1 of TIQs, such as 1-benzyl-TIQ, are discussed in a separate section from TIQs and 6,7-DHTIQs, because the methylation of the former may be catalyzed in a different manner from the latter.

4.1   MPTP analogs

Because of structural similarity to MPTP, desmethylated analogs of paraquat, that are not charged species, have been tested as substrates for N-methyltransferase. Godin and Crooks (1989) have examined the *in vivo* methylation of 4,4'-bispyridyl (desmethylparaquat) in rabbits and guinea pigs (Fig. 3a). The mono-methylated compound, N-methyl-4,4'-bispyridyl, was found in the urine of rabbit, but di-methylated metabolite, paraquat, was not observed. However, both mono- and di-methylated compounds were significantly excreted in the urine of guinea pig. In *in vitro* studies, ANMTs from rabbit liver methylated 4,4'- and 3,3'-bispyridyl but not 2,2'-bispyridyl to form mono-methylated pyridiniums (Crooks et al., 1988). Desmethylation of paraquat can occur *via* bacterium, and the products have been identified in the milk and urine of cow and sheep after paraquat administration (Calderbank and Slade, 1976). The effects of desmethylated paraquat on brain function are not well known.

A number of pyridines structurally related to MPTP exists the environment, especially in foods (Snyder and D'Amato, 1985). Of hundreds of such compounds, 4-phenyl-1,2,3,6-tetrahydropyridine (PTP), desmethylated MPTP, and 4-phenylpyridine (PPP), desmethylated MPP$^+$, are of special interest. PPP and PTP are also present in foods and industrial sources (Snyder and D'Amato, 1985; Ansher et al., 1986a). If they are substrates for N-methyltransferase in the brain after blood-brain barrier penetration, neurotoxic MPP$^+$ would be formed (Fig. 3). N-Methylation of these two compounds are catalyzed by an N-methyltransferase, possibly ANMT, in the cytosolic fraction from brains of humans, monkeys, rabbits, mice and rats; K_m values ranged from 200 to 800 μM (Ansher et al., 1986). Structural studies showed that 3- and 4-phenylpyridine are methyl acceptors, but 2-phenylpyridine is inactive, and the same result is apparent with bispyridyls (Ansher et al., 1986; Crooks et al., 1988) as described above. In contrast to the 4,4'-bispyridyl study, the

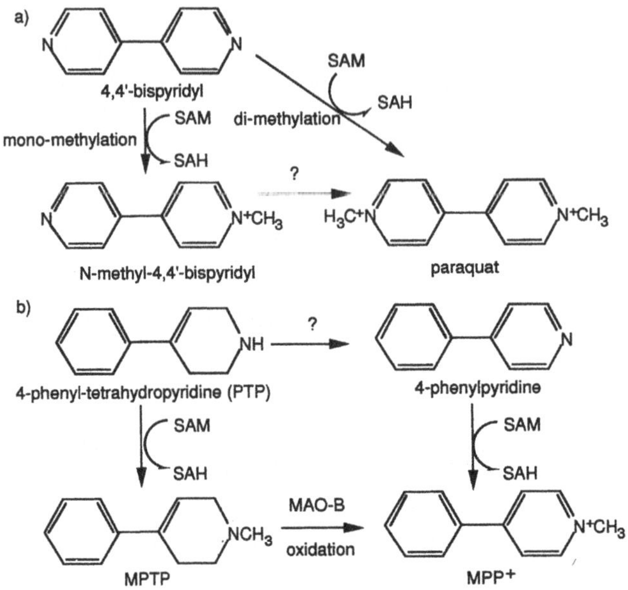

Fig. 3   N-Methylation of MPTP analogs to pyridinium ions: a) N-Methylation of bispyridyls, and
b) PTP and 4-phenylpyridine to pyridinium cations.

in vivo methylation of PPP has not been confirmed by the analysis of urine in guinea pig
and rabbit after the administration of this compound (Godin and Crooks, 1989). This lack
of excretion does not necessarily rule out methylation of PPP *in vivo,* since PPP does produce the depletion of dopamine-related biochemical markers in a manner similar to that of
MPP$^+$ in PC12 cultures and in intact mice (Snyder and D'Amato, 1985).

4.2   βCs and their tetrahydro forms (THβCs)

βCs are proposed as endogenous and/or exogenous protoxins underlying idiopathic Parkinson's disease (Collins, 1994). The methyltransferase activities for 2[β] and 9[indole] nitrogens of βCs to directly form quaternary cations have been identified in the brains of guinea
pig (Collins et al., 1992; Matsubara et al., 1992b) and human (Matsubara et al., 1993), but
is very low in rat. The enzyme activities were originally found in the nuclei fraction of
guinea pig. Recently, the enzyme activity has been shown to be dominantly present in the
cytosolic fraction of bovine brain (Gearhart et al., 1997). This localization discrepancy may
be dependent on the preparation method for the enzyme source, or species differences. The
reaction requires SAM as a methyl donor and displays low micro-molar, K_m values for both
2[β]- and 9[indole]-nitrogens. The involvement of a single enzyme is considered, because
the two N-methyltransferases with βC substrate have similar subcellular activity patterns,
regional brain distributions, and K_m and V_{max} values. In human brain, however, 2[β]-N-
methylation activity is significantly higher than 9[indole]-N-methylation activity (Matsubara et al., 1993). These data indicate that this process involves sequential N-methylation
of βCs, first on the 2[β]- and then on the 9[indole]-nitrogen, to produce the 2,9-dimethy-
lated βC cations (2,9-Me$_2$βC$^+$s). The initial methylation on the 2[β]-nitrogen in the βC

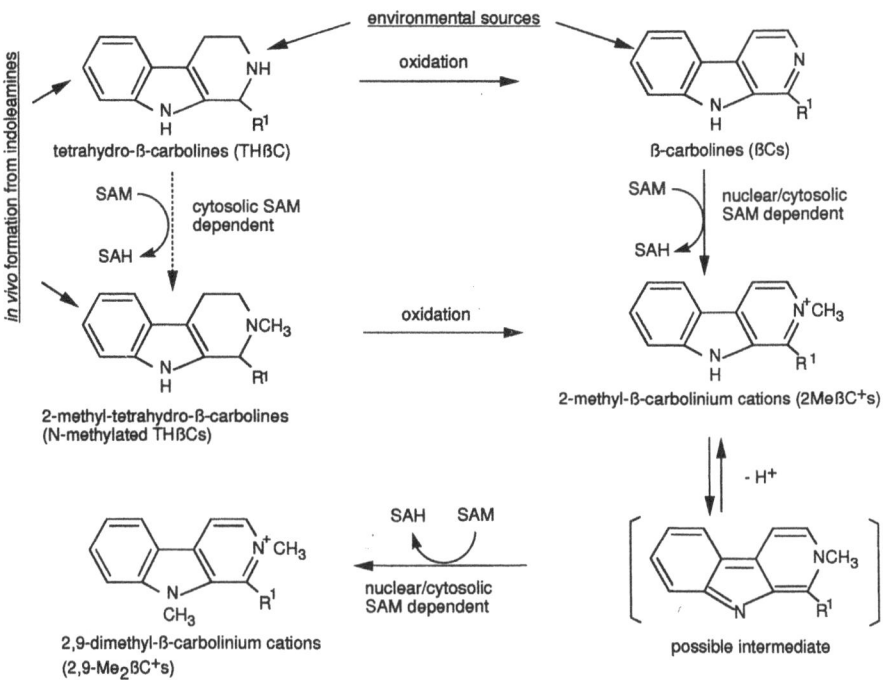

Fig. 4 Metabolic bioactivation routes to form neurotoxic βC⁺s in mammalian brain. R¹ = H: norharman; R¹ = CH₃: harman.

structure results in the neutral base intermediate (Fig. 4) and enhances nucleophilicity of the 9[indole]-nitrogen moiety before the attack on SAM. The enzyme(s) catalyzed βC N-methylation, "β-carboline N-methyltransferase(s)", needs to be established more firmly, however. A possible bioactivation route to produce potentially neurotoxic 2,9-Me₂βC⁺s, which mirror MPP⁺ in mitochondrial toxicity (Collins et al., 1992), is summarized in Fig. 4.

The methyltransferase activity for the tetrahydropyridyl nitrogen of THβCs to form 2[β]-N-methylated THβC is also present in the guinea pig and rat brain and is concentrated in the cytosolic fraction with milli-molar K_m values, but methylation of 9[indole]-nitrogen of THβCs is not observed in any brain fraction (Matsubara et al., 1992a). The most likely reason is that 2[β]-N-methylated THβCs, which are tertiary amines, do not display increased nucleophilicity of the 9[indole]-nitrogen. THβCs apparently are substrates for a different SAM-dependent N-methylation system than the βCs, possibly ANMT. However, a route from 2[β]-N-methylated THβCs to quaternary βC cations by an oxidation reaction is possible *in vivo*.

Further support for *in vivo* methylation of βCs has been provided by the evidence of 2[β]-N-methylated βCs (2-MeβC⁺s) and 2,9-Me₂βC⁺s in human brain and CSF (Matsubara et al., 1993; Matsubara et al., 1995). The 2-MeβC⁺s contents significantly increases with the progression of the Parkinson's disease, but 2,9-Me₂βC⁺s contents decreases as the disease is exacerbated, and they are not found in any of the control samples (Matsubara et al., 1995). Also, simple βCs, precursors of βC⁺s, are equally present in the CSF of parkinsonians and controls. If these observations reflect the etiology of Parkinson's disease, some genetic factors appearing in the N-methylation steps would be involved in Parkinson's disease. Also, 2-MeβC$^+$s might possibly be generated in certain localized brain sites, before accumulating in the nigrostriatal dopaminergic neurons to eventually undergo 9[indole]-N-methylation.

4.3   TIQ and 6,7-DHTIQ

TIQ and 6,7-DHTIQ derivatives constitute the second class of endogenous candidate protoxins or toxins capable of causing idiopathic Parkinson's disease. Originally, pharmacological and biosynthetic interest in mamalian 6,7-DHTIQs, as well as in THβCs, came from their postulated formation and roles in alcoholism (see the review of Myers, 1989). If present at elevated concentrations of these substances in the brain, they might promote central mechanisms inducing alcohol drinking behavior. 6,7-DHTIQs are catecholamine-origin condensation products. The carbon atom bearing the methyl group at the position 1 of 1-methyl-6,7-DHTIQ (salsolinol) is chiral, and occurrence of the R-enantiomer is reported to predominate in humans (Dostert et al., 1990), it is postulated that (R)-salsolinol is formed when dopamine condenses with pyruvate, forming 1-carboxy-salsolinol, which is then decarboxylated. However, Collins and Cheng (1988) reported in an *in vitro* study that decarboxylation of 1-carboxy-salsolinol results in the formation of the dihydro-isoquinoline species, but not in salsolinol. TIQ formation mechanisms have been further advanced by the finding of an enzyme catalyzing the reaction of phenethylamine with aldehydes or α-keto acids (Makino et al., 1990; Tasaki et al., 1993; Haber et al., 1995). Non-enzymatic cyclization based on the Pictet-Spengler reaction does not (Whaley and Govindachari, 1951) or hardly occurs with phenethylamines (personal communication from Dr. S. Ohta).

Both of TIQs and 6,7-DHTIQs can be N-methylated, and this can be followed by oxidation of the N-methylated TIQ and 6,7-DHTIQ products to corresponding isoquinolinium ions. The possible activation routes of TIQs and 6,7-DHTIQs are shown in Fig. 5. There is evidence of their N-methylation in the central nervous system of mammals. Naoi et al. (1989) have found N-methylation activities of TIQ in the human brain *in vitro*. In terms of subcellular localization, the enzyme activity is greatest in the cytosolic and microsomal fractions and lowest in the nuclei fraction, and the optimal pH of the reaction is 8.25. Further evidence of the methylation was obtained using GC/MS by Niwa et al (1990), who administered TIQ to monkeys and then identified N-methyl TIQ in the brain. However, a negative result was also reported by Kikuchi et al. (1991) who systematically administered ^{14}C-labeled TIQ and 1-methyl-TIQ to rats and searched for their metabolites in urine and tissues. They failed to detect neither N-methylated metabolites of both compounds, nor their quaternary ions in the brain, although they identified a small amount of N-methylated TIQ and 1-methyl-TIQ in the urine. The reason for the discrepancy in the results from these two studies is unclear, but might be due to the sensitivities of the assays employed.

After the oxidation of TIQs and 6,7-DHTIQs to isoquinolines, they can be methylated by either NNMT (Alston and Abeles, 1988) or ANMT (Crooks et al., 1988). In the case of 6,7-DHTIQs, Maruyama et al. (1992) demonstrated the N-methylation of (R)-salsolinol in various regions of rat brain using *in vivo* microdialysis with HPLC/ECD. Methylation activity was found to be highest in the nigra, but lower in the striatum. Niwa et al. (1992) further confirmed the chemical structure of N-methyl-salsolinol in the human brain by GC/MS. From these observations, Naoi et al. (1994) have proposed that salsolinol is methylated and subsequently oxidized within the nigrostriatal neurons after its accumulation into the nerves *via* dopamine transporter. N-Methylated salsolinol has been recently found as

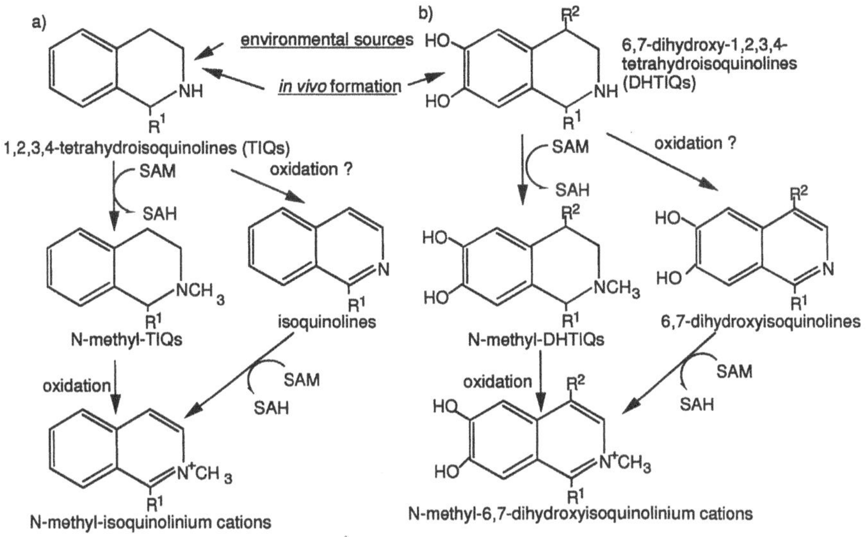

Fig. 5 Metabolic conversions of tetrahydroisoquinolines to quarternary amines. a) TIQs, and b) 6,7-DHTIQs. $R^1 = R^2 = H$: TIQ or norsalsolinol; $R^1 = CH_3$, $R^2 = H$: 1-methyl-TIQ or salsolinol; $R^1 = CH_3$, $R^2 = OH$: 4,6,7-trihydroxy-TIQ.

higher concentrations in the CSF of parkinsonian patients (Maruyama et al., 1996). However, CSF concentrations of N-methylated norsalsolinol, that also could be a product catalyzed by N-methyltransferase in the brain, appear to decrease as the Parkinson's disease progresses. This is explained as due to a compensatively activated dopaminergic system or the loss of N-methylation activity in the nigrostriatal neurons (Moser et al., 1995). The same phenomenon may be occurring in the $2,9-Me_2\beta^+$s (Matsubara et al., 1995).

The product from formaldehyde condensation with norepinephrine, 4,6,7-trihydroxy-TIQ, could be a substrate for both PNMT and ANMT, but it has not yet been examined. When N-methylated, this compound is reported to be a potent toxin to dopaminergic neurons (Liptrot et al., 1993; Liptrot et al., 1994).

4.4   1-Aromatic substitution of TIQs

1-Benzyl-TIQ, postulated as an endogenous compound underlying Parkinson's disease, has been found at higher concentrations in the CSF of parkinsonian patients (Kotake et al., 1995). An interesting monamine-oxidase B (MAO-B, EC 1.4.3.4)-dependent formation route to 1-benzyl- and 1-methyl-TIQs has been proposed by Ohta and co-workers (Fig. 6). It is suggested to explain the protective and degenerative mechanism in dopaminergic neurons mediated by MAO-B. The former substance is a dopaminergic toxin, but the latter has anti-parkinsonian properties (Tasaki et al., 1991, 1993). Two early studies reported by Davis's group (Cashaw et al., 1974; Meyerson and Davis, 1975) suggest possible N-methylation of 1-benzyl-TIQ in mammalian tissues, although these works were particularly concerned with morphinan biosynthesis. These investigators isolated and identified two isomeric tetrahydroxyberbines after the incubation of tetrahydropapaveroline (THP), one of 1-benzyl-TIQ analogs, with SAM in the soluble fraction from rat liver and brain (Fig. 2).

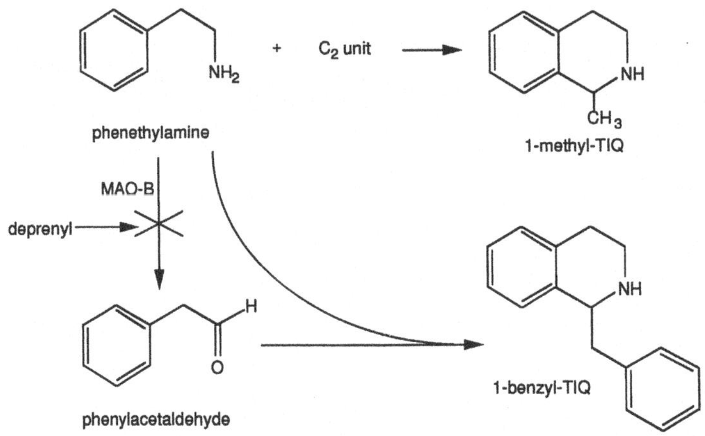

Fig. 6 MAO-B-dependent formation of 1-Benzyl-TIQ and 1-methyl-TIQ.

Two berbines also were found in the urine of rat injected with THP, as well as in the urine of a parkinsonian patient taking L-dopa. Kametani et al. (1977) stated that tetrahydroberberine is formed through the intermediate, N-methyl-THP. Indeed, incorporation of radioactivity in the product was observed after the incubation of THP with [^{14}CH$_3$]-SAM. The responsible N-methyltransferase was purified from rat liver using gel filtration and ion exchange chromatography. It is entirely soluble and has a molecular mass of 27500 daltons. The pH optimum is between 7.7 and 8.0. However, whether this enzyme coincides with tetrahydrobenzylisoquinoline N-methyltransferase confirmed in plants is unclear.

Recently, 1-phenyl-TIQ and its N-methylated product were also identified in the brain of a parkinsonian patient (Kajita et al., 1995). This methylation could have been catalyzed by the same enzyme as that for 1-benzyl-TIQ or ANMT.

5. Possible Formation of Azaheterocyclics via SAM-Dependent N-methylation

Heterocyclic amines are known to be synthesized endogenously, and two formation routes are considered to be possible (Melchior and Collins, 1982; Matsubara, 1996). The first is the Pictet-Spengler condensation of monoamines with aldehydes or α-keto acids. As a second route, monoamines could undergo SAM-dependent methylation on the primary amine, followed by cytochrome P450-mediated oxidation of the N-methyl group, followed by cyclization of the resultant imine to the TIQ or THβC (Fig. 7). The first (with α-keto acids) and/or second paths, which obviate the need for free aldehydes, is possibly the primary route, since endogenous free aldehydes, acetaldehyde and formaldehyde are absent or nearly so in the mammalian brain even after alcohol intake. Indeed, N-methyl-dopamine has been identified in the human brain (Kajita et al., 1993), and tryptamine is known to be a good substrate for ANMTs to form N-methyl-tryptamine and N,N-dimethyl-tryptamine (Crooks et al., 1986). In addition, after the perfusion with N-methyl-dopamine, N-methyl-norsalsolinol has been observed in the dialysate (Kajita et al., 1994). Thus, especially with

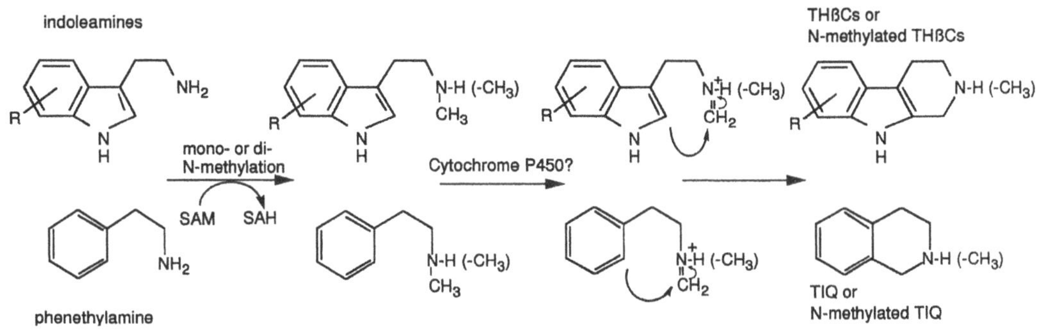

Fig. 7   Possible SAM-dependent formation route of TIQs and THβCs.

nor-compounds, the SAM-dependent second path is the most likely biosynthetic pathway for certain THβCs and TIQs.

Alternatively, formation of 1-carboxylated THβC has been seen after intracerebroventricular injection of tryptamine and pyruvic acid (Susilo and Rommelspacher, 1987). In the 6,7-DHTIQ series, the 1-carboxylic compound is decarboxylated to a dehydro-heterocyclic amine, but not to the tetrahydro-form (Collins and Cheng, 1988), and 1,2-dehydrosalsolinol is dominant in human urine (Dostert et al., 1990). In the first route, the cyclization of monoamines with aldehydes or α-keto acids is also possibly enzyme-catalyzed, either in the formation of the Schiff base or the cyclization step, or both (Makino et al., 1990; Tasaki et al., 1993; Haber et al., 1995). The condensation of acetaldehyde with exogenous 5-HT to form 6-hydroxy-THβC in brainstem homogenates also appeared to be catalyzed, since the reaction is much slower without brain tissue or in boiled tissue samples (Saheb and Dajani, 1973). Barker et al. (1981) have also argued that the formation of formaldehyde-derived THβCs in brain is an enzyme-regulated or catalyzed process.

Although developments in support of the bioactivation of azaheterocyclics have been made during the past decade, as summarized in this chapter, much remains to be done to establish more firmly the role of N-methylation of endogenous and environmental protoxins in the etiology of idiopathic Parkinson's disease.

Acknowledgment

I express my special thanks to Dr. Michael A. Collins at Loyola University of Chicago and Dr. Shigeru Ohta at Hiroshima University for their critical comments, and Dr. Chiaki Fuke at Ryukyu University for providing paraquat information.

References

Aksoy S., Brandriff B.F., Ward A., Little P.F., and Weinshilboum R.M. (1995) Human nicotinamide N-methyltransferase gene: molecular cloning, structural characterization and chromosomal localization. Genomics 29:555–561.

Aksoy S., Raftogianis R., and Weinshilboum R. (1996) Human histamine N-methyltransferase gene: structural characterization and chromosomal location. Biochem. Biophys. Res. Commun. 219:548–554.

Alston T.A., and Abeles R.H. (1988) Substrate specificity of nicotinamide methyltransferase isolated from porcine liver. Arch. Biochem. Biophys. 260:601–608.

Ansher S.S., Cadet J.L., Jakoby W.B., and Baker J.K. (1986a) Role of N-methyltransferases in the neurotoxicity associated with the metabolites of 1-methyl-4-phenyl-1,2,3,6-tetrahydropyridine (MPTP) and other 4-substituted pyridines present in the environment. Biochem. Pharmacol. 35:3359–3363.

Ansher S.S., and Jakoby W.B. (1986b) Amine N-methyltransferases from rabbit liver. J. Biol. Chem. 261:3996–4001.

Baldessarini R.J. (1987) Neuropharmacology of S-adenosyl-L-methionine. Am. J. Med. 83:95–103.

Barker S.A., Harrison R.E.W., Monti J.A., Brown G.B., and Christian S.T. (1981) Identification and quantitation of 1,2,3,4-tetrahydro-β-carboline, 2-methyl-1,2,3,4-tetrahydro-β-carboline, and 6-methoxy-1,2,3,4-tetrahydro-β-carboline as *in vivo* constituents of rat brain and adrenal gland. Biochem. Pharmacol. 30:9–17.

Beart P.M., Prosser D., and Louis W.J. (1979) Adrenaline and phenylethanolamine-N-methyltransferase in rat medullary and anterior hypothalamic-preoptic nuclei. J. Neurochem. 33:947–950.

Cabrero C., Duce A.M., Ortiz P., Alemany S., and Mato J.M. (1988) Specific loss of the high-molecular-weight form of S-adenosyl-L-methionine synthetase in human liver cirrhosis. Hepatology 8:1530–1534.

Calderbank A., and Slade P. (1976) Diquat and paraquat in herbicides. In: Chemistry Degradation and Mode of Action (Kearney P.C., and Kaufman D.D., eds.), pp. 501–540. Marcel Dekker, New York.

Cashaw J.L., McMurtrey K.D., Brown H., and Davis V.E. (1974) Identification of catecholamine-derived alkaloids in mammals by gas chromatography and mass spectrometry. J. Chromatogr. 99:567–573.

Charlton C.G., and Crowell B., Jr. (1992) Parkinson's disease-like effects of S-adenosyl-L-methionine: effects of L-dopa. Pharmacol. Biochem. Behav. 43:423–431.

Charlton C.G., and Mack J. (1994) Substantia nigra degeneration and tyrosine hydroxylase depletion caused by excess S-adenosylmethionine in the rat brain. Support for an excess methylation hypothesis for parkinsonism. Mol. Neurobiol. 9:149–161.

Collins M.A., and Cheng B.Y. (1988) Oxidative decarboxylation of salsolinol-1-carboxylic acid to 1,2-dehydrosalsolinol: evidence for exclusive catalysis by particulate factors in rat kidney. Arch. Biochem. Biophys. 263:86–95.

Collins M.A., Neafsey E.J., Matsubara K., Cobuzzi Jr R.J., and Rollema H. (1992) Indole-N-methylated β-carbolinium ions as potential brain-bioactivated neurotoxins. Brain Res. 570:154–160.

Collins M.A., (1994) Potential parkinsonian protoxicants within and without. Neurobiol. Aging 15:277–278.

Crooks P.A., Godin C.S., Nwosu C.G., Ansher S.S., and Jakoby W.B. (1986) Reevaluation of the products of tryptamine catalyzed by rabbit liver N-methyltransferases. Biochem. Pharmacol. 35:1600–1603.

Crooks P.A., Godin C.S., Damani L.A., Ansher S S., and Jakoby W.B. (1988) Formation of quaternary amines by N-methylation of azaheterocycles with homogeneous amine N-methyltransferases. Biochem. Pharmacol. 37:1673–1677.

Crowell B.G., Jr., Benson R., Shockley D., and Charlton C.G. (1993) S-Adenosyl-L-methionine decreases motor activity in the rat: similarity to Parkinson's disease-like symptoms. Behav. Neural. Biol. 59:186–193.

Cumming P., and Vincent S.R. (1992) Inhibition of histamine-N-methyltransferase (HNMT) by fragments of 9-amino-1,2,3,4-tetrahydroacridine (tacrine) and by beta-carbolines. Biochem. Pharmacol. 44:989–992.

Dostert P., Benedetti M.S., Bellotti V., Allievi C., and Dordain G. (1990) Biosynthesis of salsolinol, a tetrahydroisoquinoline alkaloid, in healthy subjects. J. Neural. Transm. (General Section) 81:215–223.

Fleming L., Mann J.B., Bean J., Briggle T., and Sanchez-Ramos J.R. (1994) Parkinson's disease and brain levels of organochlorine pesticides. Ann. Neurol. 36:100–103.

Fuhr N., and Kownatzki E. (1986) Inhibition of rat kidney histamine-N-methyltransferase by biogenic amines. Pharmacology 32:114–20.

Fukushima T., Tawara T., Isobe A., Hojo N., Shiwaku K., and Yamane Y. (1995) Radical formation site of cerebral complex I and Parkinson's disease. J. Neurosci. Res. 42: 385–390.

Gahl W.A., Finkelstein J.D., Mullen K.D., Bernardini I., Martin J.J., Backlund P., Ishak K.G., Hoofnagle J.H., and Mudd S.H. (1987) Hepatic methionine adenosyltransferase deficiency in a 31-year-old man. Am. J. Human Gen. 40:39–49.

Gairola C., Godin C.S., Houdi A.A., and Crooks P.A. (1988) Inhibition of histamine N-methyltransferase activity in guinea-pig pulmonary alveolar macrophages by nicotine. J. Pharm. Pharmacol. 40:724–726.

Gearhart D.A., Neafsey E.J., and Collins M.A. (1997) Characterization of brain β-carbo-line-2-N-methyltransferase, an enzyme that may play a role in idiopathic Parkinson's disease. Neurochem. Res. 22:113–1210.

Gharib A., Sarda N., Chabannes B., Cronenberger L., and Pacheco H. (1982) The regional concentrations of S-adenosyl-L-methionine, S-adenosyl-L-homocysteine, and adeno-sine in rat brain. J. Neurochem. 38:810–815.

Gitomer W.L., and Tipton K.F. (1986) Purification and kinetic properties of ox brain hista-mine N-methyltransferase. Biochem. J. 233:669–676.

Godin C.S., Crooks P.A., and Damani L.A. (1986) N-methylation of phenylpyridines and bispyridyls as a potential toxication route: tissue distribution of azaheterocycle N-methyltransferase activity in the rabbit. Toxicol. Lett. 34:217–222.

Godin C.S., and Crooks P.A. (1989) N-methylation as a toxication route for xenobiotics. II. *In vivo* formation of N,N'-dimethyl-4,4'-bipyridyl ion (paraquat) from 4,4'-bipyridyl in the guinea pig. Drug Metab. Dispos. 17:180–185.

Green S., Buttrum S., Molloy H., Steventon G., Sturman S., Waring R., Pall H., and Williams A. (1991) N-Methylation of pyridines in Parkinson's disease. Lancet 338: 120–121.

Haber H., Collins M.A., and Melzig M.F. (1995) The *in vitro* formation of 1,3-dimethyl-1,2,3,4-tetrahydroisoquinoline, a neurotoxic metabolite of amphetamines. In: Alz-heimer's and Parkinson's Disease: Recent Advances (Hanin I., Yoshida M., and Fisher A., eds.), pp. 589–597. Plenum, New York.

Hoffman J.L. (1994) Bioactivation by S-adenosylation, S-methylation, or N-methylation. Adv. Pharmacol. 27:449–477.

Kajita M., Niwa T., Takeda N., Yoshizumi H., Tatematsu A., Watanabe K., and Nagatsu T. (1993) Presence of N-methyldopamine in parkinsonian and normal human brains. J. Chromatogr. 613:1–8.

Kajita M., Niwa T., Maruyama W., Nakahara D., Takeda N., Yoshizumi H., Tatematsu A.,

Watanabe K., Naoi M., and Nagatsu T. (1994) Endogenous synthesis of N-methylnorsalsolinol in rat brain during *in vivo* microdialysis with epinine. J. Chromatogr. 654: 263–269.

Kajita M., Niwa T., Fujisaki M., Ueki M., Niimura K., Sato M., Egami K., Naoi M., Yoshida M., and Nagatsu T. (1995) Detection of 1-phenyl-N-methyl-1,2,3,4-tetrahydroisoquinoline and 1-phenyl-1,2,3,4-tetrahydroisoquinoline in human brain by gas chromatography-tandem mass spectrometry. J. Chromatogr. 669:345–351.

Kametani T., Ohata Y., Takemura M., Ihara M., and Fukumoto K. (1977) Biotransformation of reticuline into coreximine, scoulerine, pallidine, and isoboldine with rat liver enzyme. Bio-organic Chem. 6:249–256.

Kaneda N., Ichinose H., Kobayashi K., Oka K., Kishi F., Nakazawa A., Kurosawa Y., Fujita K., and Nagatsu T. (1988) Molecular cloning of cDNA and chromosomal assignment of the gene for human phenylethanolamine N-methyltransferase, the enzyme for epinephrine biosynthesis. J. Biol. Chem. 263:7672–7677.

Kikuchi K., Nagatsu Y., Makino Y., Mashino T., Ohta S., and Hirobe M. (1991) Metabolism and penetration through blood-brain barrier of parkinsonism-related compounds. 1,2,3,4-Tetrahydroisoquinoline and 1-methyl-1,2,3,4-tetrahydroisoquinoline. Drug Metab. Dispos. 19:257–262.

Koike G., Jacob H.J., Krieger J.E., Szpirer C., Hoehe M.R., Horiuchi M., and Dzau V.J. (1995) Investigation of the phenylethanolamine N-methyltransferase gene as a candidate gene for hypertension. Hypertension 26:595–601.

Koller W., Vetere-Overfield B., Gray C., Alexander C., Chin T., Dolezal J., Hassanein R., and Tanner C. (1990) Environmental risk factors in Parkinson's disease. Neurology 40: 1218–1221.

Kotake Y., Tasaki Y., Makino Y., Ohta S., and Hirobe M. (1995) 1-Benzyl-1,2,3,4-tetrahydroisoquinoline as a parkinsonism-inducing agent: a novel endogenous amine in mouse brain and parkinsonian CSF. J. Neurochem. 65:2633–2638.

Kunz G.L., Hoffman J.L., Chia C.S., and Stremel B. (1980) Separation of rat liver methionine adenosyltransferase isozymes by hydrophobic chromatography. Arch. Biochem. Biophys. 202:565–572.

Liptrot J., Holdup D., and Phillipson O. (1993) 1,2,3,4-Tetrahydro-2-methyl-4,6,7-isoquinolinetriol depletes catecholamines in rat brain. J. Neurochem. 61:2199–2206.

Liptrot J., Holdup D., and Phillipson O. (1994) 1,2,3,4-Tetrahydro-2-methyl-4,6,7-isoquinolinetriol inhibits tyrosine hydroxylase activity in rat striatal synaptosomes. J. Neural. Transm. (General Section) 96:51–62.

Luchins D., Ban T.A., and Lehmann H.E. (1978) A review of nicotinic acid, N-methylated indoleamines and schizophrenia. Int. Pharmacopsychiat. 13:16–33.

Makino Y., Tasaki Y., Ohta S., and Hirobe M. (1990) Confirmation of the enantiomers of 1-methyl-1,2,3,4-tetrahydroisoquinoline in the mouse brain and foods applying gas chromatography/mass spectrometry with negative ion chemical ionization. Biomed. Environ. Mass Spectr. 19:415–419.

Maruyama W., Nakahara D., Ota M., Takahashi T., Takahashi A., Nagatsu T., and Naoi M. (1992) N-Methylation of dopamine-derived 6,7-dihydroxy-1,2,3,4-tetrahydroisoquinoline, (R)-salsolinol, in rat brains: *in vivo* microdialysis study. J. Neurochem. 59: 395–400.

Maruyama Y., Abe T., Tohgi H., Dostert P., and Naoi M. (1996) A dopaminergic neurotoxin, (R)-N-methylsalsolinol, increases in parkinsonian cerebrospinal fluid. Ann. Neurol. 40:119–122.

Matsubara K., Collins M.A., and Neafsey E.J. (1992a) Mono-N-methylation of 1,2,3,4-tetrahydro-β-carbolines in brain cytosol: Absence of indole methylation. J. Neurochem. 59:505–510.

Matsubara K., Neafsey E.J., and Collins M.A. (1992b) Novel S-adenosylmethionine-dependent indole-N-methylation of β-carbolines in brain particulate fractions. J. Neurochem. 59:2240–2245.

Matsubara K., Collins M.A., Akane A., Ikebuchi J., Neafsey E.J., Kagawa M., and Shiono H. (1993) Potential bioactivated neurotoxicants, N-methylated β-carbolinium ions, are present in human brain. Brain Res. 610:90–96.

Matsubara K., Kobayashi S., Kobayashi Y., Yamashita K., Koide H., Hatta M., Iwamoto K., Tanaka O., and Kiumura K. (1995) β-Carbolinium cations, endogenous MPP[+] analogs, in the lumber cerebrospinal fluid of parkinsonian patients. Neurology 45: 199–202.

Matsubara K. (1996) Occurrence of neurotoxic β-carbolinium cations in mammalian central nervous system. Biogenic Amines 12:161–169.

Matsui Y., Kubo Y., and Iwata N. (1987) S-adenosyl-L-methionine prevents ischemic neuronal death. Eur. J. Pharmacol. 144:211–216.

Melchior C., and Collins M.A. (1982) The route and significance of endogenous synthesis of alkaloids in animals. Crit. Rev. Toxicol. 9:313–356.

Meyerson L.R., and Daivs V.E. (1975) Purification and characterization of a benzyltetrahydroisoquinoline methyltransferase from rat liver. Fed. Proc. 34:508.

Morano A., Jimenez-Jimenez F.J., Molina J.A., and Antolin M.A. (1994) Risk factors for Parkinson's disease: case-control study in the province of Caceres, Spain. Acta Neurol. Scand. 89:164–170.

Moser A., Scholz J., Nobbe F., Vieregge P., Bohme V., and Bamberg H. (1995) Presence of N-methyl-norsalsolinol in the CSF: correlations with dopamine metabolites of patients with Parkinson's disease. J. Neurol. Sci. 131:183–189.

Myers R.D. (1989) Isoquinolines, beta-carbolines and alcohol drinking: Involment of opioid and dopaminergic mechanisims. Experientia 45:436–443.

Naoi M., Matsuura S., Takahashi T., and Nagatsu T. (1989) A N-methyl-transferase in human brain catalyses N-methylation of 1,2,3,4-tetrahydroisoquinoline, a precursor of a dopaminergic neurotoxin, N-methylisoquinolinium ion. Biochem. Biophys. Res. Commun. 161:1213–1219.

Naoi M., Maruyama W., Niwa T., and Nagatsu T. (1994) Novel toxins and Parkinson's disease: N-methylation and oxidation as metabolic bioactivation of neurotoxin. J. Neural. Transm. 41 (Suppl):197–205.

Nestoros J.N., Ban T.A., and Lehmann H.E. (1977) Transmethylation hypothesis of schizophrenia: methionine and nicotinic acid. Int. Pharmacopsych. 12:215–246.

Niwa T., Yoshizumi H., Tatematsu A., Matsuura S., Yoshida M., Kawachi M., Naoi M., and Nagatsu T. (1990) Endogenous synthesis of N-methyl-1,2,3,4-tetrahydroisoquinoline, a precursor of N-methylisoquinolinium ion, in the brains of primates with parkinsonism after systemic administration of 1,2,3,4-tetrahydroisoquinoline. J. Chromatogr. 533:145–151.

Niwa T., Maruyama W., Nakahara D., Takeda N., Yoshizumi H., Tatematsu A., Takahashi A., Dostert P., Naoi M., and Nagatsu T. (1992) Endogenous synthesis of N-methylsalsolinol, an analogue of 1-methyl-4-phenyl-1,2,3,6-tetrahydropyridine, in rat brain during *in vivo* microdialysis with salsolinol, as demonstrated by gas chromatography-mass spectrometry. J. Chromatogr. 578:109–115.

Rajput A.H., Uitti R.J., Stern W., Laverty W., O'Donnell K., O'Donnell D., Yuen W.K., and Dua A. (1987) Geography, drinking water chemistry, pesticides and herbicides and the etiology of Parkinson's disease. Can. J. Neurol. Sci. 14:414–418.

Rini J., Szumlanski C., Guerciolini R., and Weinshilboum R.M. (1990) Human liver nicotinamide N-methyltransferase: ion-pairing radiochemical assay, biochemical properties and individual variation. Clin. Chim. Acta. 186:359–374.

Saheb S.E., and Dajani R.M. (1973) 1-Methyl-6-hydroxy-tetrahydro-β-carboline: a possible product of ethanol and tryptophan metabolism. Comp. Gen. Pharmacol. 4:225–227.

Sano A., Endo N., and Takitani S. (1992) Fluorometric assay of rat tissue N-methyltransferases with nicotinamide and four isomeric methylnicotinamides. Chem. Pharm. Bull. 40:153–156.

Sano A., Endo N., and Takitani S. (1993) Fluorometric assay of rat brain N-methyltransferase with 4-methylnicotinamide. Biol. Pharm. Bull. 16:304–306.

Sato H., Hariyama H., and Moriguchi K. (1988) S-Adenosyl-L-methionine protects the hippocampal CA1 neurons from the ischemic neuronal death in rat. Biochem. Biophys. Res. Commun. 150:491–496.

Seidler A., Hellenbrand W., Robra B.P., Vieregge P., Nischan P., Joerg J., Oertel W.H., Ulm G., and Schneider E. (1996) Possible environmental, occupational, and other etiologic factors for Parkinson's disease: a case-control study in Germany. Neurology 46:1275–1284.

Seifert R., Hoshino J., and Kroger H. (1984) Nicotinamide methylation. Tissue distribution, developmental and neoplastic changes. Biochim. Biophys. Acta. 801:259–264.

Semchuk K.M., Love E.J., and Lee R.G. (1993) Parkinson's disease: a test of the multifactorial etiologic hypothesis. Neurology 43:1173–1180.

Snyder S.H., and D'Amato R.J. (1985) Predicting Parkinson's disease. Nature 317:198–199.

Surtees R., and Hyland K. (1990) Cerebrospinal fluid concentrations of S-adenosylmethionine, methionine, and 5-methyltetrahydrofolate in a reference population: cerebrospinal fluid S-adenosylmethionine declines with age in humans. Biochem. Med. Metab. Biol. 44:192–199.

Susilo R., and Rommelspacher H. (1987) Formation of a β-carboline (1,2,3,4-tetrahydro-1-methyl-β-carboline-1-carboxylic acid) following intracerebroventricular injection of tryptamine and pyruvic acid. Naunyn-Schmiedeberg's Arch. Pharmacol. 335:70–76.

Tanner C.M., and Langston J.W. (1990) Do environmental toxins cause Parkinson's disease? A critical review. Neurology 40 (suppl):17–30.

Tasaki Y., Makino Y., Ohta S., and Hirobe M. (1991) 1-Methyl-1,2,3,4-tetrahydroisoquinoline, decreasing in 1-methyl-4-phenyl-1,2,3,6-tetrahydropyridine-treated mouse, prevents parkinsonism-like behavior abnormalities. J. Neurochem. 57:1940–1943.

Tasaki Y., Makino Y., Ohta S., and Hirobe M. (1993) Biosynthesis of 1-methyl-1,2,3,4-tetrahydroisoquinoline (1MeTIQ), a possible antiparkinsonism agent. Adv. Neurol. 60:231–233.

Trolin C.G., Lofberg C., Trolin G., and Oreland L. (1994) Brain ATP: L-methionine S-adenosyltransferase (MAT), S-adenosylmethionine (SAM) and S-adenosylhomocysteine (SAH): regional distribution and age-related changes. Eur. Neuropsychopharmacol. 4:469–477.

Whaley W.M., and Govindachari T.R. (1951) The Pictet-Spengler synthesis of tetrahydroisoquinolines and related compounds. Org. React. 6:151–190.

Yu P.H. (1978) Radioenzymatic estimation of S-adenosylmethionine in rat brain regions and subcellular fractions. Analyt. Biochem. 86:498–504.

Chapter 9

Tyrosine Hydroxylase: Biochemical Properties and Short-term Regulation in vitro and in vivo

Yoko Hirata

Contents in Brief

Tyrosine hydroxylase (TH, EC 1.14.16.2, tyrosine 3-monooxygenase) catalyzes the first step in the biosynthesis of catecholamines (dopamine, noradrenaline and adrenaline) (Fig. 1), hydroxylating tyrosine to L-3,4-dihydroxyphenylalanine (L-dopa) (Nagatsu et al. 1964). Since it is a rate-limiting step, the regulation of its activity as well as amounts of enzyme protein play a central role in controlling the synthesis of catecholamines. These are known to be involved in many diseases, including neurological disorders (Parkinson's disease, dystonia, manic depressive illness, schizophrenia), hypertension and diabetes mellitus. The physiological importance of TH has been evidenced by recent studies showing that targeted disruption of the TH gene results in mid-gestational lethality: about 90% of mutant embryos die between embryonic days 11.5 and 15.5, apparently of cardiovascular failure (Zhou et al., 1995; Kobayashi et al., 1995).

1. Basic Properties of TH

TH is a mixed-function oxidase that uses molecular oxygen and tyrosine as substrates, and L-erythro-tetrahydrobiopterin (BH_4) as a cofactor. It is coupled *in vivo* with dihydropteridine reductase (DPR, EC 1.6.99.7), which reduces the quinonoid L-erythro-dihydrobiopterin (qBH_2) formed during the hydroxylation reaction back to BH_4 (Fig. 2). The BH_4

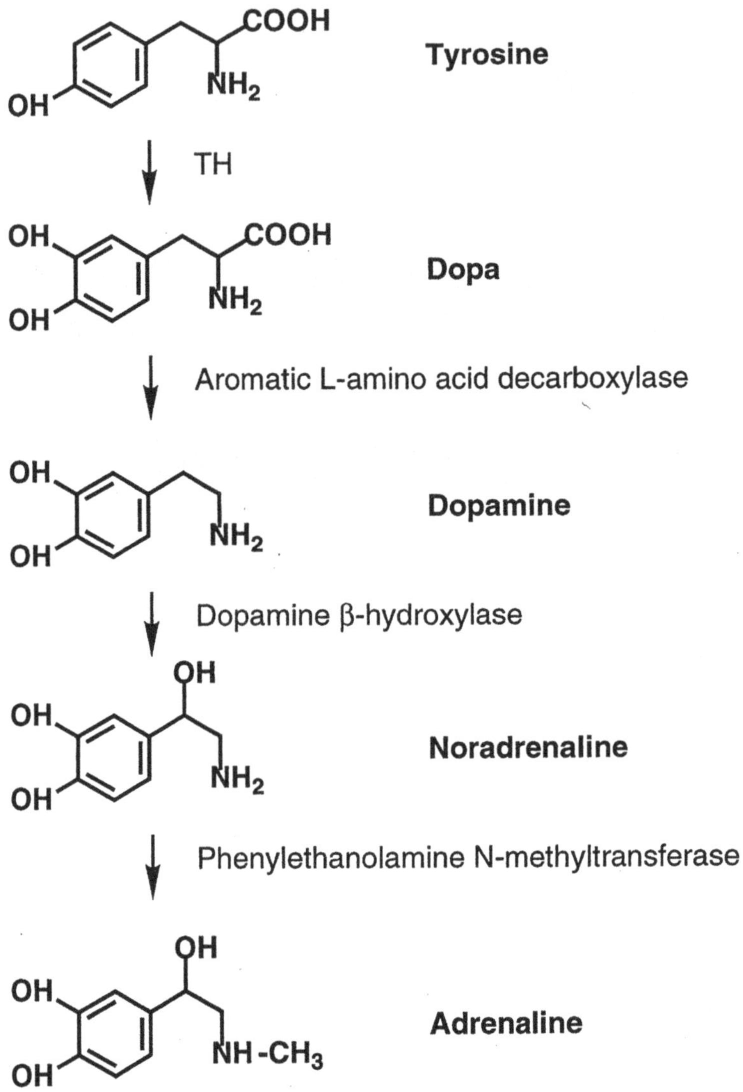

Fig. 1   Catecholamine biosynthetic pathway

concentration within catecholamine-containing neurons and the adrenal *medulla* is below the enzyme's Michaelis constant (K_m), and thus hydroxylase activity should normally be limited by the availability of the cofactor. Tetrahydrobiopterin plays many important roles as a cofactor for pterin-requiring monooxygenases and nitric oxide synthase. It is synthesized from GTP by (i) GTP cyclohydrolase I (EC 3.5.4.16), (ii) 6-pyruvoyltetrahydropterin synthase (EC 4.6.1.10), and (iii) sepiapterin reductase (EC 1.1.1.153).

TH oxidizes only the L-tyrosine, naturally occurring amino acid, and to a lesser extent L-phenylalanine. D-Tyrosine, tyramine, and L-tryptophan do not serve as substrates. An alternative synthetic pathway may be of significance in patients affected with phenylke-

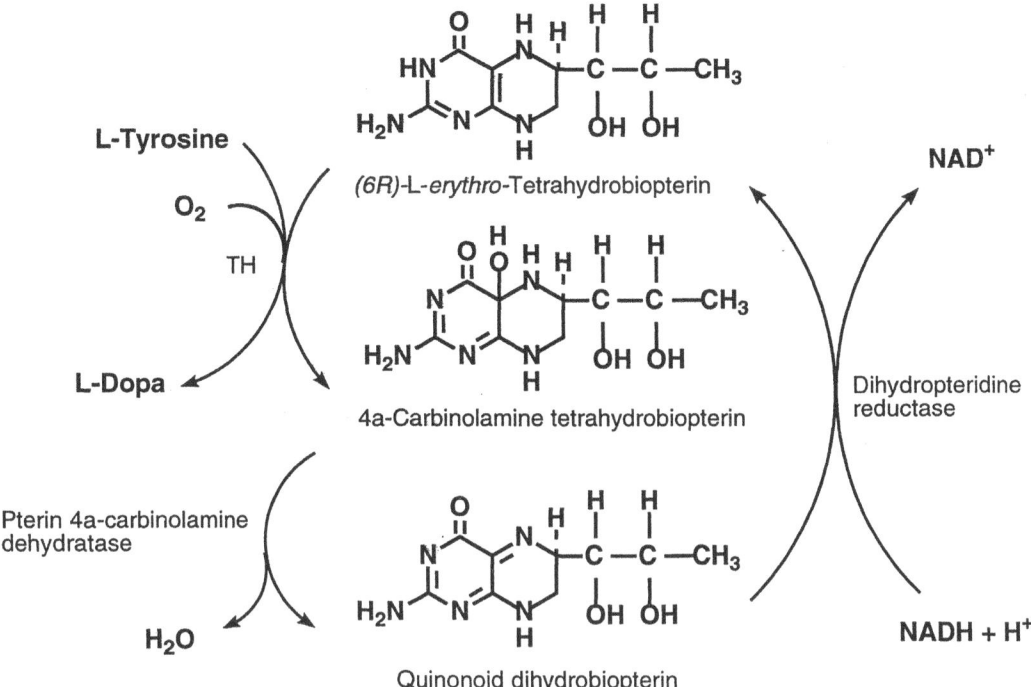

Fig. 2   The TH reaction in relation to cycling of the tetrahydrobiopterin cofactor

tonuria, in which phenylalanine hydroxylase activity is depressed. In contrast to cofactor BH_4, TH is virtually saturated by endogenous tyrosine at normal plasma concentrations, and thus tyrosine does not limit the rate of catecholamine synthesis.

TH requires Fe^{2+} for activity. Human TH in crude tissue extracts is activated by exogenously added Fe^{2+}. Values for the stoichiometry of iron binding to TH purified from bovine adrenal *medulla* are in the range of 0.6–0.8 mol per subunit (Haavik et al., 1988). More recent studies using recombinant human TH, purified as a metal-free apoenzyme, showed the enzyme to be rapidly activated by the incorporation of stoichiometric amounts of Fe^{2+} (Haavik et al., 1991).

Effective inhibitors of TH include amino acid analogues such as α-methyl-p-tyrosine, α-methyl-3-iodotyrosine and 3-iodotyrosine which compete with the substrate tyrosine. In general, α-methyl-amino acids are more potent than the unmethylated analogues, and the action of inhibitors is potentiated by substituting a halogen at the 3 position of the benzene ring. Catechol derivatives, such as dopamine, noradrenaline and adrenaline are competitive inhibitors of the pterin cofactor.

TH is present in peripheral and central catecholaminergic neurons and in chromaffin cells of adrenal *medulla*. It is primarily a soluble enzyme, localized in the cytosol, but *in vitro* some is recovered in a particulate form bound to membrane or cytoskeleton elements, and transient association may occur *in vivo*. Interactions with membrane constituents, such as phosphatidylserine, or with polyanions, such as heparin sulfate, have been shown to alter its kinetic characteristics.

2. Structure and Function

TH is a member of the family of aromatic amino acid hydroxylases, including phenylalanine hydroxylase (EC 1.14.16.1) and tryptophan hydroxylase (EC 1.14.16.4), that share many physical, structural and catalytic properties. A detailed comparison of these enzymes was provided in a recent review (Hufton et al., 1995).

TH is a 240 kDa tetramer composed of four subunits of approx. 60 kDa each. Analysis of mRNA and genomic DNA has revealed that only a single form of TH is found in most species, including rats, mice and cows, but that two to four splice variants of TH exist in humans and higher primates (Grima et al., 1985, 1987; Kaneda et al., 1987; Ichinose et al., 1993). The 60 kDa (498 amino acid) rat protein is composed of an inhibitory regulatory domain at the N-terminus and a catalytic domain at the C-terminus (Fig. 3). In fact, the phosphorylation sites have been identified in the N-terminal region, and the removal of up to 165 amino acids of this domain increases the activity (Walker et al., 1994). The catalytic core of rat TH is included in the region stretching from amino acid #165 to #479 (Walker et al., 1994) and the C-terminal domain of rat TH (343 amino acids) is fully active (Lohse and Fitzpatrick, 1993). The iron-binding sites have been identified as amino acid residues His^{331} and His^{336} that are conserved in phenylalanine hydroxylase (Ramsey et al., 1995). Both lie within the proposed pterin-binding region (Hufton et al., 1995). The C-terminal 20 amino acids of TH containing a putative leucine zipper, which have coiled coil characteristics, may form an intersubunit binding region (Lohse and Fitzpatrick, 1993; Vrana et al., 1994). There is essentially no information available on the three-dimensional structure of the TH, largely due to difficulties in the crystallization of the protein.

3. Assays for TH

Two types of assays have been performed to study TH: (i) assessment of enzyme activity in homogenates or cell extracts, or (ii) determination of the rate of tyrosine hydroxylation in synaptosomes, tissue slices or cultured cells. For the former, TH activity was first detected with a radio-isotopic assay in which L-$[^{14}C]$-dopa formation from L-$[^{14}C]$-tyrosine was measured (Nagatsu et al., 1964). Later a non-radio-isotopic assay was developed by the introduction of high-performance liquid chromatography with electrochemical detection (HPLC-ECD) (Nagatsu et al., 1979). The practical methods have been described in detail in *Methods in Biogenic Amine Research* (Nagatsu, 1983).

To measure TH activity in homogenates or cell extracts, sufficient amounts of substrate, a pterin cofactor, a tetrahydropterin-regenerating system and an H_2O_2-destroying system such as catalase are added to the reaction mixture. The concentration of the pterin cofactor and the pH are important because in many cases the activation of TH is caused by a decrease in the enzyme K_m for a cofactor, and in some cases increases in activity are more prominent when the enzyme is assayed at a physiological pH (around pH 7.0) although the pH optimum is around 6. As the cofactor, 6,7-dimethyltetrahydropterin or 6-methyltetrahydropterin are generally used, both of these having a higher K_m than the natural cofactor tetrahydrobiopterin.

For determination of tyrosine hydroxylation and thus the rate of dopa synthesis in intact tissue, synaptosomes, tissue slices or cultured cells have been employed. A radiometric technique is available based on the formation of labeled catecholamine products from radioactive precursors, L-tyrosine or L-phenylalanine (Anagnoste et al., 1974). The introduction of HPLC-ECD allows measurement of the conversion of endogenous tyrosine to dopa under the inhibition of L-aromatic amino acid decarboxylase (Hirata and Nagatsu, 1985). Furthermore, *in vivo* hydroxylation of tyrosine in the brain of conscious rats can be monitored by microdialysis-HPLC (Westerink et al., 1990).

4. Regulation of TH

TH is subject to short- and long-term regulation; the former occurs at post-translational levels (feedback inhibition, allosteric regulation, and enzyme phosphorylation) and the latter at transcriptional as well as at translational levels (transcriptional regulation, alternative RNA splicing, RNA stability, translational regulation, and enzyme stability) (see Nagatsu, 1995; Kumer and Vrana, 1996). In this review, we will focus on short-term regulation of TH.

4.1 Feedback inhibition

Catecholamines, the end product of the TH reaction, inhibit the enzyme activity competitively with a pterin cofactor (Nagatsu et al., 1964). The question of whether the feedback inhibition of TH activity observed *in vitro* is of physiological significance has been extensively studied. High affinity binding of catecholamines results in the inhibition of TH activity (Okuno and Fujisawa, 1985), and it has been demonstrated that dopamine forms an inhibitory complex with Fe(III) within the active site of the enzyme, characterized as a blue-green chromophore (Andersson et al., 1988; Almas et al., 1992; Ribeiro et al., 1992). Furthermore, catecholamines inactivate the enzyme reversibly by converting the active/labile form to an inactive/stable form (Okuno and Fujisawa, 1991). The phosphorylation of TH at Ser[40] by PKA produces an activated form of the enzyme which is less sensitive to dopamine. Interestingly enough, recombinant TH which is free of inhibiting catecholamines shows a very high specific activity, a pH optimum close to 7 and no significant activation by PKA (Ribeiro et al., 1992). These results suggest that the high-affinity binding of catecholamine products is an important post-translational modification that determines the state of enzyme activation and the response to phosphorylation.

4.2 Enzyme phosphorylation and activation *in vitro*

It has been shown that TH is directly phosphorylated *in vitro* by several different protein kinases, such as protein kinase A (PKA) (Vulliet et al., 1980), protein kinase C (PKC) (Albert et al., 1984), cGMP-dependent protein kinase (PKG) (Roskoski et al., 1987), Ca^{2+}/calmodulin dependent protein kinase II (CaM-PKII) (Yamauchi and Fujisawa, 1981), proline-directed protein kinase (PDPK) (Vulliet et al., 1989), MAP kinases (ERK 1 and 2) (Haycock et al., 1992) and MAP kinase-activated protein kinases 1 and 2 (MAPKAP kinases-1 and -2) (Sutherland et al., 1993). As shown in Fig. 3, the main phosphorylation sites of TH *in vitro* have been identified as Ser[8], Ser[19], Ser[31] and Ser[40].

Ser[8] has been found to be phosphorylated by PDPK, designated by the recognition sequence specificity (-X-Ser/Thr-Pro-X-) (Vulliet et al., 1989), which was originally copurified with TH (Campbell et al., 1986) and subsequently identified to be a dimeric complex of p34cdc2 and p58cyclin A (Hall et al., 1992). Although the phosphorylation of Ser[8] within dopaminergic nerve terminals is enhanced by treatment with okadaic acid, a specific

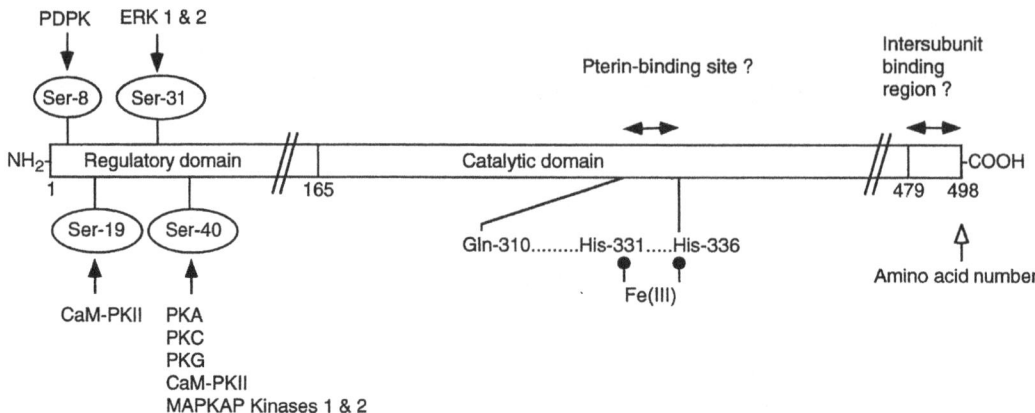

Fig. 3   Schematic diagram of rat TH showing phosphorylation sites and important structures

inhibitor of phosphatase, its significance has yet to be elucidated (Haycock and Haycock, 1991).

Ser[31] is phosphorylated by ERK1 and ERK2 (also termed MAP kinase 1 and MAP kinase 2) with the increase in TH activity produced by ERK1 being much smaller than that produced by PKA, in spite of equivalent phosphorylation of Ser[40] by the latter (Haycock et al., 1992). Sutherland et al. (1993) further showed the four alternatively spliced forms of human TH to be phosphorylated at Ser[31] by MAP kinase, but at markedly different rates (TH-3 = TH-4 > TH-1 >> TH-2). The TH-2, TH-3 and TH-4 contain insertions between residues 30 and 31 of TH-1, creating different sequences around Ser[31]. Another example of diversity in the regulation of human TH isoforms has been identified. The insertion of the four additional amino acids in TH-2 between Met[30] and Ser[31] of TH-1 generates a consensus sequence for CaM-PKII (-RXXS-). In fact, the putative phosphorylation site generated by alternative splicing (Ser[31]) was found to be phosphorylated by CaM-PKII only in the TH-2 case (Le Bourdelles et al., 1991). It seems likely that each of the isoforms may respond in a unique manner to the same physiological stimulus, thus providing more intricate regulation of TH activity in humans and higher primates.

Of the phosphorylation sites, Ser[40] seems to be the most important for the regulation of TH activity. Several kinases can phosphorylate Ser[40], but their effects on the TH activity differ in spite of modification of same serine residue. It is generally accepted that phosphorylation at Ser[40] by PKA produces a reduction in the K_m for pterin cofactors and an increase in the inhibitory constant (K_i) for catecholamine feedback inhibitors. Funakoshi et al. (1991) have suggested the existence of an allosteric effect, based on the observation of a linear relationship between the activation and phosphorylation of the enzyme by PKA. They clearly showed that PKA can phosphorylate all the subunits (approximately 1 mol of phosphate/mol of TH subunit), whereas PKC and CaM-PKII can only phosphorylate two of four subunits at Ser[40], based on exact estimation of TH amounts. Furthermore, PKA activates TH in the presence of saturated amounts of the pterin cofactor when PKC and CaM-PKII do not produce significant activation. The results suggest that the four Ser[40] residues do not behave identically, although TH is composed of four identical subunits. CaM-PKII additionally phosphorylates almost all the Ser[19] sites, and this appears to cause activation of the enzyme via involvement of the 14-3-3 activator protein (Yamauchi and Fujisawa, 1981). In this context, it should be noted that formation of complexes between another aromatic amino acid hydroxylase, tryptophan hydroxylase, and the 14-3-3 protein is dependent on enzyme phosphorylation (Furukawa et al., 1993). Similarities in structure and function between TH and tryptophan hydroxylase (Hufton et al., 1995) suggest that TH may be regulated by a similar mechanism.

Sutherland et al. (1993) have demonstrated that MAPKAP kinase-1 phosphorylates the human TH isoforms TH-1, TH-2, TH-3, TH-4 at Ser^{40} while MAPKAP kinase-2 targets Ser^{19} and Ser^{40}. The resultant activation correlates with the extent of phosphorylation of Ser^{40}. Substitution of Ser^{40} with Leu or Tyr also causes activation of TH and loss of the effect of PKA, suggesting that Ser^{40} exerts an inhibitory effect on the catalytic function, and modification at this site may produce a conformational change, which leads to increased enzymatic activity (Wu et all., 1992).

Little is known about phosphatase control of TH, although protein phosphatase 2A dephosphorylates the enzyme after phosphorylation with PKA, and incubation of adrenal chromaffin cells with okadaic acid, a specific inhibitor, increases phosphorylation and activity (Haavik et al., 1989). Thus, type 2A phosphatase may play an important role in regulating TH *in vivo*. The possibility that other phosphatases could be involved in dephosphorylation at Ser^8, Ser^{19} and/or Ser^{31} remains to be assessed.

In closing this section, I would like to stress that although *in vitro* studies using purified materials have been invaluable in characterizing the factors with potential for TH regulation, further *in vivo* studies are necessary to determine how the enzyme is controlled under physiological conditions. Experiments *in vitro* are very much dependent on a number of variables and especially the enzyme preparations. As previously noted, the activity of TH at neutral pH is suppressed by binding of catecholamines and iron (see *Feedback inhibition*) and the enzyme isolated from various tissues was found to contain significant amounts of both of these (Haavik et al., 1988; Anderson et al., 1988).

4.3 Regulation of TH by protein phosphorylation and by dopamine autoreceptor in dopaminergic nerve terminals

Figure 4 shows a schematic model of the short-term regulation of dopamine biosynthesis via regulation of TH activity in dopaminergic nerve terminals. Acute regulation of TH by nerve activity and by neurotransmitters in the sympathetic nervous system has been discussed in the literature (Zigmond et al., 1989).

Several lines of evidence suggest that cyclic AMP analogues, such as dibutyryl cyclic AMP, or depolarization with high K^+ increase dopamine synthesis in rat striatal synaptosomes or slices (Anagnoste et al., 1974). Sodium nitroprusside, which activates guanylate cyclase and enhances cyclic GMP biosynthesis, stimulates TH activity in rat striatal synaptosomes and in PC12 cells (Roskoski and Roskoski, 1987). CaM-PK II has been directly implicated in TH regulation in rat striatal slices or PC12 cells through the use of specific inhibitors of calmodulin such as W-7 and trifluoperazine, or of CaM-PK II itself such as KN-62 (Hirata and Nagatsu, 1985; Lee et al., 1985; Ishii et al., 1991). Haycock and Haycock (1991) have demonstrated that the TH in the rat striatum is phosphorylated in response to physiological stimuli. Thus, electrical stimulation of the medial forebrain bundle was found to increase ^{32}P incorporation into TH at Ser^{19}, Ser^{30} and Ser^{40}. These results suggest that second messengers such as cyclic AMP, cyclic GMP or Ca^{2+} and their cognate protein kinases activate the enzyme. Growth factors such as NGF regulate TH activity via the second-messenger-independent serine/threonine protein kinases. Thus NGF activates the intrinsic tyrosine kinase activity of proto-oncogene product Trk, a component of the high-

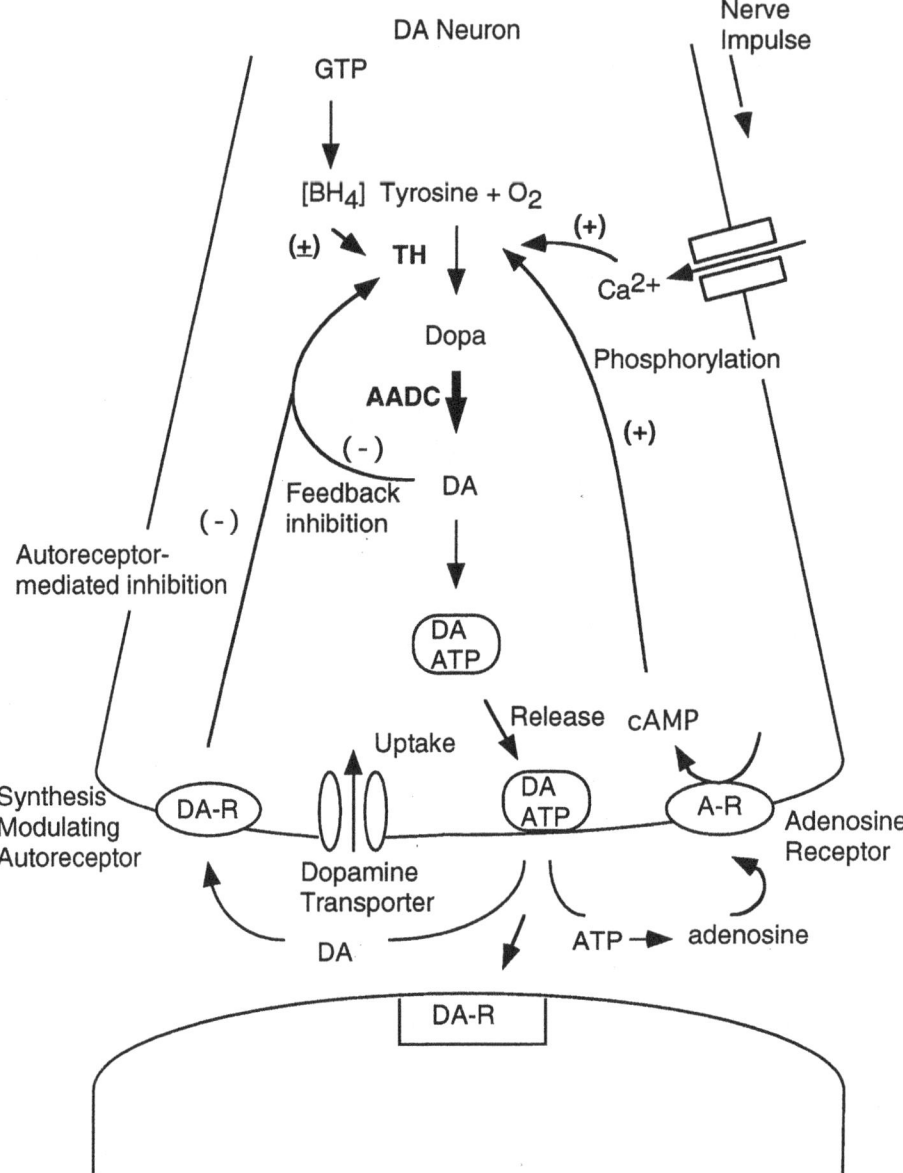

Fig. 4 Schematic model of the short-term regulation of dopamine biosynthesis via TH activity in dopaminergic nerve terminals

affinity NGF receptor, resulting in activation of the MAP kinase cascade (Greene and Kaplan, 1995). Indeed, treatment of PC12 cells with NGF increases the phosphorylation of TH at the Ser[31] *in situ* and the catalytic activity of ERKs (Haycock et al., 1992). It is possible that several neurotrophic factors regulate TH activity by similar mechanisms in the central nervous system.

Dopamine synthesis in most mesencephalic dopamine neurons is modulated by autoreceptors generally classified as D2 dopamine receptors. They exist on most portions of dopamine cells, including the soma, dendrites, and nerve terminals. The stimulation of autoreceptors by dopamine or dopamine agonists inhibits striatal TH activity and release of dopamine from nerve terminals (Roth and Elsworth, 1995). Which signal transduction pathway is involved with these synthesis-modulating autoreceptors is not clear, but a link to pertussis toxin-sensitive G proteins has been suggested (Bean et al., 1988).

As discussed above, TH activity is regulated by various mechanisms that provide redundancy and diversity in the control of catecholamine biosynthesis. It should be noted that catecholamines are not only essential neurotransmitters or hormones but are also themselves toxic substances. Catecholamines can form reactive quinones and oxygen radicals that damage proteins and DNA (Stokes et al., 1996). Dopamine-derived 1-methyl-6,7-dihydroxy-1,2,3,4-tetrahydroisoquinoline (salsolinol) and related compounds have selective toxicity to the dopamine neurons in the *substantia nigra* (Naoi et al., 1996) (see also Part A of this volume). Therefore it is important that only the amounts of catecholamines actually needed for physiological requirements be supplied.

References

Albert K.A., Helmer-Matyjek E., Nairn A.C., Muller T.H., Haycock J.W., Greene L.A., Goldstein M., and Greengard P. (1984) Calcium/phospholipid-dependent protein kinase (protein kinase C) phosphorylates and activates tyrosine hydroxylase. Proc. Natl. Acad. Sci. USA 81:7713–7717.

Almas B., Le Bourdelles B., Flatmark T., Mallet J., and Haavik J. (1992) Regulation of recombinant human tyrosine hydroxylase isozymes by catecholamine binding and phosphorylation. Structure/activity studies and mechanistic implications. Eur. J. Biochem. 209:249–255.

Anagnoste B., Shirron C., Friedman E., and Goldstein M. (1974) Effect of dibutyryl cyclic adenosine monophosphate on ^{14}C-dopamine biosynthesis in rat brain striatal slices. J. Pharmacol. Exp. Ther. 191:370–376.

Andersson K.K., Cox D.D., Que L. Jr., Flatmark T., and Haavik J. (1988) Resonance Raman studies on the blue-green-colored bovine adrenal tyrosine 3-monooxygenase (tyrosine hydroxylase). Evidence that the feedback inhibitors adrenaline and noradrenaline are coordinated to iron. J. Biol. Chem. 263:18621–18626.

Bean A.J., Shepard P.D., Bunney B.S., Nestler E.J., and Roth R.H. (1988) The effects of pertussis toxin on autoreceptor-mediated inhibition of dopamine synthesis in the rat striatum. Mol. Pharmacol. 34:715–718.

Campbell D.G., Hardie D.G., and Vulliet P.R. (1986) Identification of four phosphorylation sites in the N-terminal region of tyrosine hydroxylase. J. Biol. Chem. 261:10489–10492.

Funakoshi H., Okuno S., and Fujisawa H. (1991) Different effects on activity caused by phosphorylation of tyrosine hydroxylase at serine 40 by three multifunctional protein kinases. J. Biol. Chem. 266:15614–15620.

Furukawa Y., Ikuta N., Omata S., Yamauchi T., Isobe T., and Ichimura T. (1993) Demonstration of the phosphorylation-dependent interaction of tryptophan hydroxylase with the 14-3-3 protein. Biochem. Biophys. Res. Commun. 194:144–149.

Greene L.A., and Kaplan D.R. (1995) Early events in neurotrophin signalling via Trk and p75 receptors. Curr. Opin. Neurobiol. 5:579–587.

Grima B., Lamouroux A., Blanot F., Faucon Biguet N., and Mallet J. (1985) Complete coding sequence of rat tyrosine hydroxylase mRNA. Proc. Natl. Acad. Sci. USA 82:617–621.

Grima B., Lamouroux A., Boni C., Julien J.-F., Javoy-Agid F., and Mallet J. (1987) A single human gene encoding multiple tyrosine hydroxylases with different predicted functional characteristics. Nature 326:707–711.

Haavik J., Andersson K.K., Petersson L., and Flatmark T. (1988) Soluble tyrosine hydroxylase (tyrosine 3-monooxygenase) from bovine adrenal *medulla:* large-scale purification and physicochemical properties. Biochim. Biophys. Acta 953:142–156.

Haavik J., Schelling D.L., Campbell D.G., Andersson K.K., Flatmark T., and Cohen P. (1989) Identification of protein phosphatase 2A as the major tyrosine hydroxylase phosphatase in adrenal *medulla* and *corpus striatum:* evidence from the effects of okadaic acid. FEBS Lett. 251:36–42.

Haavik J., Le Bourdelles B., Martinez A., Flatmark T., and Mallet J. (1991) Recombinant human tyrosine hydroxylase isozymes. Reconstitution with iron and inhibitory effect of other metal ions. Eur. J. Biochem. 199:371–378.

Hall F.L., Braun R.K., Mihara K., Fung Y.K., Berndt N., Carbonara-Hall D.A., and Vulliet P.R. (1992) Characterization of the cytoplasmic proline-directed protein kinase in proliferative cells and tissues as a heterodimer comprised of p34cdc2 and p58cyclin A. J. Biol. Chem. 266:17430–17440.

Haycock J.W., and Haycock D.A. (1991) Tyrosine hydroxylase in rat brain dopaminergic nerve terminals. Multiple-site phosphorylation *in vivo* and in synaptosomes. J. Biol. Chem. 266:5650–5657.

Haycock J.W., Ahn N.G., Cobb M.H., and Krebs E.G. (1992) ERK1 and ERK2, two microtubule-associated protein 2 kinases, mediate the phosphorylation of tyrosine hydroxylase at serine-31 *in situ.* Proc. Natl. Acad. Sci. USA 89:2365–2369.

Hirata Y., and Nagatsu T. (1985) Evidence for the involvement of Ca^{2+}-calmodulin and cyclic AMP in the regulation of the tyrosine hydroxylase system in rat striatal tissue slices. Biochem. Pharmacol. 34:2637–2643.

Hufton S.E., Jennings I.G., and Cotton R.G.H. (1995) Structure and function of the aromatic amino acid hydroxylases. Biochem. J. 311:353–366.

Ichinose H., Ohye T., Fujita K., Yoshida M., Ueda S., and Nagatsu T. (1993) Increased heterogeneity of tyrosine hydroxylase in humans. Biochem. Biophys. Res. Commun. 195:158–165.

Ishii A., Kiuchi K., Kobayashi R., Sumi M., Hidaka H., and Nagatsu T. (1991) A selective Ca^{2+}/calmodulin-dependent protein kinase II inhibitor, KN-62, inhibits the enhanced phosphorylation and the activation of tyrosine hydroxylase by 56 mM K^+ in rat pheochromocytoma PC12h cells. Biochem. Biophys. Res. Commun. 176:1051–1056.

Kaneda N., Kobayashi K., Ichinose H., Kishi F., Nakazawa A., Kurosawa Y., Fujita K., and Nagatsu T. (1987) Isolation of a novel cDNA clone for human tyrosine hydroxylase: alternative RNA splicing produces four kinds of mRNA from a single gene. Biochem. Biophys. Res. Commun. 146:971–975.

Kobayashi K., Morita S., Sawada H., Mizuguchi T., Yamada K., Nagatsu I., Hata T., Watanabe Y., Fujita K., and Nagatsu T. (1995) Targeted disruption of the tyrosine hydroxylase locus results in severe catecholamine depletion and perinatal lethality in mice. J. Biol. Chem. 270:27235–27243.

Kumer S.C., and Vrana K.E. (1996) Intricate regulation of tyrosine hydroxylase activity and gene expression. J. Neurochem. 67:443–462.

Le Bourdelles B., Horellou P., Le Caer J.-P., Denefle P., Latta M., Haavik J., Guibert B., Mayaux J.-F., and Mallet J. (1991) Phosphorylation of human recombinant tyrosine hydroxylase isoforms 1 and 2: An additional phosphorylated residue in isoform 2, generated through alternative splicing. J. Biol. Chem. 266:17124–17130.

Lee K.Y., Seeley P.J., Muller T.H., Helmer-Matyjek E., Sabban E., Goldstein M., and Greene L.A. (1985) Regulation of tyrosine hydroxylase phosphorylation in PC12 pheochromocytoma cells by elevated K⁺ and nerve growth factor. Evidence for different mechanisms of action. Mol. Pharmacol. 28:220–228.

Lohse D.L., and Fitzpatrick P.F. (1993) Identification of the intersubunit binding region in rat tyrosine hydroxylase. Biochem. Biophys. Res. Commun. 197:1543–1548.

Nagatsu T., Levitt M., and Udenfriend S. (1964) Tyrosine hydroxylase. The initial step in norepinephrine biosynthesis. J. Biol. Chem. 239:2910–2917.

Nagatsu T., Oka K., and Kato T. (1979) Highly sensitive assay for tyrosine hydroxylase activity by high-performance liquid chromatography. J. Chromatogr. 163:247–252.

Nagatsu T. (1983) Analysis of monooxygenases in catecholamine biosynthesis: tyrosine hydroxylase and dopamine-β-hydroxylase. In: Methods in Biogenic Amine Research (Parvez S., Nagatsu T., Nagatsu I., and Parvez H., eds.), pp. 329–357. Elsevier Science Publishers B.V.

Nagatsu T. (1995) Tyrosine hydroxylase: human isoforms, structure and regulation in physiology and pathology. In: Essays in Biochemistry, Vol. 30 (Apps D.K. and Tipton K.F., eds.), pp. 15–35. Portland Press, London.

Naoi M., Maruyama W., Dostert P., Hashizume Y., Nakahara D., Takahashi T., and Ota M. (1996) Dopamine-derived endogenous 1(R),2(N)-dimethyl-6,7-dihydroxy-1,2,3,4-tetrahydroisoquinoline, N-methyl-(R)-salsolinol, induced parkinsonism in rat: biochemical, pathological and behavioral studies. Brain Res. 709:285–295.

Okuno S., and Fujisawa H. (1985) A new mechanism for regulation of tyrosine 3-monooxygenase by end product and cyclic AMP-dependent protein kinase. J. Biol. Chem. 260:2633–2635.

Okuno S., and Fujisawa H. (1991) Conversion of tyrosine hydroxylase to stable and inactive form by the end products. J. Neurochem. 57:53–60.

Ramsey A.J., Daubner S.C., Ehrlich J.I., and Fitzpatrick P.F. (1995) Identification of iron ligands in tyrosine hydroxylase by mutagenesis of conserved histidinyl residues. Protein Sci. 4:2082–2086.

Ribeiro P., Wang Y., Citron B.A., and Kaufman S. (1992) Regulation of recombinant rat tyrosine hydroxylase by dopamine. Proc. Natl. Acad. Sci. USA 89:9593–9597.

Roskoski R. Jr., and Roskoski L.M. (1987) Activation of tyrosine hydroxylase in PC12 cells by the cyclic GMP and cyclic AMP second messenger systems. J. Neurochem. 48:236–242.

Roskoski R. Jr., Vulliet P.R., and Glass D.B. (1987) Phosphorylation of tyrosine hydroxylase by cyclic GMP-dependent protein kinase. J. Neurochem. 48:840–845.

Roth R.H., and Elsworth J.D. (1995) Biochemical pharmacology of midbrain dopamine neurons. In: Psychopharmacology: The Fourth Generation of Progress (Bloom F.E. and Kupfer D.J., eds.), pp. 227–243. Raven Press, New York.

Stokes A.H., Brown B.G., Lee C.K., Doolittle D.J., and Vrana K.E. (1996) Dopamine covalently modifies DNA in a tyrosinase-enhanced manner. In: Neurodegenerative Diseases: Molecular and Cellular Mechanisms and Therapeutic Advances (Fiskum G., ed.), pp. 299–304. Plenum Press, New York.

Sutherland C., Alterio J., Campbell D.G., Le Bourdelles B., Mallet J., Haavik J., and Cohen P. (1993) Phosphorylation and activation of human tyrosine hydroxylase *in vitro* by mitogen-activated protein (MAP) kinase and MAP-kinase-activated kinases 1 and 2. Eur. J. Biochem. 217:715–722.

Vrana K.E., Walker S.J., Rucker P., and Liu X. (1994) A carboxyl terminal leucine zipper is required for tyrosine hydroxylase tetramer formation. J. Neurochem. 63:2014–2020.

Vulliet P.R., Langan T.A., and Weiner N. (1980) Tyrosine hydroxylase: A substrate of cyclic AMP-dependent protein kinase. Proc. Natl. Acad. Sci. USA 77:92–96.

Vulliet P.R., Hall F.L., Mitchell J.P., and Hardie D.G. (1989) Identification of a novel proline-directed serine/threonine protein kinase in rat pheochromocytoma. J. Biol. Chem. 264:16292–16298.

Walker S.J., Liu X., Roskoski R., and Vrana K.E. (1994) Catalytic core of rat tyrosine hydroxylase: terminal deletion analysis of bacterially expressed enzyme. Biochim. Biophys. Acta 1206:113–119.

Westerink B.H.C., De Vries J.B., and Duran R. (1990) Use of microdialysis for monitoring tyrosine hydroxylase activity in the brain of conscious rats. J. Neurochem. 54:381–387.

Wu J., Filer D., Friedhoff A.J., and Goldstein M. (1992) Site-directed mutagenesis of tyrosine hydroxylase. J. Biol. Chem. 267:25754–25758.

Yamauchi T., and Fujisawa H. (1981) Tyrosine-3-monooxygenase is phosphorylated by Ca^{2+}-calmodulin dependent protein kinase followed by activation by activator protein. Biochem. Biophys. Res. Commun. 100:807–813.

Zhou Q-Y., Qualfe C.J., and Palmiter R.D. (1995) Targeted disruption of the tyrosine hydroxylase gene reveals that catecholamines are required for mouse fetal development. Nature 374:640–643.

Zigmond R.E., Schwarzschild M.A., and Rittenhouse A.R. (1989) Acute regulation of tyrosine hydroxylase by nerve activity and by neurotransmitters via phosphorylation. Ann. Rev. Neurosci. 12:415–461.

Chapter 10

Tyrosine Hydroxylase and Endogenous Neurotoxins

Joachim Scholz and Andreas Moser

Contents in Brief

Tyrosine hydroxylase (L-tyrosine, tetrahydropteridine, oxygen: oxidoreductase (3-hydroxylating), EC 1.14.16.2) (TH) is the rate-limiting enzyme in catecholamine synthesis (Nagatsu et al., 1964). TH uses molecular oxygen and L-tyrosine as substrates. Since the K_m value for tyrosine is 10 µmol/L, the enzyme is virtually saturated under physiological conditions by the high tissue concentrations of endogenous tyrosine. (6R)-L-erythro-5,6,7,8-tetrahydrobiopterin (($6R$)BH$_4$) and iron are essential cofactors for the enzyme. TH catalyzes the formation of L-3,4-dihydroxyphenylalanin (dopa), the first step in dopamine (DA) synthesis (Fig. 1). The enzyme is localized in the cytosol of catecholaminergic cells.

1. Tyrosine Hydroxylase

1.1. Genetic aspects: Transcription and translation

Human TH cDNA and genomic DNA have been isolated and the nucleotide sequences have been determined (for review, see Nagatsu et al., 1993). Analysis of human DNA suggests the existence of a single gene per haploid DNA. 14 exons and 13 introns, together spanning approximately 8.5 kb, have been identified in the genomic DNA. Alternative splicing of the human TH pre-mRNA results in four mRNA species. They differ by the insertion or deletion of two sequences containing 12 bp and 81 bp, respectively (Fig. 2). Thus, four TH isoforms are generated, designated as type 1 to type 4. Type 1 is the shortest and is similar to the TH protein of various animal species. TH isoforms 1 and 2 represent the major species in both human *substantia nigra* (SN) and adrenal *medulla*. Recently, different splicing junctions with the skipping of exon 3 of the pre-mRNA were identified (Fig. 2) (Dumas et al.,

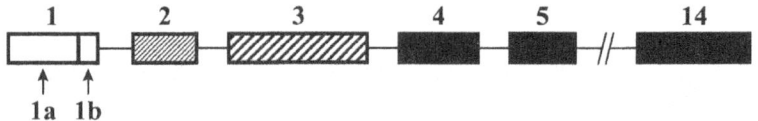

Fig. 1 The synthesis of dopa from L-tyrosine catalyzed by TH.

Human TH pre-mRNA

Alternative splicing

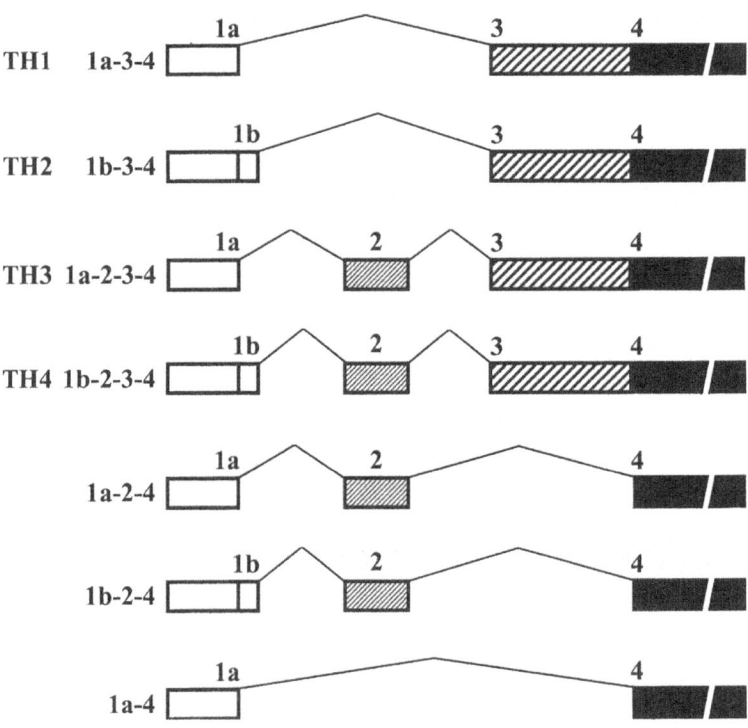

Fig. 2 Splicing patterns in the human TH pre-mRNA including the four previously described mRNA types and the recently identified species (according to Dumas et al., 1996). The boxes and lines represent exons and introns, respectively.

1996). The corresponding three additional TH isoforms were found in the adrenal *medulla* with a proportion of 4–6%. They were not detected in the SN. Remarkably, patients suffering from progressive supranuclear palsy showed significantly higher levels, that is 11–34% (Dumas et al., 1996). These findings indicate an impaired regulation in the alternative splicing. Further studies will have to demonstrate whether the abundance of the newly identified TH isoforms in the adrenal *medulla* is specific to this neurodegenerative disorder.

Previously, it has been suggested that multiplicity of TH mRNA exists only in primates. Two types corresponding to the human types 1 and 2 had been described in *Macaca iris* and *Macaca fuscata* (Ichikawa et al., 1990). They were found in the brain and in the adrenal *medulla*. Only single transcripts had been isolated and characterized from mouse (Ichikawa et al., 1991), quail (Fauquet et al., 1988), and cow (D'Mello et al., 1988). However, two isoforms of TH mRNA are generated by alternative splicing also in *Drosophila* (Birman et al., 1994). Recently, the group of Mallet and co-workers reported the presence of a second rat TH mRNA species. They identified a second transcript with deletion of exon 2 in the pre-mRNA in the adrenal *medulla,* but not in the catecholaminergic nuclei of the brain. The corresponding putative protein lacks a sequence of 33 amino acids in the N-terminal region (Lanièce et al., 1996).

1.2. Molecular structure

Rat, bovine and also human TH are tetrameric proteins of about 240 kDa molecular mass. Each of the four homogenous protein subunits has a molecular mass of about 60 kDa. The subunits possess a C-terminal catalytic domain and a regulatory domain at the N-terminal region. Heptad repeats of leucin residues at the C-terminal amino acid sequence are suggested to be involved in the tetramer formation. A leucine zipper motif seems to mediate the assembly of subunit dimers to the final tetramer (Vrana et al., 1994). Furthermore, C-terminal hydrophobic interactions presumably form a coiled-coil protein structure (Fig. 3). The mechanism of the dimer formation still remains to be elucidated.

At the catalytic domain, the active enzyme protein binds the substrates tyrosine and oxygen, the pterin cofactor $(6R)BH_4$ and iron. A complex interaction exists between TH activity and the cofactor $(6R)BH_4$. $(6R)BH_4$ is suggested to have an allosteric regulatory effect on TH and beyond that to change the substrate affinity of the enzyme (Minami et al., 1991). Phosphorylation at different serin residues of the N-terminal regulatory domain results in TH activation. Phosphorylation at Ser^{40} by the cAMP-dependent protein kinase A plays an important role in short-term regulation of TH activity (Vuillet et al., 1980). Other kinases catalyze phosphorylation at Ser^8, Ser^{19}, and Ser^{31} (Campbell et al., 1986; Haycock and Haycock, 1991). Phosphatase 2A dephosphorylates the enzyme protein after phosphorylation by protein kinase A (Haavik et al., 1989). An increase in TH activity is also mediated by the cGMP second messenger system (Roskoski et al., 1987). Nerve growth factor seems to have an effect on short-term activation of the enzyme and, furthermore, to enhance TH protein expression (Guroff, 1993). Finally, TH enzyme activity is submitted to feedback-inhibition by catecholamines (Okuno and Fujisawa, 1991).

1.3. Investigation of tyrosine hydroxylase expression

To investigate the interaction of neurotoxins with TH expression, we recently developed a quantitative method to label TH protein in homogenate of the rat brain by means of

A

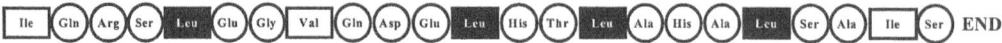

Ile Gln Arg Ser Leu Glu Gly Val Gln Asp Glu Leu His Thr Leu Ala His Ala Leu Ser Ala Ile Ser END

B

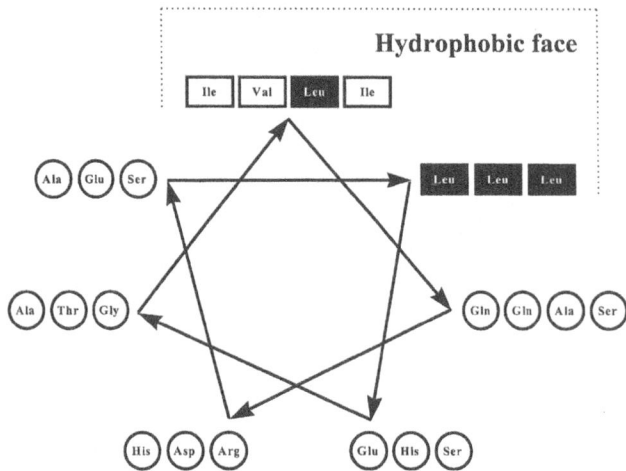

Fig. 3 (A) Amino acid sequence at the C-terminus of rat TH. Amino acids represented by squares are part of a 4-3 repeat presumably involved in hydrophobic interactions to form a coiled-coil protein structure. Heptad repeats of leucine residues are represented as filled squares. (B) Schematic draw of the C-terminal TH protein structure representing the leucine zipper motif and hydrophobic interactions suggested to be essential in the tetramer formation. (Modified from Vrana et al., 1994)

immunofluorescence. Immunolabeling was performed according to the method of Weissman and Pujol (Weissman et al., 1989) with certain modifications. In brief, rat brain is prepared in an ice-cold 5 mmol/L potassium phosphate buffer, pH 6.0. After 1:5 w/v mixture with the same buffer containing 0.2% Triton X-100, the tissue is homogenated. The homogenated tissue is centrifuged at 10 000 g at 4°C. Supernatant of control animals serves as protein source for standard dilutions. It is thoroughly mixed with increasing amounts of supernatant from centrifuged rat cerebellum homogenate in order to maintain constant protein concentrations in each standard. Finally, 1 µl of each dilution is deposited onto nitrocellulose sheets (Immobilon HAHY-NC, Millipore) and incubated as described below. Nonspecific binding sites are saturated by 30 min incubation with a 50 mmol/L Tris-buffered saline, pH 7.4, containing 1% bovine serum albumin (TBS/BSA). Subsequently, the nitrocellulose sheets are incubated at room temperature for 18 h together with a monoclonal anti-TH antibody (Boehringer) diluted 1:2000 in TBS/BSA. The tissues are washed in TBS/BSA three times for 10 min each and incubated in TBS/BSA containing protein A labeled with fluorescein isothiocyanate (ICN) (1:400) at room temperature for 2 h. The sheets are successively rinsed for 10 min with TBS/BSA, TBS and 500 mmol/L TBS. The dried sheets are mounted on glasses. A 1% w/v solution of mowiol 40–88 (Aldrich) protects the immunofluorescent labeling from fading. The labeled tissue is examined through a fluorescence microscope. The resulting images are digitalized and analyzed by a special

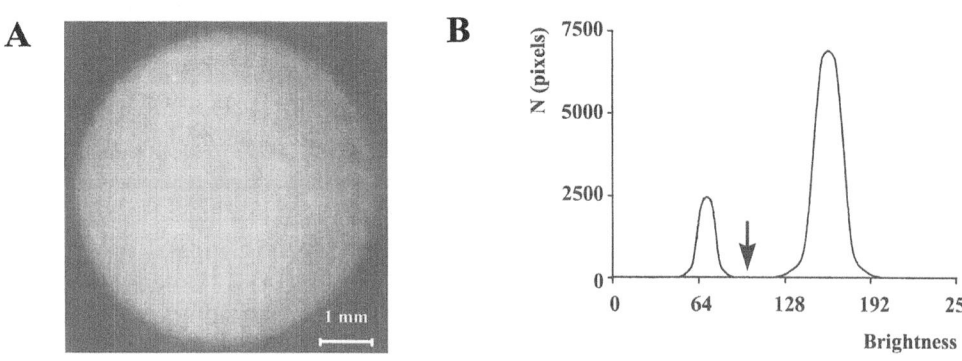

Fig. 4 (A) TH protein in homogenated striatal tissue immunolabeled with protein A fluorescent isothiocyanate conjugated, visualized by fluorescence microscopy. The digitalized signals appear on a gray-tone scale ranging from 1 to 256. (B) Schematic histogram showing brightness of pixels in the digitalized fluorescence signal. A threshold (*arrow*) is set to separate spectra of the background and the specific fluorescent signal, respectively.

software. Setting a threshold is necessary to separate specific immunofluorescence from the background (Fig. 4). Integration of brightness for area and comparison with the standard series permit quantification of the fluorescence signal.

Quantification of TH protein *in situ* by means of autoradiography has been described by Weissmann et al. (1989) and Raisman-Vozari et al. (1991). TH quantification has become possible even at the cellular level (Blanchard et al., 1993), and *in situ* hybridization of TH mRNA allows further insights in the process of protein expression.

1.4. An assay of tyrosine hydroxylase enzyme activity

The *nucleus accumbens* has been described as one of the rat brain regions with a high TH concentration (Hirata et al., 1983). We measured a basal TH activity of 20.1 ± 5.9 pmol dopa/min/mg protein. Brains were prepared in an ice-cold solution of 0.1 mol/L sodium phosphate buffer, pH 7.4. Tissues were homogenized by 3×10 strokes with 10 μl 0.1 mol/L phosphate buffer per mg tissue weight. The primary homogenate was diluted 1:4 using the same phosphate buffer. The enzyme assay was performed according to Naoi et al. (1988) with some modifications. The assay was composed of 20 μl homogenate containing approximately 40 μg protein, 2 mmol/L ferrous ammonium sulfate, 10 μg bovine catalase, 50 μmol/L NSD 1015 as inhibitor of dopa decarboxylase (aromatic L-amino acid decarboxylase, EC 4.1.1.28), 10 mmol/L sodium acetate buffer, pH 6.0, previously gassed with oxygen for 10 min. After a preincubation period of 5 min, the assay was started by the addition of 0.1 mmol/L L-tyrosine and 10 μmol/L 6,7-dimethyl-5,6,7,8-tetrahydropterin (DMPH$_4$) as cofactor. After 10 min, incubation was terminated by the addition of 33 ml/L perchloric acid containing 50 nmol/L L-α-methyl-dopa as internal chromatography standard. Both incubation and preincubation were performed at 37 °C. Dopa was measured by means of high performance liquid chromatography (HPLC) with electrochemical detection. A C18 column (Eurospher RP 18, particle size 5 μm, column size 250×4.0 mm) and a precolumn (column size 35×4.0 mm) were used. The mobile phase consisted of a degassed solution of 0.3 mmol/L disodium-EDTA, 0.52 mmol/L 1-sodium-octansulfonate,

115 ml/L methanol and 0.1 mol/L citrate buffer, pH 3.0. All chromatography was performed at 30°C. The separations were achieved under isocratic conditions. The detector cell operated at +0.8 V. Non-enzymatic formation of dopa was determined using 0.1 mmol/L D-tyrosine as substrate and 0.1 mmol/L α-methyl-L-p-tyrosine (αMpT) as known inhibitor of TH. Enzymatic dopa formation was calculated by total dopa synthesis minus non-enzymatic formation.

2. The Effect of Neurotoxins on Tyrosine Hydroxylase

2.1. Models of neurotoxicity involving tyrosine hydroxylase

A variety of experimental models has been developed using changes in TH expression as parameter of neurotoxicity in catecholaminergic cells. The loss of TH enzyme activity serves as an additional marker of toxic effects.

6-OH-dopamine and αMpT are the two neurotoxins used in the major part of previous studies. Other compounds with a distinct effect on TH enzyme activity in catecholaminergic neurons are 3-iodotyrosine and α-methyl-3-iodotyrosine.

In recent years, a model of neurotoxicity with high selectivity for dopaminergic neurons in the SN has been established based on the effects of 1-methyl-4-phenyl-1,2,3,6-tetrahydropyridine (MPTP). Hirata and Nagatsu (1985) described an inhibitory effect of MPTP on TH enzyme activity. TH inhibition by MPTP and its toxic metabolite 1-methyl-4-phenylpyridinium ion (MPP$^+$) has been confirmed in a series of studies. In regard of MPP$^+$, TH inhibition is suggested to result from interference with the cofactor $(6R)BH_4$ (Maruyama and Naoi, 1994) and, moreover, with the enzyme activation through phosphorylation (Kiuchi et al., 1988).

2.2. Quinoline and isoquinoline derivatives

Booth et al. (1989) published one of the first comparative studies of the neurotoxicity of quinoline and isoquinoline derivatives. Using an *in vivo* microdialysis technique, they measured the striatal DA release after perfusion of the test compound. The effects of quinoline, isoquinoline, their N-methylated quaternary salts, N-methylquinolinium ion (1-MQ$^+$) and N-methylisoquinolinium ion (2-MIQ$^+$), and the corresponding 1,2,3,4-tetrahydro-analogues tetrahydroquinoline, tetrahydroisoquinoline (TIQ), N-methyl-tetrahydroquinoline and N-methyl-tetrahydroisoquinoline (2-MTIQ) were studied. Only 1-MQ$^+$ and 2-MIQ$^+$ were found to produce significant changes in DA release. These authors concluded that N-methylation is essential for the neurotoxicity of quinoline and isoquinoline derivatives. This conclusion is supported by the fact that methylated isoquinolines have also been described to severely interfere with DA degradation by monoamine oxidase (monoamine: oxygen oxidoreductase (deaminating), EC 1.4.3.4) (Naoi et al., 1987, 1988; for more details, see Chapter 11). Booth et al. (1989), however, did not investigate whether the reduction of DA release was a result of a decreased transmitter synthesis. Since we have demonstrated that TIQ is able to modulate DA release in slices of the rat caudate-putamen by inhibiting the DA reuptake transporter system of presynaptic dopaminergic membranes (Scholz et al., 1996), it appears not to be justified to deduce the evidence of DA synthesis from changes in the transmitter release.

The reduction of DA concentrations in basal ganglia induced by local or systemic application of quinoline and isoquinoline derivatives *in vivo* has provided the first evidence of their toxic effects on catecholamine synthesis. Nagatsu and Yoshida (1988) subcutaneously injected TIQ (50 mg/kg per day, for 11 days) in marmosets. They found a reduction of DA concentrations in the substantia nigra to 28.4 and 31.5 % of control animals, respectively. Intrastriatal DA concentrations differed considerably, but maximal reduction reached 43.5% of controls. In an experimental condition with chronic TIQ application to squirrel monkeys, intranigral DA was measured to be 23%, 25% and 53% of control, respectively. Intrastriatal changes were not reproducible (Yoshida et al., 1990). In both studies, the biochemical changes correlated with parkinsonism observed in the treated animals. Naoi et al. (1996) demonstrated an even more pronounced, substantial loss of DA in the rat basal ganglia after intrastriatal injection of the isoquinoline derivative 1,2-dimethyl-6,7-dihydroxy-1,2,3,4-tetrahydroisoquinoline (1,2-DDTIQ) and its oxidation product 1,2-dimethyl-6,7-dihydroxyisoquinolinium ion (1,2-DDIQ$^+$). DA concentration in the striatum was less than 50 % for both compounds, whereas a complete loss of DA was observed in the substantia nigra after intrastriatal injection of 100 nmol 1,2-DDTIQ or 1,2-DDIQ$^+$, respectively (Naoi et al., 1996). The authors also reported parkinsonian symptoms in the treated rats. Taken together, these results might indicate a reduction in DA synthesis. On the other hand, an increased metabolism of DA would likewise result in decreases of DA concentrations.

There are, however, some arguments against the hypothesis that DA is decreased just because of an increased metabolism in the presence of quinoline or isoquinoline derivatives. First, the concentration of 3,4-dihydroxyphenylacetic acid (DOPAC) as one of the main metabolites in DA oxidation was decreased in the model of Naoi et al. (1996), whereas homovanillic acid (HVA) was found to be increased. Furthermore, studies on the effect of quinoline and a series of isoquinoline derivatives on monoamine oxidase type A and B have demonstrated inhibition of the enzyme (for details and references, see Chapter 11). Finally, *in vivo* experiments with short-term measurements of catecholamines showed an increase of DA in the *corpus striatum* and in the SN as well. Maruyama et al. (1992) found an increase in DA from 1.73 ± 0.49 to 356 ± 177 nmol/L after 120 min intrastriatal microdialysis of 1 mmol/L 1-methyl-6,7-dihydroxy-1,2,3,4-tetrahydroisoquinoline (salsolinol, 1-MDTIQ) in rats. The concentrations of DOPAC and HVA decreased to 24.3 ± 26.7% and 33.5 ± 8.98% of baseline values, respectively.

In conclusion, microdialysis of isoquinoline derivates, first, seems to stimulate DA release. This effect lasts for minutes to a few hours. Measurements several days after systemic administration of TIQ and its methylated and hydroxylated derivatives showed that DA formation decreases under baseline levels. Similar results with a biphasic effect on DA concentrations have been described for MPTP (Burns et al., 1983).

The effects of TIQ derivatives on DA synthesis have been studied in more detail by Weiner and Collins (1978). They assayed homogenates of the whole rat brain together with 1-MDTIQ, 3-carboxy-salsolinol, 4,6,7-trihydroxy-1,2,3,4-tetrahydroisoquinoline and tetrahydropapaveroline (1-(3′,4′-dihydroxybenzyl)-6,7-dihydroxy-1,2,3,4-tetrahydroisoquinoline). Only 1-MDTIQ and to a lesser extent 3-carboxy-salsolinol significantly inhibited TH-activity *in vitro*. K_i was calculated 1.38 × 10^{-5} mol/L. The authors suggested a type of enzyme inhibition competitive to the synthetic pteridine cofactor used in their TH assay. After intraperitoneal administration of 1-MDTIQ (50 mg/kg), no effect on dopa synthesis was observed *in vivo* (Weiner and Collins, 1978). TH inhibition by 1-MDTIQ was recently confirmed by the studies of Minami et al. (1992) and Maruyama et al. (1993). In contrast to the statement of Booth et al. (1989), these results demonstrated that tetrahydro-derivatives of quinolines have a neurotoxic potential and interfere with DA synthesis. In a more recent study, Maruyama et al. (1993) compared the effect of TIQ derivatives on tyrosine hydroxylation. In this assay, the authors added different 6,7-dihydroxylated TIQ derivatives to the culture medium of rat pheochromocytoma PC12h cells and described 2-MDTIQ to be the most potent inhibitor with an IC_{50} of about 10 μmol/L (Maruyama et al., 1993).

1-MDTIQ, 2-MDTIQ and 1,2-DDTIQ at concentrations of pmol/L have been identified in the cerebrospinal fluid (CSF) or the brains of patients with Parkinson's disease (PD) (Niwa et al., 1991; Moser and Kömpf, 1992; Maruyama et al., 1996). These TIQ derivatives, structurally related to MPTP, might represent the products of a condensation reaction with DA in an impaired DA metabolism (Moser et al., 1995). PD results from the degeneration of dopaminergic neurons in the SN and a subsequent imbalance of neurotransmitters in the basal ganglia. Thus, it might be crucial for the pathophysiological understanding of the disease to know whether there is an interference of these compounds with DA synthesis.

As mentioned above, TH inhibition by 1-MDTIQ had been described in several studies (Weiner and Collins, 1978; Minami et al., 1992; Maruyama et al., 1993). When Maruyama et al. (1993) reported an inhibitory effect of 2-MDTIQ on TH in cultured rat pheochromocytoma cells, the question was raised whether 2-MDTIQ has a similar effect on DA synthesis in brain tissue. Therefore, we assayed homogenated tissue of the rat *nucleus accumbens* together with 2-MDTIQ and measured tyrosine hydroxylation. 2-MDTIQ dose-dependently inhibited dopa formation (Fig. 5). TH activity was decreased to 50% at approximately 10 μmol/L 2-MDTIQ. Enzyme activity was completely blocked at 0.1 mmol/L. In the diagram according to Lineweaver and Burk, a noncompetitive type of inhibition was suggested. Since the degree of enzyme inhibition by 10 μmol/L 2-MDTIQ did not change with different $DMPH_4$ concentrations, the inhibitory mechanism seemed to be independent of the TH cofactor (Scholz et al., 1997). Interestingly, Maruyama et al. (1993) had reported the same IC_{50} in their assay using cultured rat pheochromcocytoma PC12h cells. Furthermore, Hirata and Nagatsu (1985) had examined the inhibition of TH by MPTP in tissue slices of the *corpus striatum* and the *nucleus accumbens* of the rat and also found an IC_{50} of 10 μmol/L. Consequently, 2-MDTIQ showed the same inhibitory potential in our assay compared to MPTP in their study.

An inhibitory effect on TH activity has been described for a series of other TIQ derivatives. When compared with 2-MDTIQ, a weaker inhibitory effect was observed with 2-MIQ^+, 6,7-dihydroxy-1,2,3,4-tetrahydroisoquinoline, 2-MTIQ, and 1,2-DDTIQ (Naoi et al., 1989; Maruyama et al., 1993; Naoi et al., 1996). For striatal tissue of the rat, an inhibitory effect of 1,2,3,4-tetrahydro-2-methyl-4,6,7-isoquinolinetriol (2-MTTIQ) was reported by Liptrot et al. (1994). The IC_{50} of this TIQ derivative was 4 μmol/L. Since there are several reports of TH inhibition by 6,7-hydroxylated TIQ derivatives including our own results, we cannot support the assumption of the latter authors that 4,6,7-hydroxylation of methylated TIQ derivatives is essential for an effective inhibition of TH. Moreover, we found no evidence for an interaction of 2-MDTIQ with the TH cofactor $(6R)BH4$ as discussed by these authors. In their assay, however, a higher concentration of the cofactor, 50 mmol/L, was used to reverse the decrease in TH activity caused by 2-MTTIQ. A reversal of TH inhibition by very high tetrahydrobiopterin concentrations was also reported for 2-MIQ^+ (Naoi et al., 1989). Weiner and Collins (1978) even suggested a competitive interaction of 1-MDTIQ and the pteridine cofactor used in their assay. A complex interaction of 1-MDTIQ with the natural cofactor $(6R)BH_4$ was described by Minami et al. (1992). According to these authors, 1-MDTIQ interferes with TH affinity towards the cofactor. An interaction of TIQ derivatives with $(6R)BH_4$ would be of special importance since $(6R)BH_4$

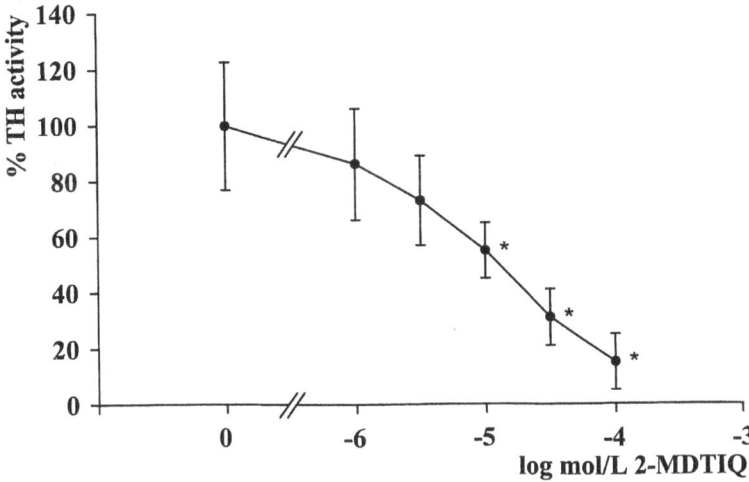

Fig. 5 TH activity in the presence of 2-MDTIQ. Molar 2-MDTIQ concentrations are given as logarithms. TH activity is represented as percentage of basal activity. Basal TH activity was 20.1 ± 5.9 pmol DOPA/min/mg protein (=100%). Values represent means ± standard deviations obtained from 6 determinations for each experimental condition. Statistical analysis used ANOVA for testing differences from basal TH activity, *p-value < 0.05.

seems to influence the conformation of the tetrameric protein TH (Minami et al., 1991; Minami et al., 1992).

Recently, inhibition of TH was described for 1-benzyl- (1-BDTIQ) and 1-phenyl-6,7-dihydroxy-1,2,3,4-tetrahydroisoquinoline (1-PDTIQ). A competitive type of inhibition was discussed. K_i was 5 μmol/L and 3 μmol/L for 1-BDTIQ and 1-PDTIQ, respectively. The authors suggested that these TIQ derivatives may represent the products of a non-enzymatic condensation of DA with organic solvents (Smargiassi et al., 1994). 1-BDTIQ has also been described in the CSF of patients with PD and in a control group consisting of patients suffering from other neurological diseases (Kotake et al., 1995). 1-BDTIQ was found at three times higher concentrations in patients with PD, mean value 1.17 ± 0.35 ng/ml, than in controls, but the difference was not statistically significant.

There are several reports of *in vivo* administration of TIQ derivatives to primates and other animals which demonstrated a clinical effect by producing parkinsonian syndromes. In two studies with subcutaneous application of TIQ in squirrel monkeys or common marmosets, respectively, a remarkable decrease in TH activity was found in the SN when the brains of the treated animals were examined *post mortem*. No significant changes were measured in the *corpus striatum* even after 60 days of treatment with 20 mg/kg TIQ. A neuronal loss in the *substantia nigra pars compacta* (SNc) was not observed (Nagatsu and Yoshida, 1988; Yoshida et al., 1990).

In contrast, repeated subcutaneous injections of TIQ in C57BL/6J mice resulted in a significant reduction of TH-immunoreactive neurons in the SNc as well as in the ventral tegmental area (VTA). The cell size was reduced, but no cell death was observed (Ogawa et al., 1989). The authors concluded that TIQ led to a diminished TH production in dopaminergic neurons of the mesencephalon before cell death occurred. Fukuda (1994) reported a dose-dependent decrease in TH-immunoreactive neurons in the SN of C57BL/6J mice after intraperitoneal treatment with 2-MTIQ. Within the SNc, the changes were more pronounced in the central portion. 2-MTIQ doses of 16 mg/kg led to a loss of nerve cells in the medial portion of the SNc, whereas a specific loss of TH-immunoreactive neurons was observed both, in the medial and also in the central portion, even at lower doses. A reduction in TH-positive cells was also seen in the VTA and in the *locus ceruleus* (Fukuda, 1994). A loss of TH-immunoreactivity without significant cell death was observed in the SN but not the VTA of Wistar rats continuously treated with local injections of 1,2-DDTIQ into the *corpus striatum* (Naoi et al., 1996).

2.3. β-Carbolines

Besides TIQ derivatives, β-carbolines (βC) represent another class of heterocyclic compounds assumed to be endogenously formed neurotoxins related to biochemical changes in PD (see Chapter 5). Collins and Neafsey (1985) and Ohkubo et al. (1985) first suggested βC as possible neurotoxins in the context of PD because of their structural similarity to MPTP. Endogenous formation from condensation of tryptamine or related substituted indoleamines with naturally occurring aldehydes of α-ketoacids was discussed. Recently, norharman, 2-methyl-norharmanium ion, harman, and to a lesser extent 2-methylharmanium ion have been identified in the CSF of patients with PD and controls by means of HPLC/fluorescence detection. Significant differences between patients and controls were found for 2,9-dimethyl-norharmanium ion and 2,9-dimethylharmanium ion, but the latter was detected only at a neglegible level. All concentrations were in the range of fmol/ml (Matsubara et al., 1995a).

The assumption that βC interfere with the dopaminergic metabolism was further supported by the observation of significant reductions in rat striatal concentrations of DA, DOPAC and HVA following intranigral injections of 40 nmol 2,9-dimethyl-norharman (2,9-DNH), 2-methylharman, 2,9-dimethylharman (2,9-DHA). Norharman, 2-methyl-norharman, and 2-methylharmaline were effective only in a higher dose of 200 nmol. When compared with 40 nmol MPP$^+$, which caused a DA reduction to 0.6% of controls, the most effective among the βC derivatives were 2,9-DHA with a decrease to 37% and 2,9-DNH with 42% of controls (Neafsey et al., 1995). However, Perry et al. (1986, 1987) found no changes in DA or metabolites after systemic treatment of mice and marmosets with 2-methyl-1,2,3,4-tetrahydro-β-carboline.

There is only few data about βC with structural analogy to MPTP and their effect on TH activity. A rapid reduction of striatal dopa formation was seen after stereotactical application of N-methyl-β-carbolinium ion (2-MβC$^+$) in rats (Matsubara et al., 1995b). In this study, a marked reversible decrease to 10% of the basal dopa level was observed with 1 mmol/L 2-MβC$^+$. A direct interaction of 2-MβC$^+$ with the enzyme was suggested because of the rapid reduction of TH activity. In contrast, MPP$^+$ lead to a graduate but irreversible inhibition of tyrosine hydroxylation. These results are partially conflicting with pharmacological studies on benzodiazepine inverse agonists with a βC structure like 2-methyl-β-carboline-3-carboxyamide (FG-7142). There are several reports describing an increase in DA release in the prefrontal cortex but not in the *corpus striatum* (for example Bradberry et al., 1991). The enzyme activity of TH was found to be significantly increased in the rat prefrontal cortex *in vivo* and *in vitro*, whereas no changes in TH activity *in vivo* could be observed in the caudate-putamen or the *nucleus accumbens* (Knorr et al., 1989). Examination of TH activity in rat striatal slices *in vitro,* however, demonstrated a decrease in dopa formation. As a hypothesis, TH stimulation in the prefrontal cortex *in vivo* was at least to some extent mediated through benzodiazepine receptors on dopaminergic cells in the VTA and subsequent activition of prefrontal afferents. The precise mechanism whereby FG-7142 has different effects on prefrontal and striatal TH activity in the *in vitro* experiments remained unclear (Knorr et al., 1989).

3. Summary

TH represents a complex enzyme system. From the expression of the different protein isoforms over the formation of the tetrameric structure to the enzymatic function itself, any alteration by neurotoxins is suggested to severely impair tyrosine hydroxylation, the rate-limiting step of catecholamine synthesis. TIQ derivatives and βC are possible candidates for endogenously synthesized neurotoxins in the context of PD. 1-MDTIQ, 2-MDTIQ, 1,2-DDTIQ and different βC derivatives have been identified in patients with PD. They are of striking structural similarity to MPTP, a toxic compound that caused severe parkinsonian syndromes in humans. Inhibition of TH enzyme activity by TIQ derivatives has been confirmed in various experimental conditions. 2-MDTIQ and 2-MTTIQ appear to be the most potent inhibitors *in vitro*. There is evidence of an interference with the cofactor $(6R)BH_4$, but the results are somewhat conflicting and the mechanism of enzyme inhibition by TIQ derivatives has to be the subject of further studies. *In vivo* experiments have demonstrated the reduction of TH expression in dopaminergic neurons caused by TIQ, 2-MTIQ, and 1,2-DDTIQ, but no cell death occurred. There is only few data on the effect of βC derivatives on TH. MPTP analogue βC derivatives were reported to reduce DA levels in the rat basal ganglia and TH inhibition has been shown for 2-MβC$^+$. In contrast, stimulation of TH activity in the prefrontal cortex has been described for benzodiazepine receptor inverse agonists with a βC structure. Thus, further research work is necessary to understand these contradictory results.

List of abbreviations

αMpT	α-Methyl-L-p-tyrosine
βC	β-Carboline
1-BDTIQ	1-Benzyl-6,7-dihydroxy-1,2,3,4-tetrahydroisoquinoline
bp	Base pair
cAMP	3'5'-Cyclic adenosine monophosphate
cGMP	3'5'-Cyclic guanosine monophosphate
cDNA	Complementary deoxyribonucleic acid
CSF	Cerebrospinal fluid
DA	Dopamine
1,2-DDIQ$^+$	1,2-Dimethyl-6,7-dihydroxyisoquinolinium ion
1,2-DDTIQ	1,2-Dimethyl-6,7-dihydroxy-1,2,3,4-tetrahydroisoquinoline
2,9-DHA	2,9-Dimethylharman
DMPH$_4$	6,7-Dimethyl-5,6,7,8-tetrahydropterin
DNA	Deoxyribonucleic acid

2,9-DNH	2,9-Dimethyl-norharman
dopa	L-3,4-Dihydroxyphenylalanin
DOPAC	3,4-Dihydroxyphenylacetic acid
FG-7142	2-Methyl-β-carboline-3-carboxyamide
HVA	Homovanillic acid
kb	Kilobase
kDa	Kilodalton
2-MβC$^+$	N-Methyl-β-carbolinium ion
1-MDTIQ	1-Methyl-6,7-dihydroxy-1,2,3,4-tetrahydroisoquinoline (salsolinol)
2-MDTIQ	2-Methyl-6,7-dihydroxy-1,2,3,4-tetrahydroisoquinoline
2-MIQ$^+$	N-Methylisoquinolinium ion
MPP$^+$	1-Methyl-4-phenylpyridinium ion
MPTP	1-Methyl-4-phenyl-1,2,3,6-tetrahydropyridine
1-MQ$^+$	N-Methylquinolinium ion
mRNA	Messenger ribonucleic acid
2-MTIQ	N-Methyl-tetrahydroisoquinoline
2-MTTIQ	1,2,3,4-Tetrahydro-2-methyl-4,6,7-isoquinolinetriol
PD	Parkinson's disease
1-PDTIQ	1-Phenyl-6,7-dihydroxy-1,2,3,4-tetrahydroisoquinoline
(6R)BH$_4$	(6R)-L-erythro-5,6,7,8-tetrahydrobiopterin
SN	*Substantia nigra*
SNc	*Substantia nigra pars compacta*
TH	Tyrosine hydroxylase
TIQ	1,2,3,4-Tetrahydroisoquinoline
VTA	Ventral tegmental area
w/v	Weight/volume

References

Birman S., Morgan B., Anzvino M., and Hirsh J. (1994) A novel and major isoform of tyrosine hydroxylase in Drosophila is generated by alternative RNA processing. J. Biol. Chem. 269:1–9.

Blanchard V., Raisman-Vozari R., Savasta M., Hirsch E., Javoy-Agid F., Feuerstein C., and Agid Y. (1993) Cellular quantification of tyrosine hydroxylase in the rat brain by immunoautoradiography. J. Neurochem. 61:617–626.

Booth R.G., Castagnoli N., and Rollema H. (1989) Intracerebral microdialysis neurotoxicity studies of quinoline and isoquinoline derivatives related to MPTP/MPP$^+$. Neurosci. Lett. 100:306–312.

Bradberry C.W., Lory J.D., and Roth R.H. (1991) The anxiogenic beta-carboline FG 7142 selectively increases dopamine release in rat prefrontal cortex as measured by microdialysis. J. Neurochem. 56:748–752.

Burns R.S., Chiueh C.C., Markey S.P., Ebert M.H., Jacobowitz D.M., and Kopin I.J. (1983) A primate model of parkinsonism: selective destruction of dopaminergic neurons in the pars compacta of the substantia nigra by N-methyl-4-phenyl-1,2,3,6-tetrahydropyridine. Proc. Natl. Acad. USA 80:4546–4550.

Campbell D.G., Hardie D.G., and Vuillet P.R. (1986) Identification of four phosphorylation sites in the *N*-terminal region of tyrosine hydroxylase. J. Biol. Chem. 261:10489–10492.

Collins M.A., and Neafsey E.J. (1985) β-Carboline analogs of *N*-methyl-4-phenyl-1,2,5,6-tetrahydropyridine (MPTP): endogenous factors underlying idiopathic parkinsonism? Neurosci. Lett. 55:179–184.

D'Mello S.R., Weisberg E.P., Stachowiak M.K., Turzai L.M., Gioio A.E., and Kaplan, B.B. (1988) Isolation and nucleotide sequence of a cDNA clone encoding bovine adrenal tyrosine hydroxylase: comparative analysis of tyrosine hydroxylase gene products. J. Neurosci. Res. 19:440–449.

Dumas S., Le Hir H., Bodeau-Péan S., Hirsch E., Thermes C., and Mallet J. (1996) New species of human tyrosine hydroxylase mRNA are produced in variable amounts in adrenal medulla and are overexpressed in progressive supranuclear palsy. J. Neurochem. 67:19–25.

Fauquet M., Grima B., Lamouroux A., and Mallet J. (1988) Cloning of quail tyrosine hydroxylase amino acid homology with other hydroxylases discloses functional domains. J. Neurochem. 50:142–148.

Fukuda T. (1994) 2-Methyl-1,2,3,4-tetrahydroisoquinoline does dose-dependently reduce the number of tyrosine hydroxylase-immunoreactive cells in the substantia nigra and locus ceruleus of C57BL/6J mice. Brain Res. 639:325–328.

Guroff G. (1993) The influence of nerve growth factor on the level and activity of tyrosine hydroxylase. In: Tyrosine Hydroxylase (Naoi M. and Parvez S.H., eds.), pp. 177–191. VSP, Utrecht.

Haavik J., Schelling D.L., Campbell D.G., Andersson K.K., Flatmark T., and Cohen P. (1989) Identification of protein phosphatase 2A as the major tyrosine hydroxylase phosphatase in adrenal medulla and corpus striatum: evidence from the effects of okadaic acid. FEBS Lett. 251:36–42.

Haycock J.W., and Haycock D.A. (1991) Tyrosine hydroxylase in rat brain dopaminergic nerve terminals: multiple-site phosphorylation in vivo and in synaptosomes. J. Biol. Chem. 266:5650–5657.

Hirata Y., Togari A., and Nagatsu T. (1983) Studies on tyrosine hydroxylase system in rat brain slices using high-performance liquid chromatography with electrochemical detection. J. Neurochem. 40:1585–1589.

Hirata Y., and Nagatsu T. (1985) Inhibition of tyrosine hydroxylation in tissue slices of the rat corpus striatum by 1-methyl-4-phenyl-1,2,3,6-tetrahydropyridine. Brain Res. 337: 193–196.

Ichikawa S., Ichinose H., and Nagatsu T. (1990) Multiple mRNAs of monkey tyrosine hydroxylase. Biochem. Biophys. Res. Comm. 173:1331–1336.

Ichikawa S., Sasaoka T., and Nagatsu T. (1990) Primary structure of mouse tyrosine hydroxylase deduced from its cDNA. Biochem. Biophys. Res. Comm. 176:1610–1616.

Kiuchi K., Hagiwara M., Hidaka H., and Nagatsu T. (1988) Effect of the 1-methyl-4-phenylpyridinium ion on phosphorylation of tyrosine hydroxylase in rat pheochromocytoma PC12h cells. Neurosci. Lett. 89:209–15.

Knorr A.M., Deutch A.Y., and Roth R.H. (1989) The anxiogenic β-carboline FG-7142 increases *in vivo* and *in vitro* tyrosine hydroxylation in the prefrontal cortex. Brain Res. 495:355–361.

Kotake Y., Tasaki Y., Makino Y., Ohta S., and Hirobe M. (1995) 1-Benzyl-1,2,3,4-tetrahydroisoquinoline as a parkinsonism-inducing agent: a novel endogenous amine in mouse brain and parkinsonian CSF. J. Neurochem. 65:2633–2638.

Lanièce P., Le Hir H., Bodeau-Péan S., Charon Y., Valentin L., Thermes C., Mallet J., and Dumas S. (1996) A novel rat tyrosine hydroxylase mRNA species generated by alternative splicing. J. Neurochem. 66:1819–1825.

Liptrot J., Holdup D., and Phillipson O. (1994) 1,2,3,4-Tetrahydro-2-methyl-4,6,7-isoquinolinetriol inhibits tyrosine hydroxylase activity in rat striatal synaptosomes. J. Neural. Transm. [Gen. Sect.] 96:51–62.

Maruyama W., Nakahara D., Ota M., Takahashi T., Takahashi A., Nagatsu T., and Naoi M. (1992) N-methylation of dopamine-derived 6,7-dihydroxy-1,2,3,4-tetrahydroisoquinoline, (R)-salsolinol, in rat brains: in vivo microdialysis study. J. Neurochem. 59: 395–400.

Maruyama W., Takahashi T., Minami M., Takahashi A., Dostert P., Nagatsu T., and Naoi M. (1993) Cytotoxicity of dopamine-derived 6,7-dihydroxy-1,2,3,4-tetrahydroisoquinolines. Adv. Neurol. 60:224–230.

Maruyama W., and Naoi M. (1994) Inhibiton of tyrosine hydroxylase by a dopamine neurotoxin, 1-methyl-4-phenylpyridinium ion: depletion of allostery to the biopterin cofactor. Life Sci. 55:207–212.

Maruyama W., Narabayashi H., Dostert P., and Naoi M. (1996) Stereospecific occurrence of a parkinsonism-inducing catechol isoquinoline, N-methyl(R)salsolinol, in the human intraventricular fluid. J. Neural Transm. 103:1069–1076.

Matsubara K., Kobayashi S., Kobayashi Y., Yamashita K., Koide H., Hatta M., Iwamato K., Tanaka O., and Kimura K. (1995a) β-Carbolinium cations, endogenous MPP[+] analogs, in the lumbar cerebrospinal fluid of patients with Parkinson's disease. Neurology 45: 2240–2245.

Matsubara K., Idzu T., Kobayashi Y., Nakahara D., Maruyama W., Kobayashi S., Kimura K., and Naoi M. (1995b) N-Methyl-4-phenylpyridinium and an endogenously formed analog, N-methyl-β-carbolinium, inhibit striatal tyrosine hydroxylation in freely moving rats. Neurosci. Lett. 199:199–202.

Minami M., Takahashi T., Maruyama W., Takahashi A., Nagatsu T., and Naoi M. (1991) Allosteric effect of tetrahydrobiopterin cofactors on tyrosine hydroxylase activity. Life Sci. 50:15–20.

Minami M., Takahashi T., Maruyama W., Takahashi A., Dostert P., Nagatsu T., and Naoi M. (1992) Inhibition of tyrosine hydroxylase by R and S enantiomers of salsolinol, 1-methyl-6,7-dihydroxy-1,2,3,4-tetrahydroisoquinoline. J. Neurochem. 58:2097–2101.

Moser A., and Kömpf D. (1992) Presence of methyl-6,7-dihydroxy-1,2,3,4-tetrahydroisoquinolines, derivatives of the neurotoxin isoquinoline, in parkinsonian lumbar CSF. Life Sci. 50:1885–1891.

Moser A., Scholz J., Nobbe F., Vieregge P., Böhme V., and Bamberg H. (1995) Presence of N-methyl-norsalsolinol in the CSF: correlations with dopamine metabolites of patients with Parkinson's disease. J. Neurol. Sci. 131:183–189

Nagatsu T., Levitt M., and Udenfried S. (1964) Tyrosin hydroxylase. The initial step in norepinephrine biosynthesis. J. Biol. Chem. 239:2910–2917.

Nagatsu T., and Yoshida M. (1988) An endogenous substance of the brain, tetrahydroisoquinoline, produces parkinsonism in primates with decreased dopamine, tyrosine hydroxylase and biopterin in the nigrostriatal regions. Neurosci. Lett. 87:178 182.

Nagatsu T., Kaneda N., Kobayashi K., Ichinose H., Sasaoka T., Kiuchi K., Fujita K., and

Kurosawa Y. (1993) The human tyrosine hydroxylase gene. In: Tyrosine Hydroxylase (Naoi M. and Parvez S. H., eds), pp. 177–191. VSP, Utrecht.

Naoi M., Takahashi T., and Nagatsu T. (1988) Simple assay procedure for tyrosine hydroxylase activity by high-performance liquid chromatography employing coulometric detection with minimal sample preparation. J. Chromatogr. 427:229–238.

Naoi M., Takahashi T., Parvez H., Kabeya R., Taguchi E., Yamaguchi K., Hirata Y., Minami M., and Nagatsu T. (1989) *N*-Methylisoquinolinium ion as an inhibitor of tyrosine hydroxylase, aromatic L-amino acid decarboxylase and monoamine oxidase. Neurochem. Int. 15:315–320.

Naoi M., Maruyama W., Dostert P., Hashizume Y., Nakahara D., Takahashi T., and Ota M. (1996) Dopamine-derived endogenous 1(*R*),2(*N*)-dimethyl-6,7-dihydroxy-1,2,3,4-tetrahydroisoquinoline, *N*-methyl-(*R*)-salsolinol, induced parkinsonism in rat: biochemical, pathological and behavioral studies. Brain Res. 709:285–295.

Neafsey E.J., Albores R., Gerhart D., Kindel G., Raikoff K., Tamayo P., and Collins M.A. (1995) Methyl-β-carbolinium analogs of MPP$^+$ cause nigrostriatal toxicity after substantia nigra injections in rat. Brain Res. 675:279–288.

Niwa T., Takeda N., Yoshizumi H., Tatematsu A., Yoshida M., Dostert P., Naoi M., and Nagatsu T. (1991) Presence of 2-methyl-6,7-dihydroxy-1,2,3,4-tetrahydroisoquinoline and 1,2-dimethyl-6,7-dihydroxy-1,2,3,4-tetrahydroisoquinoline, novel endogenous amines, in parkinsonian and normal human brains. Biochem. Biophys. Res. Comm. 177:603–609.

Ogawa M., Araki M., Nagatsu I., Nagatsu T., and Yoshida M. (1989) The effect of 1,2,3,4-tetrahydroisoquinoline (TIQ) on mesencephalic dopaminergic neurons in C57BL/6J mice: Immunohistochemical studies—Tyrosine hydroxylase. Biogenic Amines 6:427–436.

Ohkubo S., Hirano T., and Oka K. (1985) Methyltetrahydro-β-carbolines and Parkinson's disease. Lancet I:1272–1273.

Okuno S., and Fujisawa H. (1991) Conversion of tyrosine hydroxylase to stable and inactive form by end products. J. Neurochem. 57:53–60.

Perry T.L., Yong V.W., Wall R.A., and Jones K. (1986) Paraquat and two endogenous analogues of the neurotoxic substance N-methyl-4-phenyl-1,2,3,6-tetrahydropyridine do not damage dopaminergic nigrostriatal neurons in the mouse. Neurosci. Lett. 69:285–289.

Perry T.L., Jones K., Hansen S., and Wall R.A. (1987) 4-Phenylpyridine and three other analogues of 1-methyl-4-phenyl-1,2,3,6-tetrahydropyridine lack dopaminergic nigrostriatal neurotoxicity in mice and marmosets. Neurosci. Lett. 75:65–70.

Raisman-Vozari R., Hirsch E., Javoy-Agid F., Vassort C., Savasta M., Feuerstein C., Thibault J., and Agid Y (1991) Quantitative autoradiography of tyrosine hydroxylase immunoreactivity in the rat brain. J. Neurochem. 57:1212–1222.

Roskoski R. Jr., and Roskoski L.M. (1987) Activation of tyrosine hydroxylase in PC12h cells by the cyclic GMP and cyclic AMP second messenger systems. J. Neurochem. 48:236–242.

Scholz J., Sippel K., and Moser A. (1996) The effect of tetrahydroisoquinoline on striatal dopamine release of the rat *in vitro*. J. Neurol. 243 (Suppl. 2):S75.

Scholz J., Bamberg H., and Moser A. (1997) *N*-Methyl-norsalsolinol, an endogenous neurotoxin, inhibits tyrosine hydroxylase activity in the rat brain nucleus accumbens *in vitro*. Neurochem. Int., in press.

Smargiassi A., Biagini C., Mutti A., Bergamaschi E., Bacchini A., Alinovi R., and Cavazzini S. (1994) Multiple interferences on catecholamine metabolism by tetrahydroisoquinolines (TIQs). Neurotoxicology 15:765–767.

Vrana K.E., Walker S.J., Rucker P., and Liu X. (1994) A carboxyl terminal leucin zipper is required for tyrosine hydroxylase tetramer formation. J. Neurochem. 63:2013–2020.

Vuillet P.R., Langan T.A., and Weiner N. (1980) Tyrosine hydroxylase: a substrate of cyclic AMP-dependent protein kinase. Proc. Natl. Acad. Sci. USA 77:92–96.

Weiner C.D., and Collins M.A. (1978) Tetrahydroisoquinolines derived from catecholamines or dopa: effects on brain tyrosine hydroxylase activity. Biochem. Pharmacol. 27:2699–2703.

Weissmann D., Labatut R., Richard F., Rousset C., and Pujol J.F. (1989) Direct transfer into nitrocellulose and quantitative radioautographic anatomical determination of brain tyrosine hydroxylase protein concentration. J. Neurochem. 53:793–799.

Yoshida M., Niwa T., and Nagatsu T. (1990) Parkinsonism in monkeys produced by chronic administration of an endogenous substance of brain, tetrahydroisoquinoline: the behavioral and biochemical changes. Neurosci. Lett. 119:109–113.

Chapter 11

Monoamine Oxidase: Interaction with Isoquinoline Derivatives

Clemens Neusch and Andreas Moser

Contents in Brief

1. MAO

1.1 Introduction

Monoamine oxidase [MAO; amine: oxygen oxidoreductase (deaminating), EC 1.4.3.4] is a flavin-adenine dinucleotide (FAD)-containing protein, which represents one of the main enzymes in the metabolism of various catecholamines and indoleamines. Originally discovered in liver as tyramine oxidase (Hare, 1928), the enzyme was found to catalyze the oxidative deamination of a number of neurotransmitter, dietary amines and xenobiotics according to the reaction:

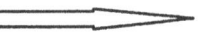

$$\boxed{R\text{-}CH_2\text{-}NH_2 \; + \; O_2 \; + \; H_2O} \quad \Longrightarrow \quad \boxed{RCHO \; + \; NH_3 \; + \; H_2O_2}$$

1.2 Classification

Based upon the substrate preference and sensitivity for specific inhibitors, MAO is divided into two types, MAO A and MAO B. MAO A is sensitive to the acetylenic inhibitor clorgyline (Johnston, 1968), while MAO B is irreversibly inhibited by deprenyl (Knoll and Magyar, 1972), but insensitive to clorgyline.

Studies on the substrate specificity *in vitro* revealed that MAO A preferentially deaminates norepinephrine, 5-hydroxytryptamine (serotonine, 5-HT), 3-O-methylepinephrine, and 3-O-methylnorepinephrine and MAO B phenylethylamine, benzylamine, *o*-tyramine, 1,4-methylhistamine, and N-*tele*-methylhistamine. Dopamine, tyramine, p-synephrine and

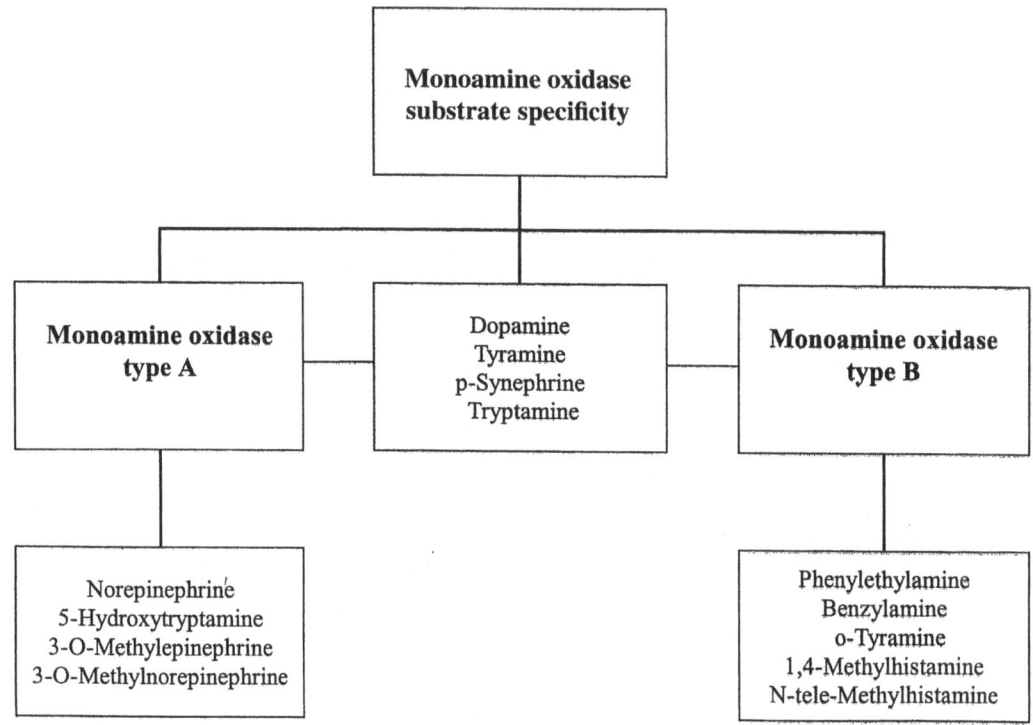

Fig. 1   Substrate specificity of monoamine oxidase. It should be noted that substrate specificity is
dependent on the substrate concentration in some cases.

tryptamine are substrates for both forms of the enzyme (see Fig. 1). Specific reversible and
irreversible inhibitors of type A and B monoamine oxidase are shown in Fig. 2.

1.3   Genetic differences

The classification according to type A and type B MAO has also been confirmed on the
genetic level. The two forms of the enzyme are coded by different genes as has been
assessed by cDNA cloning (Bach et al., 1988; Hsu et al., 1988; Lan et al., 1989). The genes,
derived from duplication of a common ancestral gene (Grimsby et al., 1991), have been
mapped on the x-chromosome between bands Xp11.23 to Xp22.1 and are closely linked
together. Both genes have similar genomic structure and consist of 15 exons with identical
exon-intron organisation (Grimsby et al., 1991).

   Studies on amino acid sequences from human liver MAO A and MAO B cDNAs have
revealed a sequence identity of 70% (Bach et al., 1988). The cDNA of type A MAO encodes
for a protein of 527 amino acids, type B MAO cDNA for a protein containing 520 amino
acids. The resulting polypeptide is either a monomer or exists as a homodimer.

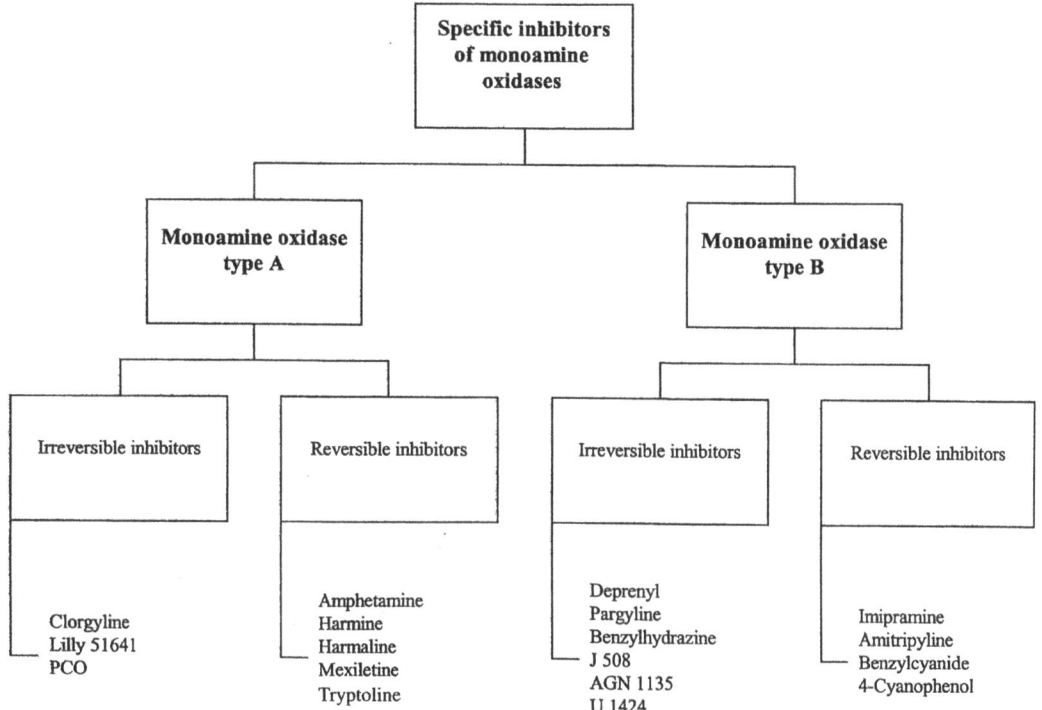

Fig. 2 Specific inhibitors of monoamine oxidase. Specificity of inhibiton is dependent on inhibitor concentration.

1.4 Occurrence

MAO A and B have been found in many organisms as well as in plants. Furthermore, they have been detected in almost all human tissues. Relatively high activities of both types of MAO are present in human liver and intestine suggesting an important role in deaminating exogenous amines. Other organs and cells, such as brain, kidney, pancreas, lung, placenta, platelets, lymphocytes and chromaffin cells, contain various amounts of both forms of the enzyme.

In humans, placenta tissue expresses predominantly MAO A (Egashira et al., 1976), whereas platelets (Donnelly and Murphy, 1977), lymphocytes (Bond and Cundall, 1977) and chromaffin cells (Youdim et al., 1984) contain primarily MAO B.

The two forms of the enzyme are differentially distributed in neuronal and nonneuronal structures. At the cellular level, studies on rat neurons have indicated that MAO A is localized preferentially in the soma of noradrenergic neurons, whereas MAO B has been found mainly in serotoninergic and serotonin-rich areas (Westlund et al., 1985). Both MAO A and MAO B are furthermore localized in a considerable amount in astroglial cells (Levitt et al., 1982).

Regarding the intracellular distribution of MAO, Tipton et al., (1967) found both isomers of the enzyme to be located in the outer mitochondrial membrane. They are tightly bound to the mitochondrial membranes, and no significant amount of soluble activity has been detected. The mode of binding to the membrane is still unknown.

In the brain, the MAO content plays a crucial role in maintaining low levels of transmitter amines and regulating transmitter concentration, whereas in peripheral organs MAO are supposed to be mainly responsible for the degradation of biogenic and exogenous amines.

Though MAO A and B activity has been detected in almost all human brain regions examined, the human brain content seems to be primarily of the B type MAO.

A study on MAO activity in human brain autopsy material was performed by Riederer and Youdim (1986). Using homogenates of different brain areas of patients who died from a non-neurological and non-psychiatric disease, their study showed the highest MAO activity toward the *substrate kynuramine* in the hypothalamus and in the *corpus striatum (caudate nucleus, putamen)* as well as in the *substantia nigra* and *globus pallidus*. Relatively high activity was found in the *locus coeruleus* and *corpus mammilare*, whereas low activity was present in the frontal cortex, hippocampus and thalamus.

Detailed information on the distribution of MAO B in human brain was obtained by a study using quantitative autoradiography with L-[^{3}H]-deprenyl as ligand (Jossan et al., 1991). High binding was observed in *caudate nucleus, putamen, cingulate gyrus* and *insula cortex*, whereas moderate to low binding was seen in *globus pallidus*, temporal and parietal cortex and thalamus. The lowest binding among the cortical regions was found in the occipital cortex and the white matter showed the lowest binding of all regions. In this study, two *postmortem* brains were used.

1.5 Reaction mechanism

The reaction catalyzed by MAO starts with dehydrogenation of the amine at the carbogennitrogen bond leading to an imine intermediate, which is subsequently hydrolysed to give an aldehyde plus ammonia (Bernheim, 1931; Tipton, 1971):

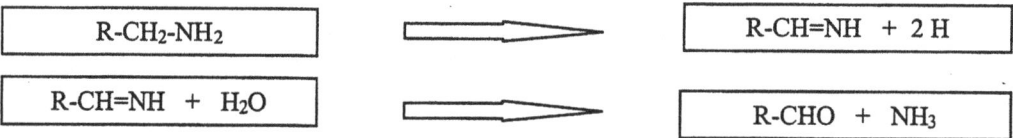

In the first step of the reaction, the oxidation of the amine reduces the flavin component of the enzyme, which itself reacts with oxygen to produce hydrogen peroxide and the starting form of the enzyme with the oxidated flavin cofactor in a second step (Youdim, 1972). This so-called double-displacement or ping-pong mechanism of the MAO is shown in the following scheme:

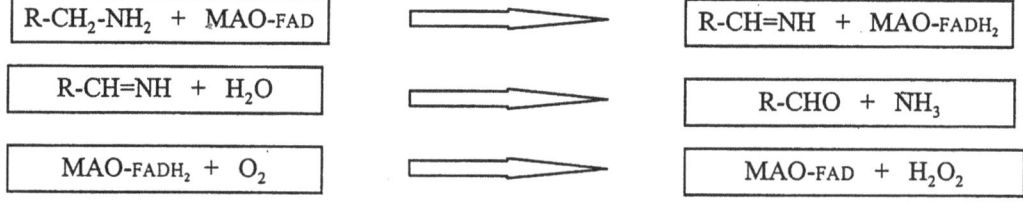

1.6 Flavin cofactor

Studies on the flavin cofactor (FAD) have shown that 100,000g protein (relative mass) contains approximately 1 mol FAD. There are inconsistent results regarding the type of linkage of the FAD molecule to the enzyme. Kearney et al. (1977) found the FAD cofactor to be covalently bound with its 8 position of the isoalloxazine ring to a cysteine residue in the enzyme by a thioether bond. On the other hand, several authors proposed the existence of a MAO requiring FAD as cofactor, which is not covalently bound to the enzyme (Yagi and Naoi, 1982). Supporting the existence of covalently bound FAD, Walker et al. (1971) were able to isolate a pentapeptide with a linkage of FAD to the amino acid cysteine.

The mechanism of enzyme inactivation by irreversible inhibitors has been examined in detail. Interaction of an irreversible inhibitor at the active site of the enzyme leads to reduction of the cofactor flavin. Subsequently, the oxidized inhibitor binds covalently to the FAD at the N-5 position of the isoalloxazine ring (Fig. 3; Salach et al., 1979).

2. Interaction Between MAO and Isoquinoline Derivatives

2.1 MPTP-model

Besides its physiological role, MAO enzymes are supposed to play an important role in pathological conditions, such as neurodegenerative diseases. 1-methyl-4-phenyl-1,2,3,6-tetrahydropyridine (MPTP) is a well known neurotoxin causing parkinsonism in humans, non-human primates and certain rodents (Burns et al., 1983). As hydrophobic agent MPTP passes the blood-brain barrier and is oxidized into 1-methyl-4-phenylpyridinium ion (MPP$^+$) via the initial oxidation product MPDP$^+$ by MAO B (Chiba et al., 1984; Fig. 4).

It has been shown that the oxidation of MPTP to MPP$^+$ is essential to elicit parkinsonism in humans (Heikkila et al., 1984). Based upon this observation, it was shown that pretreatment with a MAO B inhibitor prevented MPTP toxicity in mice (Heikkila et al., 1984) and also in monkeys (Cohen et al., 1985).

The oxidation product of MPTP, MPP$^+$ is taken into the nigrostriatal dopaminergic neuron via the high-affinity dopamine reuptake transporter. The uptake of MPP$^+$ by the

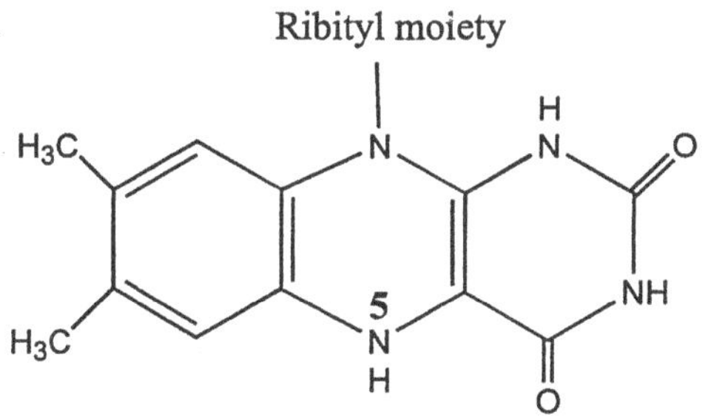

Fig. 3   Chemical structure of the flavin cofactor (flavin adenine dinucleotide, FAD).

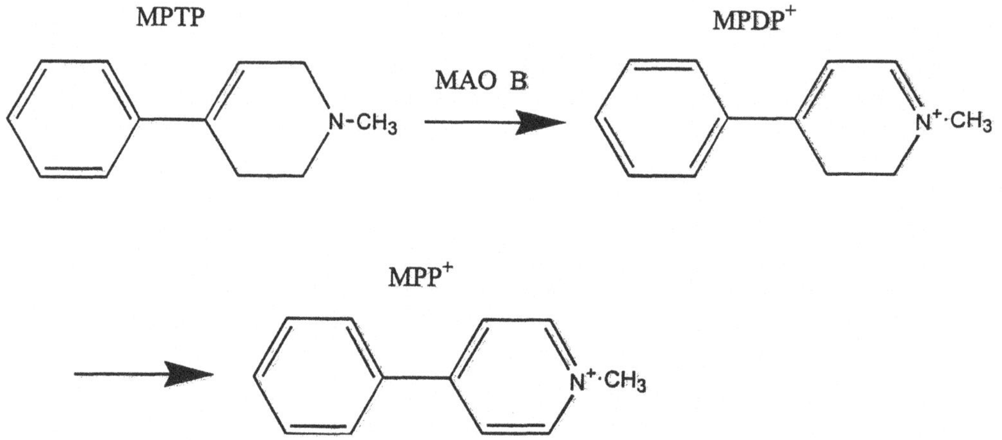

MPTP   MPDP$^+$

MPP$^+$

Fig. 4   Metabolic pathway and chemical structures of MPTP and MPP$^+$. MPTP is oxidized by monoamine oxidase into MPP$^+$ via the initial oxidative product MPDP$^+$.

dopamine transporter determines its selectivity to the dopaminergic system. Inhibition of the DA uptake system by specific uptake blocker prevents neurodegeneration induced by MPP$^+$ (Fuller and Hemrick-Lücke, 1985). The neurotoxic effects resulting from the accumulation of MPP$^+$ in the cell can be explained by different mechanisms: (1) inhibition of complex I of oxidative phosphorylation (Ramsey et al., 1991), (2) production of free radicals or peroxides during the oxidative process of MPTP/MPP$^+$ (Lambert and Bondy, 1989; Rossetti et al., 1988), (3) disturbance of intracellular calcium homeostasis (Frei and Richter, 1986; Kass et al., 1988), and (4) inhibition of tyrosine hydroxylase (Hirata and Nagatsu, 1985). Besides being a substrate for MAO, MPTP as well as MPP$^+$ inhibit MAO-A and MAO-B (Salach et al., 1984). MPTP inhibits MAO A competitively and reversibly, while MAO B inhibition by this compound is non-competitive and not completely reversible (Fuller and Hemrick-Lücke, 1985).

Since the discovery of the neurotoxic effects of MPTP, data have been accumulated to indicate that there are many naturally-occurring MPTP-like substances that probably perturb dopamine metabolism in the brain.

2.2   MPTP-like substances

Further evidence has been obtained that MPTP-like compounds might be involved in nigrostriatal degeneration and in parkinsonism in humans. Naturally-occurring compounds, which are supposed to interfere with dopamine metabolism and might contribute to neurodegeneration in Parkinson's disease, belong to one of the following groups:

—Isoquinoline derivatives
—Carboline derivatives
—TaClo derivatives
—Tryptamine derivatives
—Methyl-imidazole derivatives.

Out of them, the isoquinoline derivatives, as well as the carboline derivatives, are known to interact with monoamine oxidases. Data have been accumulated that there is an increasing number of isoquinolines and their methylated and oxidated products that potently inhibit MAO. Recent studies on this topic were performed trying to elucidate the role of isoquinoline derivatives on the monoamine catabolism and their contribution to neuropathological processes.

2.3   Isoquinoline derivatives

Recent studies on parkinsonism are focused on the isoquinoline alkaloids (Bembenek et al., 1990) and their *N*-methylated as well as oxidated products.

Isoquinoline Derivatives without Catechol Structure

- 1,2,3,4-Tetrahydroisoquinoline (TIQ)
- 1-Methyl-1,2,3,4-tetrahydroisoquinoline (1-MTIQ)
- 1-Methylisoquinolinium ion (1-MIQ$^+$)
- *N*(2)-Methyl-1,2,3,4-tetrahydroisoquinoline (NMTIQ, 2-MTIQ)
- *N*(2)-Methylisoquinolinium ion (NMIQ$^+$, 2-MIQ$^+$)
- 1,2-Dimethylisoquinolinium ion (1,2-DiMeIQ$^+$)

Isoquinoline Derivatives with Catechol Structure

- 6,7-Dihydroxy-1,2,3,4-tetrahydroisoquinoline (norsalsolinol)
- *N*(2)-Methyl-6,7-dihydroxy-1,2,3,4-tetrahydroisoquinoline (*N*-methyl-norsalsolinol, 2-MDTIQ)
- *N*(2)-Methyl-6,7-dihydroxy-isoquinolinium ion (*N*-methyl-norsalsolinium ion)
- 1-Methyl-6,7-dihydroxy-1,2,3,4-tetrahydroisoquinoline (salsolinol, 1-MDTIQ)
- 1,2-Dimethyl-6,7-dihydroxy-1,2,3,4-tetrahydroisoquinoline   (*N*-methyl-salsolinol)
- 1,2-Dimethyl-6,7-dihydroxyisoquinolinium   ion   (*N*-methyl-salsolinium   ion, DMDHIQ$^+$)

Out of these compounds, the isoquinoline derivative 1,2,3,4-tetrahydroisoquinoline (TIQ) was extensively studied. TIQ can be synthesized by non-enzymatic condensation of β-phenylethylamine with formaldehyde, but it is also present in various foods (e.g. cheese, wine). TIQ was discovered in parkinsonian human brain, and subcutaneous injection of TIQ induced L-dopa sensitive parkinsonism in monkeys with a reduction of dopamine and tyrosine hydroxylase activity in the nigro-striatal regions (Nagatsu and Yoshida, 1988; Yoshida et al., 1990).

Two enzymatic processes have been found to increase cytotoxicity of isoquinoline derivatives. *N*-Methylation of TIQ by a non-specific *N*-methyltransferase is required to chemically synthesize *N*-methyl-1,2,3,4-tetrahydroisoquinoline (NMTIQ). The *N*-methylated compound was found to be oxidized into the respective *N*-methyl-isoquinolinium ion (NMIQ$^+$) by type A and type B monoamine oxidase from human brain mitochondria (Naoi et al., 1989a; Fig. 5). Both enzymatic processes, *N*-methylation as well as oxidation, have been demonstrated to occur *in vitro* as well as *in vivo* experiments (Naoi et al., 1989a,b), suggesting an endogenous production of NMIQ$^+$. Furthermore, NMTIQ was detected in the brain of monkeys after administration of TIQ by gas chromatography-mass spectrometry

Tetrahydroisoquinoline (TIQ)   N-Methyl-TIQ (NMTIQ)

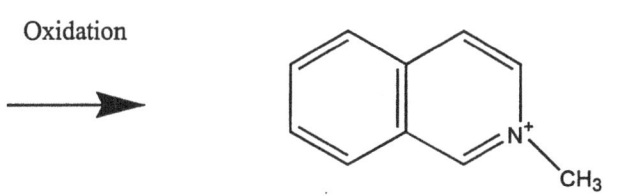

N-Methyl-Transferase

N-Methyl-isoquinolinium ion (NMIQ⁺)

Oxidation

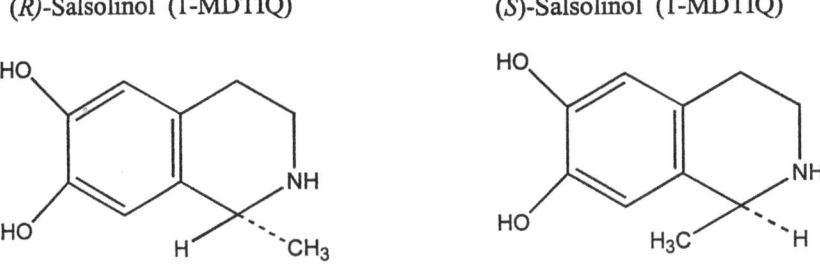

Fig. 5   Metabolic pathway and chemical structures of TIQ derivatives. TIQ is metabolized by *N*-methyltransferase into *N*-methyl-TIQ and oxidized enzymatically by monoamine oxidase or non-enzymatically into *N*-methyl-isoquinolinium ion.

(GC-MS), giving further evidence that *N*-methylation by a *N*-methyltransferase occurs *in vivo*.

The oxidative process, either enzymatic by monoamine oxidase or non-enzymatic, forming the *N*-methylisoquinolinium ion has been shown to increase the cytotoxic potential of NMTIQ as in the case of MPTP/MPP⁺. In this respect, NMIQ⁺ was found to be a more potent inhibitor of monoamine oxidase and of tyrosine hydroxylase than TIQ itself and the reduced form of the N-methylated isoquinoline (Naoi et al., 1989c). Another TIQ derivative, 1-methyl-6,7-dihydroxy-1,2,3,4-tetrahydroisoquinoline (salsolinol, 1-MDTIQ) can be formed by non-enzymatic ring cyclization of dopamine with acetaldehyde or pyruvic acid followed by decarboxylation and reduction (Niwa et al., 1991). Salsolinol was detected in urine and brain of patients treated with L-dopa. Out of the two enantiomer of salsolinol, the (*R*)- and (*S*)-enantiomer, the (*R*)-enantiomer was found to predominantly occur in human brains (Deng et al., 1995; Strolin Benedetti et al., 1989; Fig. 6).

(R)-Salsolinol (1-MDTIQ)   *(S)*-Salsolinol (1-MDTIQ)

Fig. 6   Chemical structures of (*R*)-salsolinol and (*S*)-salsolinol.

Recently, another TIQ derivative and MPTP-like compound 2-methyl-6,7-dihydroxy-1,2,3,4-tetrahydroisoquinoline (N-methyl-norsalsolinol, 2-MDTIQ) was identified in parkinsonian but not in normal lumbar cerebrospinal fluid (Moser and Kömpf, 1992), suggesting a role of isoquinoline derivatives in the Parkinson's disease.

Naoi et al. (1996) investigated the selective neurotoxicity of *N*-methyl-salsolinol and its oxidation product 1,2-dimethyl-6,7-dihydroxyisoquinolinium ion to dopaminergic neurons by injection of these compounds into the rat striatum. Injection of *N*-methyl-salsolinol and 1,2-dimethyl-6,7-dihydroxyisoquinolinium ion led to an accumulation of both compounds in the striatum. Furthermore, 1,2-dimethyl-6,7-dihydroxyisoquinolinium ion was detected in the substantia nigra followed by a marked reduction of dopamine levels in the nigro-striatal system. 1,2-dimethyl-6,7-dihydroxyisoquinolinium ion showed to be cytotoxic to neurons leading to massive necrosis and destruction of myelin structures. *N*-methyl-salsolinol was less cytotoxic but was found to be more selective to dopaminergic neurons than 1,2-dimethyl-6,7-dihydroxyisoquinolinium ion.

The mechanism by which these isoquinoline derivatives exert their neurotoxicity to the dopaminergic system and perturb the *in vivo* metabolism of monoamine is the subject of present research on Parkinson's disease (see 2.4).

2.4 Isoquinoline derivatives as MAO inhibitors

It has been proposed that some of the isoquinoline alkaloids were endogenously synthesized compounds, regulating the activity of MAO (Tasaki et al., 1991).

The *N*-methylated and oxidated product of TIQ, *N*-methyl-isoquinolinium ion proved to be a potent inhibitor of MAO with preference to MAO A (Naoi et al., 1989c). Salsolinol was measured in the urine of patients treated with L-dopa (Sandler et al., 1973) and was also identified in the human brain by GC-MS (Niwa et al., 1991; Sjoequist et al., 1982). MAO-inhibitory effects of salsolinol was suggested since perfusion of the rat *striatum* with salsolinol reduced levels of the oxidized products of dopamine (DA) and 5-hydroxytryptamine (5-HT), 3,4-dihydroxyphenylacetic acid (DOPAC), homovanillic acid (HVA) and 5-hydroxyindoleacetic acid (5-HIAA) (Maruyama et al., 1993b). These findings have been confirmed by Minami et al. (1993) who found that salsolinol, as well as its *N*-methylated derivatives (Fig. 7), and N-methyl-norsalsolinol inhibit kynuramine oxidation by type A and B MAO isolated from human brain synaptosomal mitochondria *in vitro*.

Another study showing the effects of isoquinoline derivatives on MAO activity was performed by Maruyama et al. (1995). The activity of MAO was measured fluorometrically in human brain synaptosomes using kynuramine as substrate. The samples were preincubated with either deprenyl or clorgyline to differentiate between type A and type B MAO activity. Salsolinol, *N*-methyl-salsolinol and its oxidative product *N*-methyl-salsolinium ion inhibited MAO type B non-competitively, whereas all three compounds showed to inhibit MAO A competitively.

Moser et al. (1996) described the effects of N-methyl-norsalsolinol on monoamine oxidase in membrane preparations from the *caudate nucleus* of the rat. N-methyl-norsalsolinol dose-dependently inhibited MAO activity with a marked decrease of the dopamine metabolite 3,4-dihydroxyphenylacetic aldehyde (DPAA) formation with an IC_{50} of 33 μM. The first significant inhibitory effect of *N*-methyl-norsalsolinol was seen in a concentration of 10 μM, whereas it was most effective in a concentration of 0.1 mM. These results were in agreement with Maruyama et al. (1993b) who studied the effect of norsalsolinol and its

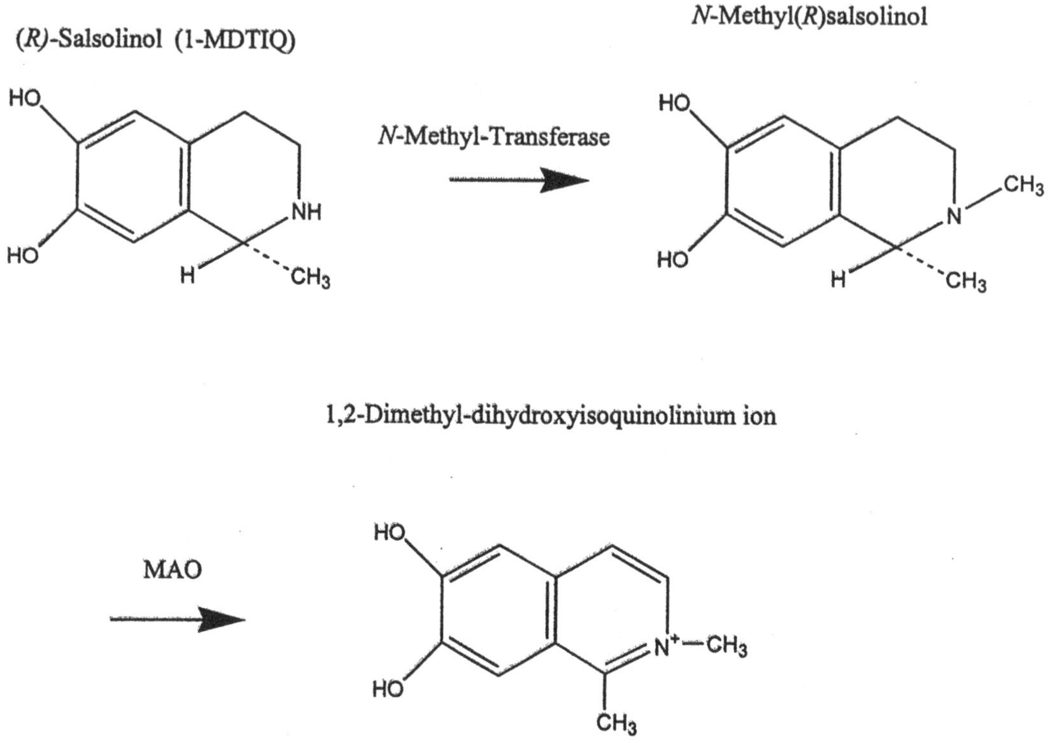

(R)-Salsolinol (1-MDTIQ)

N-Methyl(R)salsolinol

N-Methyl-Transferase

1,2-Dimethyl-dihydroxyisoquinolinium ion

MAO

Fig. 7   Chemical structures of (R)-salsolinol and its N-methylated and oxidated products. (R)-Salsolinol is N-methylated by a N-methyltransferase into N-methyl-(R)salsolinol and oxidated by a monoamino oxidase or non-enzymatically into 1,2-dimethyl-dihydroxyisoquinolinium ion.

methylated derivatives on MAO and catechol-O-methyltransferase activity by *in vivo* microdialysis in rats. Salsolinol as well as N-methyl-norsalsolinol inhibited the activity of type A MAO most markedly with a significant decline in DOPAC outflow.

2.5   Inhibition pattern of N-methyl-norsalsolinol

The mechanism by which N-methyl-norsalsolinol inhibits MAO still remains unclear. Minami et al (1993) found N-methyl-norsalsolinol to inhibit type A monoamine oxidase competitively to the substrate kynuramine, while type B oxidase was inhibited non-competitively to kynuramine with much higher K_i values than those to type A.

Moser et al. (1996) found a definite degree of inhibition by N-methyl-norsalsolinol that remained nearly constant over the incubation period of 60 min, suggesting a reversible mechanism. Since N-methyl-norsalsolinol inhibited in two phases, at low (<10 μM) and at high (>10 μM) antagonist concentrations, two different mechanisms were proposed. Addition of the cofactor NAD to the incubation did not modulate the inhibition-pattern of N-methyl-norsalsolinol. Thus, interaction of N-methyl-norsalsolinol with the NADH oxidoreductase (EC 1.6.99.3) seems unlikely.

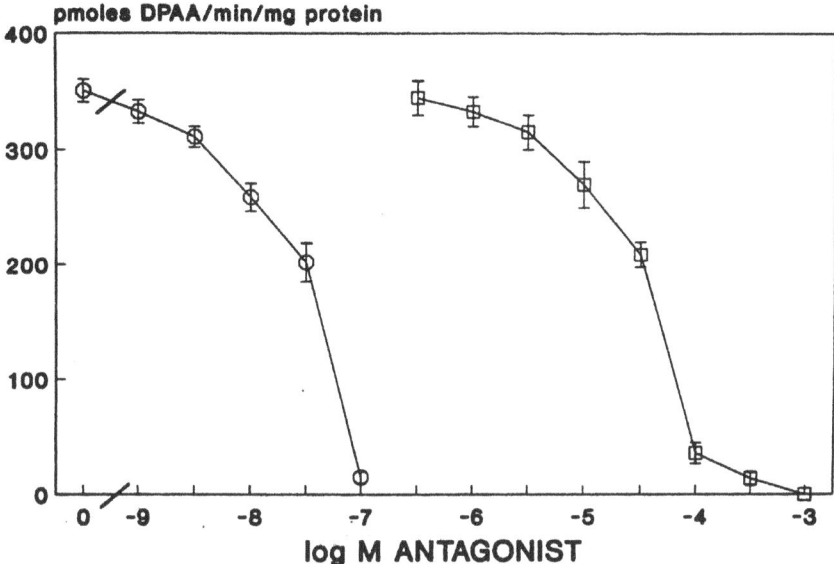

Fig. 8 The effect of clorgyline (○) and deprenyl (□) on MAO activity in pmol DPAA/min/mg protein (according to Moser et al., 1996).

In subsequent experiments, addition of type A and B inhibitors did not influence submaximal inhibition of *N*-methyl-norsalsolinol. It seems very unlikely that the mechanism of inhibition of *N*-methyl-norsalsolinol follows a simple, probably competitive, type A/B enzyme inhibition (Moser et al., 1996).

The inhibition pattern of isoquinoline derivatives is summarized in Table 1. To differentiate between type A and type B MAO, samples used in the studies were mostly incubated with deprenyl or clorgyline, respectively (Fig. 8).

2.6   Chemical structure and inhibitory activity

Studies on the structure-activity relationship of TIQ derivatives have shown that the inhibitory potency of these compounds is related to the presence and position of methyl groups. Salsolinol and *N*-methyl-norsalsolinol, both dihydroxylated TIQ derivatives with one methyl group, were found to affect MAO activity more markedly than isoquinoline derivatives with two or without methyl group (*N*-methyl-salsolinol, norsalsolinol; Maruyama et al., 1993).

At present, there are inconsistent results regarding the inhibitory potency of catechol isoquinolines versus isoquinolines without catechol structure. In an *in vivo* study using rat brain microdialysis (Maruyama et al., 1993) catechol isoquinolines were detected to be a more potent inhibitor of MAO than the corresponding isoquinolines without catechol structure. The *in vivo* effects of isoquinoline derivatives with catechol structure versus without

Table 1. Inhibition pattern of isoquinoline derivatives with respective K_i values *in vitro*.

	Competitive (K_i values)	Non-competitive (K_i values)	Mixed-type (K_i values)	Unknown mechanism
TIQ	Type A (55.4 μM)*	Type B (56.8 μM)*	n.d.	n.d.
NM-TIQ	Type A (41.2 μM)*	Type B (24.8 μM)*	n.d.	n.d.
NMIQ$^+$	Type A (40.5 μM)***	Type B (284.6 μM)*	n.d.	n.d.
1,2-DiMeIQ$^+$	Type B (8.87 μM)*	Type A (2.78 μM)*	n.d.	n.d.
(R)Sal	Type A (75.9 μM)*	Type B (63.3 μM)*	n.d.	n.d.
NM-(R)Sal	Type A (86.4 μM)*	Type B (433.3 μM)*	n.d.	n.d.
NM-Sal$^+$	Type A (9.21 μM)*	Type B (77.8 μM)*	n.d.	n.d.
Norsal	n.d.	Type B (699 μM)*	Type A (65.3 μM)**	n.d.
NM-Norsal	Type A (61.4 μM)**	Type B (289 μM)**	n.d.	Type A/B****
NM-Norsal$^+$	Type A (44.4 μM)*	Type B not inhibited	n.d.	n.d.

*Naoi et al., (1994) **Minami et al., (1993)***Naoi et al., (1987) ****Moser et al., (1996) *n.d.* no data
For abbreviations refer to section 2.3.

catechol structure on monoamine levels and their metabolites were measured in the dialysate. The inhibitory potency was assessed in measuring the decrease of 3,4-dihydroxy-phenylacetic acid (DOPAC) and homovanillic acid (HVA), both metabolites of the dopamine catabolism. Salsolinol, norsalsolinol, N-methyl-(R)salsolinol and *N*-methyl-nor-salsolinol were found to inhibit MAO more strongly than in the case of TIQ, *N*-methyl-TIQ, 1-methyl-TIQ or the *N*-methyl-isoquinolinium ion.

Since dopamine (DA) and 5-hydroxytryptamine (5-HT) are mainly substrates for MAO A in the rat brain, the inhibitory potency of the examined isoquinoline derivatives with catechol structure on DA- and 5-HT-metabolism was attributed to MAO A. Among the used dihydroxylated isoquinoline derivatives, the most potent *in vivo* inhibitor of MAO was found to be (R)SAL, followed by *N*-methyl-norsalsolinol, norsalsolinol and *N*-methyl-(R)salsolinol, while the *N*-methyl-isoquinolinium ion represented the strongest inhibitor among the TIQ derivatives. *N*-methyl-TIQ did not affect monoamine metabolite levels.

An enzyme assay to measure MAO activity using synaptosomes of the human cortex showed isoquinoline derivatives without catechol structure (TIQ, 1-methyl-TIQ, *N*-methyl-TIQ, *N*-methylisoquinolinium ion and 1,2-dimethyl-TIQ) to be *more potent* inhibitors toward MAO A than their respective catechol isoquinolines. Additionally, the isoquinolines without catechol structure were also found to have much lower K_i values toward MAO B (Naoi et al, 1994).

Naoi et al. (1994) found that the presence of the catechol structure increases the *selectivity* of inhibition. The catechol isoquinolinium ions, *N*-methyl-salsolinium ion and *N*-methyl-norsalsolinium ion showed higher affinity to type A MAO than to type B. Isoquinolines without catechol structure, such as TIQ and *N*-methyl-TIQ, inhibited type B MAO with almost the same potency as MAO A.

Oxidation of isoquinoline derivatives increases the inhibitory effect as has been demonstrated in the case of 1,2-DiMeIQ$^+$ and *N*-methyl-salsolinium ion (Naoi et al., 1994).

Furthermore, the reduced isoquinolines without catechol structure inhibited type A MAO less potently than the oxidized forms.

References

Bach A. W.J., Lan N.C., Johnson D.L., Abell C.W., Bembenek M.E., Kwan S. W., Seeberg P.H., and Shih J.C. (1988) cDNA cloning of human monoamine oxidase A and B: molecular basis of differences in enzymatic properties. Proc. Natl. Acad. Sci. USA 85: 4934–4938.

Bembenek M.E., Abell C.W., Chrisey L.A., Rowadowska M.D., Gessner W., and Brossi A. (1990) Inhibition of monoamine oxidase A and B by simple isoquinoline alkaloids: racemic and optically active 1,2,3,4-tetrahydro-3,4-dihydro, and fully aromatic isoquinolines. J. Med. Chem. 33:147–152.

Bernheim M.L.C. (1931) Tyramine oxidase II. The course of the oxidation. J. Biol. Chem. 299–301.

Bond P.A., and Cundall R.L. (1977) Properties of human monoamine oxidase (MAO) in human platelets, plasma, lymphocytes and granulocytes. Clin. Chim. Acta. 80:317–326.

Burns R.S., Chiueh C.C., Markey S.P., Ebert M.H., Jacobowitz D.M., and Kopin I.J. (1983) A primate model of Parkinsonism: selective destruction of dopaminergic neurons in the pars compacta of the substantia nigra by N-methyl-4-phenyl-1,2,3,6-tetrahydropyridine. Proc. Natl. Acad. Sci. USA 80:4546–4550.

Chiba K., Trevor A.J., and Castagnoli N. Jr. (1984) Metabolism of the neurotoxic tertiary amine, MPTP, by brain monoamine oxidase. Biochem. Biophys. Res. Commun. 120: 574–578.

Cohen G., Pasik P., Cohen B., Leist A., Mytilineou C., and Yahr M.D. (1985) Pargyline and deprenyl prevent the neurotoxicity of 1-methyl-4-phenyl-1,2,3,6-tetrahydropyridine (MPTP) in monkeys. Eur. J. Pharmac. 106:209–210.

Deng Y., Maruyama W., Dostert P., Takahashi T., Kawai M., and Naoi M. (1995) Determination of the (R)- and (S)-enantiomers of salsolinol and N-methylsalsolinol by use of a chiral HPLC column. J. Chromatogr. B. 670:47–54.

Donnelly C.H., and Murphy D.L. (1977) Substrate- and inhibitor-related characteristics of human platelet monoamine oxidase. Biochem. Pharmacol. 26: 853–858.

Egashira T. (1976) Studies on monoamine oxidase. XVIII. Enzymatic properties of placental monoamine oxidase. Jpn. J. Pharmacol. 26:493–500.

Frei B., and Richter C. (1986) N-methyl-4-phenylpyridine (MPP+) together with 6-hydroxydopamine or dopamine stimulates Ca-release from mitochondria. FEBS Lett. 198: 99–102.

Fuller R.W., and Hemrick-Luecke S.K. (1985) Effects of ammfonelic acid, alphamethyltyrosine, RO 4-1284 and haloperidol on the depletion of striatal dopamine by 1-methyl-4-phenyl-1,2,3,6-tetrahydropyridine in mice. Res. Commun. Chem. Pathol. Pharmacol. 48:17–25.

Grimsby J., Chen K., Wang L.J., Lan N.C., and Shih J.C. (1991) Human monoamine oxidase A and B genes exhibit identical exon-intron organisation. Proc. Natl. Acad. Sci. USA 88:3637–3641.

Hare M.L.C. (1928) Tyramine oxidase. A new enzyme system in liver. J. Biochem. 22:968–979.

Heikkila R., Manzino L., Cabbat F., and Duvoisin R. (1984) Protection against the dopaminergic neurotoxicity of 1-methyl-4-phenyl-1,2,3,6-tetrahydropyridine by inhibitors of mitochondrial monoamine oxidases separated from human brain synaptosomes. Neurochem. Int. 16:51–57.

Hirata Y., and Nagatsu T. (1985) Inhibition of tyrosine hydroxylation in tissue slices of the rat striatum by 1-methyl-4-phenyl-1,2,3,6-tetrahydropyridine. Brain Res. 337:193–196.

Hsu Y.P., Weyler W., Chen S., Sims K.B., Rinehart W.B., Utterback M., Powell J.F., and Breakefield X.O. (1988) Structural features of human monoamine oxidase A elucidated from cDNA and peptide sequences. J. Neurochem. 51:1321–1324.

Johnston J.P. (1968) Some observations upon a new inhibitor of monoamine oxidase in brain. Biochem. Pharmacol. 17:1285–1297.

Jossan S.S., Gillberg P.G., d'Argy R., Aquilonius S.M., Långström B., Halldin C., and Oreland L. (1991) Quantitative localization of human brain monoamine oxidase B by large section autoradiography using 1-[^{3}H]deprenyl. Brain Res. 547:69–76.

Kass G.E.N., Wright J.M., Nicotera P., and Orrenius S. (1988) The mechanisms of 1-methyl-4-phenyl-1,2,3,6-tetrahydropyridine toxicity: role of intracellular calcium. Arch. Biochem. Biophys. 260:89–797.

Kearney E.B., Salach J.I., Walker W.H., Seng R.L., Kenney W.C., Zeszotek E., and Singer T.P. (1977) The covalently bound flavin of hepatic monoamine oxidase. I. Isolation and sequence of a flavin peptide and evidence for binding at the 8 α position. Eur. J. Biochem. 24:321–327.

Knoll J., and Magyar K. (1972) Some puzzling pharmacological effects of monoamine oxidase inhibitors. Adv. Biochem. Psychopharmacol. 5:393–408.

Lambert C.E., and Bondy S.C. (1989) Effects of MPTP, MPP$^+$ and paraquat on mitochondrial potential and oxidative stress. Life Sci. 44:1277–1284.

Lan N.C., Chen C.H., and Shih J.C. (1989) Expression of functional human monoamine oxidase (MAO) A and B cDNA in mammalian cells. J. Neurochem. 52:1652–1654.

Levitt P., Pintar J., and Breakefield X. (1982) Immunocyto-chemical demonstration of monoamine oxidase B in brain astrocytes and serotonergic neurons. Proc. Natl. Acad. Sci. USA 79:6385–6389.

Maruyama W., Takahashi T., Minami M., Takahashi A., Dostert P., Nagatsu T., and Naoi M. (1993) Cytotoxicity of dopamine-derived 6,7-dihydroxy-1,2,3,4-tetrahydroisoquinolines. Adv. Neurol. 60:224–230.

Maruyama W., Nakahara D., Dostert P., Takahashi A., and Naoi M. (1993b) Naturally occurring isoquinolines perturb monoamine metabolism in the brain: studied by *in vivo* microdialysis. J. Neural. Transm. 94:91–102.

Minami M., Maruyama W., Dostert P., Nagatsu T., and Naoi M. (1993) Inhibition of type A and B monoamine oxidase by 6,7- dihydroxy-1,2,3,4-tetrahydroisoquinolines and their N-methylated derivatives. J. Neural. Transm. 92:125–135.

Moser A., and Kömpf D. (1992) Presence of methyl-6,7-dihydroxy-1,2,3,4-tetrahydroisoquinolines, derivatives of the neurotoxin isoquinoline, in parkinsonian lumbar CSF. Life Sci. 50:1885–1891.

Moser A., Scholz J., Bamberg H., and Böhme V. (1996) The effect of N-methyl-norsalsolinol on monoamine oxidase of the rat caudate nucleus *in vitro*. Neurochem. Int. 28: 109–112.

Nagatsu T., and Yoshida M. (1988) An endogenous substance of the brain, tetrahydroisoquinoline, produces parkinsonism in primates with decreased dopamine, tyrosine hydroxylase and biopterin in the nigrostriatal regions. Neurosci. Lett. 87:178–182.

Naoi M., Hirata Y., and Nagatsu T. (1987) Inhibition of monoamine oxidase by N-methyl-isoquinolinium ion. J. Neurochem. 48:709–712.

Naoi M., Matsuura S., Takahashi T., and Nagatsu T. (1989a) A N-methyltransferase in human brain catalyses N-methylation of 1,2,3,4-tetrahydroisoquinoline into N-methyl-1,2,3,4-tetrahydroisoquinoline, a precursor of a dopaminergic neurotoxin, N-methylisoquinolinium ion. Biochem. Biophys. Res. Commun. 161:1213–1219.

Naoi M., Matsuura S., Parvez H., Takahashi T., Hirata Y., Minami M., and Nagatsu T. (1989b) Oxidation of N-methyl-1,2,3,4-tetrahydroisoquinoline into N-methyliso-quinolinium ion by monoamine oxidase. J. Neurochem. 52:653–655.

Naoi M., Takahashi T., Parvez H., Kabeya R., Taguchi E., Yamaguchi K., Hirata Y., Minami M., and Nagatsu T. (1989c) N-Methylisoquinolinium ion as an inhibitor of tyrosine hydroxylase, aromatic L-amino acid decarboxylase and monoamine oxidase. Neurochem. Int. 15:315–320.

Naoi M., Maruyama W., Sasuga S., Deng Y., Dostert P., Ohta S., and Takahashi T. (1994) Inhibition of type A monoamine oxidase by 2(N)-methyl-6,7-dihydroxyisoquinolin-ium ions. Neurochem. Int. 25:475–481.

Naoi M., Maruyama W., Dostert P., Hashizume Y., Nakahara D., Takahashi T., and Ota M. (1996) Dopamine-derived endogenous 1(R),2(N)-dimethyl-6,7-dihydroxy-1,2,3,4-tetrahydroisoquinoline, N-methyl-(R)-salsolinol, induced parkinsonism in rat: biochemical, pathological and behavioral studies. Brain Res. 709:285–295.

Niwa T., Takeda N., Yoshizumi H., Tatematsu A., Yoshida M, Dostert P., Naoi M., and Nagatsu T. (1991) Presence of 2-methyl-6,7-dihydroxy-1,2,3,4-tetrahydroisoquinoline and 1,2-dimethyl-6,7-dihydroxy-1,2,3,4-tetrahydroisoquinoline, novel endogenous amines, in parkinsonian and normal human brains. Biochem. Biophys. Res. Commun. 177:603–609.

Ramsey R.R., Krueger M.J., Youngster S.K., Gluck M.R., Casida J.E., and Singer T.P. (1991) Interaction of 1-methyl-4-phenyl-pyridinium ion (MPP$^+$) and its analoges with the rotenone/piericidin binding site of NADH dehydrogenase. J. Neurochem. 56:1184–1190.

Riederer P., and Youdim M.B.H. (1986) Monoamine oxidase activity and monoamine metabolism in brains of parkinsonian patients treated with l-deprenyl. J. Neurochem. 46:1359–1365.

Rossetti Z.L., Sotgiu A., Sharp D.E., and Hadjiconstantinou. M. (1988) 1-Methyl 4-phenyl-1,2,3,6-tetrahydropyridine (MPTP) and free radicals *in vitro*. Biochem. Pharmacol. 37:4537–4574.

Salach J.I., Detmer K., and Youdim M.B.H. (1979) The reaction of bovine and rat liver monoamine oxidase with [^{14}C]-clorgyline and [^{14}C]-deprenyl. Mol. Pharmacol. 16:234–241.

Salach J.I., Singer T.P., Castagnoli N., and Trevor A. (1984) Oxidation of the neurotoxic amine 1-methyl-4-phenyl-1,2,3,6-tetrahydropyridine (MPTP) by monoamine oxidases A and B and suicide inactivation of the enzymes by MPTP. Biochem. Biophys. Res. Commun. 125:831–835.

Sandler M., Carter S.B., Hunter K.R., and Stern G.M. (1973) Tetrahydroisoquinoline alkaloids; *in vivo* metabolites of l-dopa in man. Nature 241:439–443.

Sjoequist B., Eriksson A., and Winblad B. (1982) Salsolinol and catecholamines in human brain and their relation to alcoholism. Prog. Clin. Biol. Res. 90:57–67.

Strolin Benedetti M., Dostert P., and Carminati P. (1989) Influence of food intake on the enantiometric composition of urinary salsolinol in man. J. Neural. Transm. 78:43–51.

Tasaki Y., Makino Y., Ohta S., and Hirobe M. (1991) 1-methyl-1,2,3,4-tetrahydroisoquino-line, decreasing in 1-methyl-4-phenyl-1,2,3,6-tetrahydropyridine-treated mouse, prevents Parkinsoism-liked behaviour abnormalities. J. Neurochem. 57:1940–1943.

Tipton K.F. (1967) The sub-mitochondrial localization of monoamine oxidase in rat liver and brain. Biochim. Biophys. Acta 135:910–920.

Tipton K.F. (1971) Monoamine oxidases and their inhibitors. In Aldridge WN (ed.) Mechanisms of toxicity. MacMillan London 13–27.

Walker W.H., Kearney E.B., Seng R.L., and Singer T.P. (1971) The covalently bound flavin of hepatic monoamine oxidase. 2. Identification and properties of cysteinyl flavin. Eur. J. Biochem. 24:328–331.

Westlund K., Denney R., Kochersperger L., Rose R., and Abell C. (1985) Distinct monoamine oxidase A and B population in primate brain. Science 230:180–183.

Yagi K., and Naoi M. (1982) Crystallization of a monoamine oxidase purified from pig liver mitochondria. Biochem. Int. 4:457–463.

Yoshida M., Niwa T., and Nagatsu T. (1990) Parkinsonism in monkeys produced by chronic administration of an endogenous substance of the brain, tetrahydroisoquinoline: the behavioral and biochemical changes. Neurosci. Lett. 119:109–113.

Youdim M.B.H. (1972) Multiple forms of monoamine oxidase and their properties. Adv. Biochem. Psychopharmacol. 5:67–77.

Youdim M.B.H., Banerjee D.K., and Pollard H. (1984) Isolated chromaffin cells from adrenal medulla contain primarily monoamine oxidase B. Science 224:619–620.

Chapter *12*

Toxicity and Pharmacological Effects of Salsolinol in Different Cultivated Cells

Matthias F. Melzig, Ingo Putscher, Hanka Haber, Matthias Rottmann, Josef Zipper

Contents in Brief

1. Blood-Brain Barrier

The properties of tetrahydroisoquinolines (TIQs) have been discussed for a long time, especially in regards to Parkinson's disease, penetration through the blood-brain barrier, and their possible role in the development of alcoholism. There is increasing evidence that the formation of TIQs is more common in mammalian tissues than has been assumed in the past. 1-Methyl-6,7-dihydroxy-1,2,3,4-tetrahydroisoquinoline (salsolinol), a dopamine-derived TIQ, is found in urine, cerebrospinal fluid, brain and blood (Dostert et al., 1988; Sjöquist et al., 1981; Sjöquist et al., 1983; Haber et al., 1995). Isoquinoline derivatives are widely distributed in the environment, being present in plants (Shamma and Moniot, 1978), foodstuffs, and some alcoholic beverages (Makino et al., 1988). It is believed that these substances may be able to penetrate the blood-brain barrier and to accumulate in the brain (Kikuchi et al., 1991).

In this context the question arose whether the TIQs are cytotoxic to elements of the blood-brain barrier or other barriers between blood and tissues. Because of the structural similarities to the catecholamines, TIQs might also have similar pharmacological effects. Detailed studies about the mechanisms of the pharmocological and toxicological effects of salsolinol in different tissues and cells are only rarely reported. Salsolinol and other tetrahydroisoquinolines bearing a catechol moiety have been found to be easily oxidized forming cytotoxic compounds. Especially N-methyl-salsolinol was found to be oxidized enzymatically into neurotoxic hydroxyl radicals within dopamine neurons (Maruyama et al., 1995). The toxicity of N-methylated derivatives seems to be more potent than non-methylated isoquinolines. In PC12h cells, salsolinols were proved to be accumulated in the mitochondrial fraction of the cells after 3 days in culture (Maruyama et al., 1993).

The following Chapter describes results of investigations of the cytotoxicity of salsolinol in different cell systems, and its molecular pharmacological effects on receptor binding to dopamine receptors and on hormone release of pituitary cells, to elucidate a part of the pharmacological mechanisms by which TIQs induce their pharmacological activity.

2. Technical Procedures

2.1   Materials

Racemic salsolinol and also both enantiomers were synthesized in our laboratory as described previously (Haber et al., 1993). Dopamine was purchased from SIGMA.

2.2   Cell culture

Calf aortic endothelial cells (BKEz-7) were cultivated in MEM + 10% fetal calf serum (FCS) in humidified atmosphere of 37°C at 3% CO_2. The mouse anterior pituitary tumor cell line AtT-20/D16v and the human neuroblastoma cell line SK-N-SH were routinely grown in DMEM + 10% FCS (37°C, 5% CO_2).

2.3   Cytotoxicity

The cytotoxicity of salsolinol (racemate, as well as both enantiomers) in the different cell lines was estimated by a proliferation assay using 24-multiwell plates. 50 000 cells of the different cell lines were plated per well, after 24 h the appropriate concentrations of salsolinol were added, and after 4 days the total number of cells per well was counted with the electronic cell analyzing system CASY (Schärfe System, Germany). Six parallels in three independent experiments were carried out for each salsolinol concentration. Mean ± SD was calculated from the obtained data (n = 18). The IC_{50} values were calculated after regression of the curves.

2.4   Electron microscopy

Confluent endothelial cells were incubated for 2 and 6 h with different concentrations of racemic salsolinol. After that, the cells were rinsed with phosphate buffered saline (PBS) and 0.15 mol/l cacodylate buffer (pH 7.4). Then the cells were removed from the plates with a rubber scraper and placed directly into cacodylate buffer, centrifuged at 900 × g and in dissected pellets fixed for 2 h in 25 g/l glutaraldehyde in 0.1 mol/l cacodylate buffer at 4°C. After a repeated centrifugation the pellets were stored overnight in 0.15 mol/l cacodylate buffer with 70 g/l saccharose. Then the cells were washed several times with cacodylate buffer and post-fixed in 10 g/l osmium tetraoxide in cacodylate buffer at 4°C. Subsequently, the cells were rinsed three times with 0.15 mol/l cacodylate buffer, dehydrated with ethanol, and embedded in Epon 812. Ultra-thin sections were stained with uranylacetate and lead citrate and examined with a ZEISS 902 A electron microscope.

2.5 Effect of salsolinol on the β-*endorphin release of AtT-20 cells*

These experiments were carried out with short-term as well as long-term incubation of cells with the salsolinol enantiomers. In short-term experiments, the cells were cultivated as described above for 4 days before the substances were added. The incubation time with R(+)- and S(–)-salsolinol was 4 h. The long-term experiments were performed by a 72-h incubation time with the salsolinol enantiomers, which was started 24 h after seeding the cells. The used concentrations were 10, 1, and 0.1 µmol/l salsolinol. The β-endorphin concentrations were directly estimated as β-endorphin-like immunoreactivity by radioimmunoassay. The antiserum N50 was raised against the C-terminal of the molecule and showed cross-reactivity with β-lipotropin (10%). α-Endorphin, γ-endorphin, [Leu]-enkephalin and [Met]-enkephalin did not cross-react. Iodine-labeled β-endorphin was purchased from NEN, and the assay was performed as previously described (Winkler et al., 1995). Data were obtained from two independent experiments with six parallel samples. Each sample was measured twice. The data were calculated as mean ± SD.

2.6 Effect of salsolinol on the proopiomelanocortin (POMC) gene expression

For these investigations, we used a cellular model which showed a stable POMC gene expression. The POMC mRNA level of AtT-20 cells was estimated after short-term incubation (4 h) with R(+)- and S(–)-salsolinol at a concentration of 1 µmol/l. Total cellular RNA from the salsolinol-treated cells was extracted as described by Chomczynski and Sacchi (1987) and determined photometrically. Defined amounts (1, 2, 3, and 10 µg for Dot-Blot and Northern analyses, respectively) of the total cellular RNA were blotted on Hybond N membranes (Amersham, UK), and the hybridization was performed according to Putscher et al., (1995). The data were calculated as the ratio of values of the POMC signal to the signal of the standard probe oligo-dT$_{(12-18)}$. The results obtained from the POMC measurement are the mean ± SD of four independent experiments, each one consisting of four replications. The significance of the differences between the means was evaluated by Student's *t*-test after analysis of variance (p < 0.05).

2.7 Receptor binding analysis (RBA)

The affinity of the enantiomers of salsolinol to the different types of dopamine receptors was determined by using commercially available membranes of cells transfected with distinct dopamine receptor subtypes (RBI/BIOTREND, Germany). The RBA was performed according to the instructions of the manufacturer. The following specific ligands (NEN, Germany) were used in the displacement experiments:

$D_1 + D_5$ 2 nM ^{3}H-SCH 23390
D_2 0.2 nM ^{3}H-Spiperone

D_3 0.2 nM ^{3}H-YM-09151-2
D_4 0.5 nM ^{3}H-Spiperone

All experiments were done in triplicate and repeated twice. The results were analyzed by the LIGAND program.

3. Cytotoxicity of Salsolinol

The question about the penetration of TIQs into the brain through the blood-brain barrier is controversial. Because of the fact that endothelial cells are a major component of the blood-brain barrier, we investigated the cytotoxicity of the salsolinol enantiomers in endothelial cells.

The fact that the endothelium is a metabolic, highly active tissue, lining all blood vessels and forming the capillaries is the reason for the formation of a selective interface between blood and tissues by endothelial cells. The enormous endothelial surface and the presence of a multitude of metabolically important enzymes enable endothelial cells to play a significant role in the regulation of physiological processes. In the same way, these cells are also a target of different toxic substances which affect the endothelial metabolism resulting among other things, in a disturbance of the endothelial barrier function. Despite all differences between endothelial cells isolated from blood vessels and capillaries, in different animals and different tissues, all endothelial cells cultivated *in vitro* have a high number of similarities in physiology and biochemistry. The property to form a tight barrier, tied with an extensive energy metabolism seems especially to be an unique characteristic of all endothelial cell types. Because of this, the energy metabolism is a point of attack of substances which might disturb the endothelial functions.

An injury of bovine aortic endothelial cells by salsolinol might be an indication of a disturbance of the general barrier function by TIQs. The disturbance of the specific blood-brain barrier by salsolinol is followed by an increase in the TIQ-concentration within the brain, which may then result in toxic effects on neuronal structures leading to pathological effects.

Figure 1 shows the effect of concentration of salsolinol enantiomers on the proliferation of endothelial cells. Interestingly, both enantiomers showed a different cytotoxicity: S(–)-salsolinol was more toxic with an IC_{50} of 67 µmol/l than R(+)-salsolinol with an IC_{50} of 167 µmol/l. The different toxicity of enantiomers of a defined substance indicates that a stereospecific mechanism was probably included in the toxic effect. In former experiments, it was demonstrated that racemic salsolinol was able to inhibit the respiration of isolated mitochondria of mouse brain (Suzuki et al., 1990) and also of endothelial cells (Melzig and Zipper, 1993). Up to now, we do not have data that this effect is enantioselective. The toxic effect of salsolinol was also demonstrated by morphological studies.

Figure 2 shows that salsolinol caused different changes in several cellular structures, depending on its concentration and time of incubation. The mitochondria were especially a target of toxic effects. The observed damages are visible as different degrees of loss in internal structure, vacuolation, condensation or in various forms of total degeneration.

Despite such toxic effects in the range of the IC_{50} (60–170 µmol/l), an inhibition of the activity of mitochondrial succinate dehydrogenase or cytochrom c/c_1 could not be observed. Only at concentrations higher than 1 mmol/l were both enzymes inhibited by salsolinol (Melzig and Zipper, 1993). In studies examining the influence of different isoquinoline derivatives on mitochondrial complex I, it was established that salsolinol and related compounds had an IC_{50} in the range of 4 to 9 mmol/l (McNaught et al., 1995). Nevertheless, TIQ derivatives are thought to be putative mitochondrial toxins (Suzuki et al.,

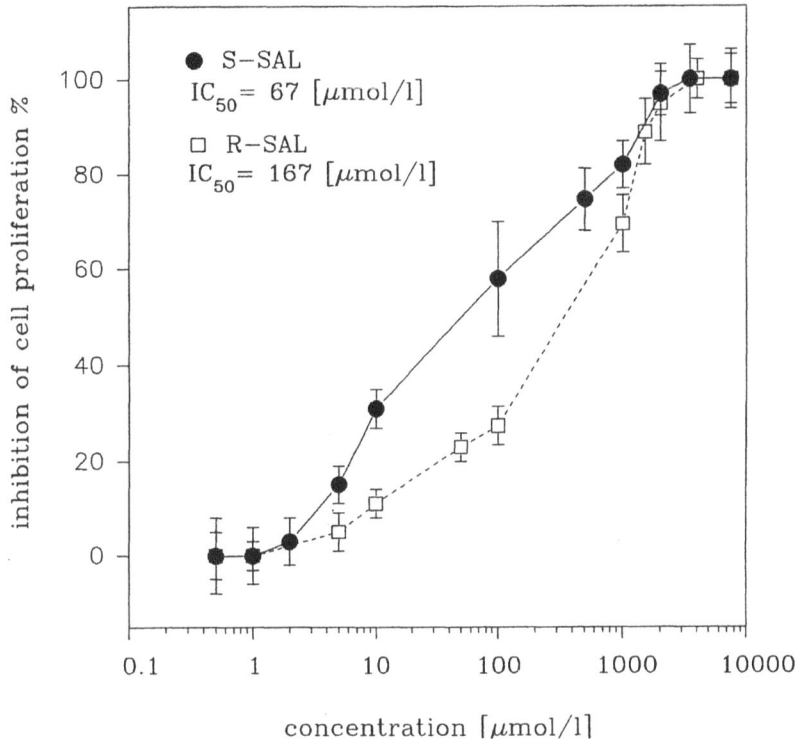

Fig. 1 Inhibition of endothelial cell proliferation by R(+)- and S(–)-salsolinol. Incubation of the cells with the TIQs was performed for 3 days followed by counting all cells. Each point of the curve is the result of six determinations in three independent experiments.

1988; 1990); the exact point of attack is not yet known. It was reported that salsolinol did not induce its cytotoxicity by membrane-directed auto-oxidation or by mechanisms requiring its uptake or bioactivation via monoamine oxidase (Willets et al., 1995).

To decide whether the cytotoxicity of salsolinol for endothelial cells was based on its endothelial-specific metabolism, we used two additional cell lines and estimated the cytotoxicity of both enantiomers of salsolinol in these cell cultures. First, we investigated the effect of salsolinol on the human neuroblastoma cell line SK-N-SH (Fig. 3). The IC_{50} values for S(–)-salsolinol were estimated with 112 μmol/l versus 335 μmol/l for R(+)-salsolinol. The data show that these cells reacted less sensitively to salsolinol than did endothelial cells, suggesting that salsolinol affected a specific pathway in endothelial cells resulting in a higher cytotoxicity. The typical morphological changes, visible in the light microscope in endothelial cells after salsolinol treatment, could not be observed in the neuroblastoma cell cultures under the same conditions. Nevertheless, in this cell line S(–)-salsolinol was also more toxic than the R(+)-enantiomer.

The third cell line we used for the cytotoxicological studies was the endocrine line AtT-20/D16v from the anterior pituitary of the mouse. This line was selected because of its ability to secrete ACTH and β-endorphin like the intact pituitary which can be stimulated via dopamine receptor interaction. AtT-20 cells do also express-dopamine D_2-receptors (Winkler et al., 1994) which might be important for the effects of salsolinol, a dopamine derived compound. Figure 4 demonstrates that in the same manner as in endothelial cells, S(–)-sal-

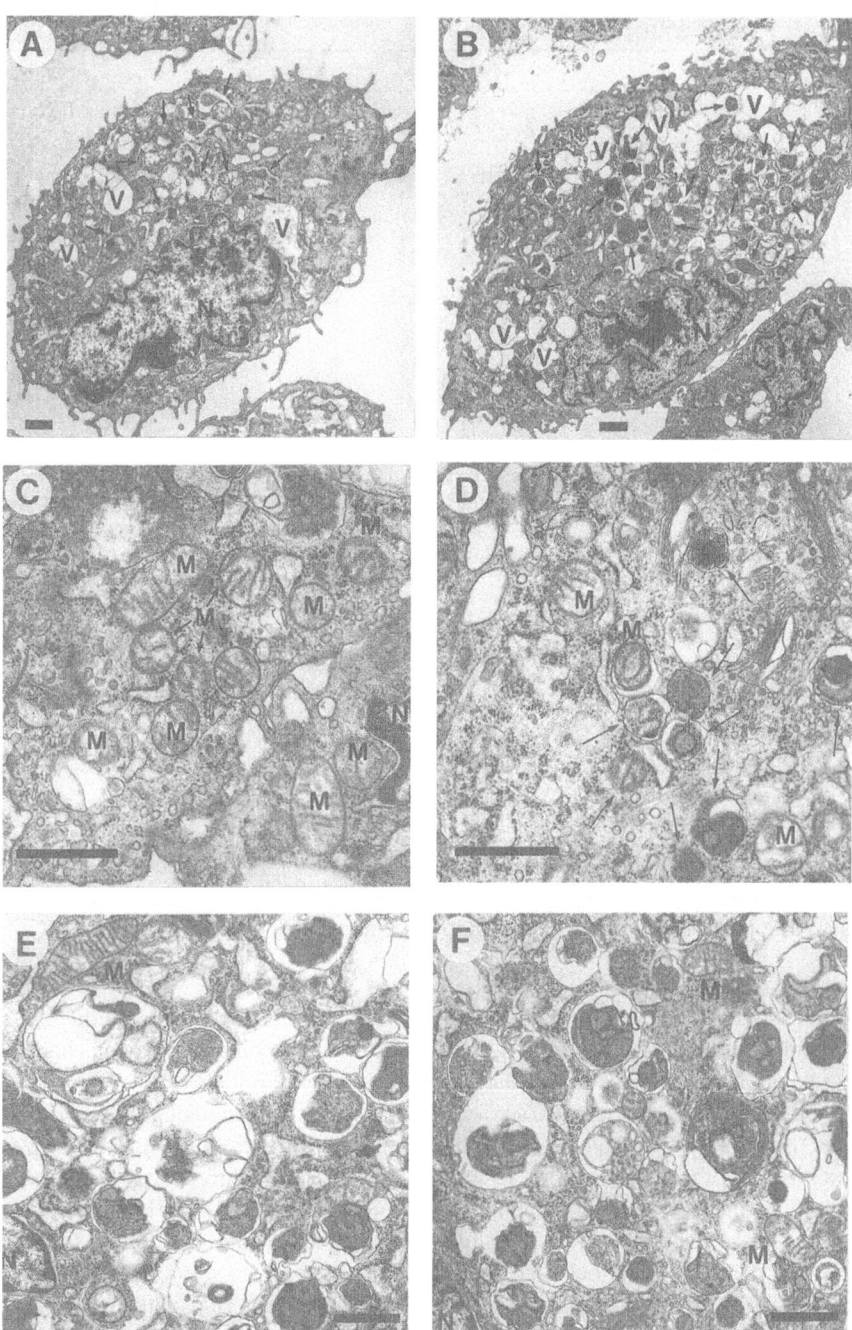

Fig. 2 (Pictures A–F). Electron micrographs showing ultrastructural damages of mitochondria in cultivated endothelial cells treated with racemic salsolinol. Bars: 1 µm. A,B: Two cells with different degrees of mitochondrial damages caused by salsolinol in a dosage of 40 µmol/l (Picture A) and 80 µmol/l (Picture B) for 6 h in each case. Vacuolated mitochondria (V) and organelle changes marked by arrows are seen in detail in the pictures C–F. C: Mitochondrial injury is characterized by disintegration or loss of cristae structures, 40 µmol/l salsolinol for 2 h. E, F: Extreme degeneration of mitochondria appearing as lysis or condensation to different extents and mainly associated with marked electron opaque deposits, 80 µmol/l salsolinol for 6 h.

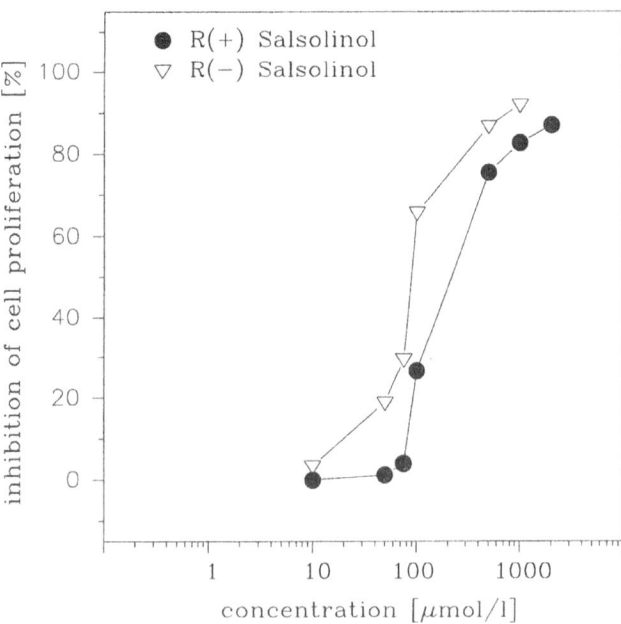

Fig. 3 Inhibition of the proliferation of the neuroblastoma cell line SK-N-SH by R(+)- and S(−)-salsolinol. Incubation of the cells with the TIQs was performed for 3 days followed by counting all cells. Each point of the curve is the result of six determinations in three independent experiments.

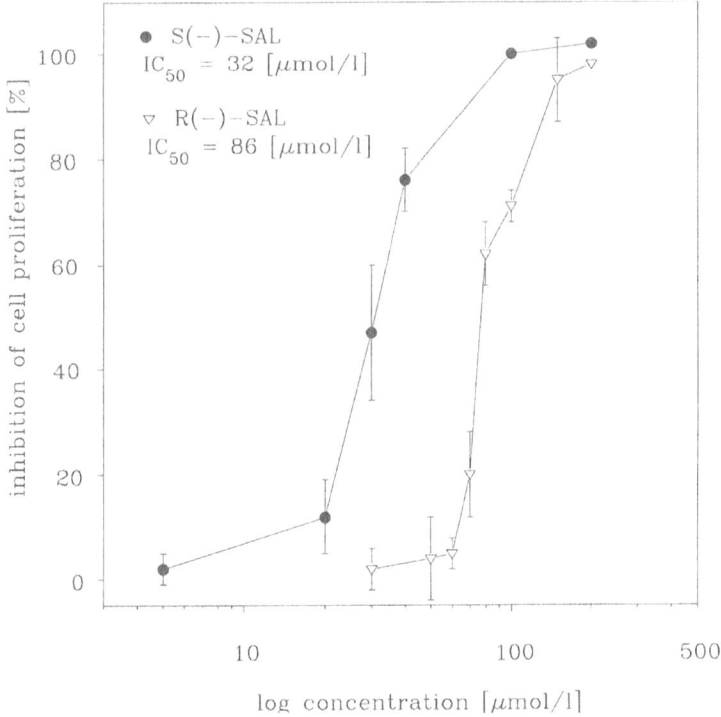

Fig. 4 Inhibition of the proliferation of AtT-20/D16v cells by R(+)- and S(−)-salsolinol. Incubation of the cells with the TIQs was performed for 3 days followed by counting all cells. Each point of the curve is the result of six determinations in three independent experiments.

solinol was more toxic (IC_{50} = 32 µmol/l) than R(+)-salsolinol (IC_{50} = 86 µmol/l). But the pituitary tumor cells were more sensitive to salsolinol in comparison to the endothelial cells. We assumed that the cytotoxic effect of salsolinol might be mediated via dopamine receptors. To prove this assumption, we estimated the cytotoxicity of dopamine, the natural ligand of dopamine receptors in both endothelial and AtT-20 cells.

Figure 5 shows that dopamine itself is less cytotoxic in both cell systems than S(–)-salsolinol, but is in the same range of concentration as the R(+)-enantiomer. This finding suggests the hypothesis that the S(–)-salsolinol cytotoxicity is induced by a specific, not dopamine receptor-mediated mechanism, whereas R(+)-salsolinol had only an nonspecific toxic effect on the investigated cells, like dopamine. The toxic effect of dopamine may be the result of the inhibition of energy metabolism. The exact mechanism by which dopamine inhibits the mitochondrial respiration chain is still under investigation. A link to NADH dehydrogenase and ADP, which could reverse the dopamine-induced inhibition of the NADH dehydrogenase activity was proposed (Ben-Shachar et al., 1995). A similar mechanism may also be discussed for salsolinol, but with a higher toxicity than that of dopamine.

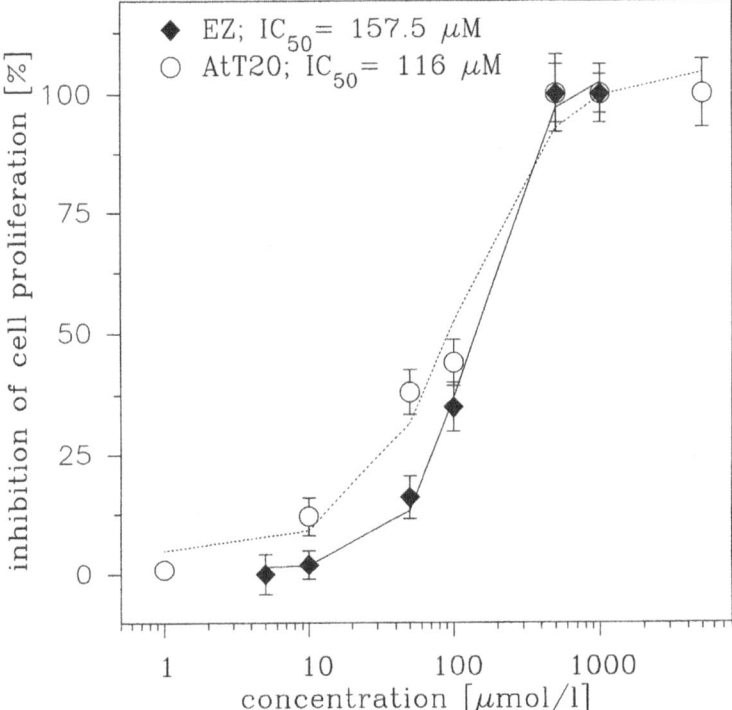

Fig. 5   Inhibition of cell proliferation by dopamine. Endothelial and AtT-20/D16v- cells were incubated for 3 days with dopamine and then all cells were counted. Each point of the curve is the result of six determinations in three independent experiments.

4. Binding Studies with Salsolinol on Dopamine Receptor Subtypes

The presence of salsolinol as a dopamine-related compound in various tissues in mammalians raised the question of whether salsolinol is able to bind to dopamine receptors. Thus, we investigated via displacement experiments, if salsolinol was able to bind to the known five dopamine receptor subtypes, in comparison to the natural ligand dopamine. To obtain unequivocal binding data at the specific subtype of the different dopamine receptor subtypes, we used in our studies the membranes of cells which were specifically transfected with only one receptor subtype. This way no cross-reactivity of binding affinities between different dopamine receptor subtypes could affect the binding analyses. Table 1 demonstrates that the S(–)-enantiomer of salsolinol showed an affinity, especially to D_1- and D_3-receptors, but its affinity was weaker than that of dopamine. Interestingly, the displacement data for S(–)-salsolinol and dopamine of the D_2-receptor are quite similar; both are rather weak competitors. With the exception of the D_3-receptor, the R(+)-salsolinol did not show a significant binding to the dopamine receptors.

The results indicated that at low concentration (1 µmol/l), both enantiomers of salsolinol were able to bind to the D_3-receptor. The physiological or toxicological significance of this binding is not clear yet and needs further molecular pharmacological investigations. Nevertheless, the binding affinity of salsolinol to the D_3-receptor is interesting because this receptor is suggested to play a crucial role in the pathogenesis of schizophrenia and other mental disorders. A strong link between dopamine receptor binding and cytotoxicity seems to be rather unlikely (dopamine binds more strongly to the dopamine receptor than salsolinol, but had a lower cytotoxicity/higher IC_{50}), despite a report about the induction of apoptosis by the dopaminergic agonist bromocriptine in AtT-20 cells (Yin et al., 1994).

A possibility that salsolinol is bound by a specific enantioselective TIQ-receptor could be an interesting hypothesis which, however, needs further investigations with radioactive-labeled TIQs in cell cultures, as well as in different tissues of the brain and the periphery.

Table 1. Inhibition of the binding of specific radioligands to dopamine receptor subtypes by the enantiomers of salsolinol and dopamine

	S(–)-salsolinol		R(+)-salsolinol		Dopamine	
	10 µmol/l	1 µmol/l	10 µmol/l	1 µmol/l	10 µmol/l	1 µmol/l
D_1	35	3	13	3	61	34
D_5	14	7	0	0	79	50
D_2	16	12	3	0	20	9
D_3	63	23	41	15	80	68
D_4	28	3	5	4	55	32

The values in the table show the inhibition of specific ligand binding in % of the different dopamine receptor subtypes by the salsolinol enantiomers in comparison to dopamine.

5. Effects of Salsolinol on POMC Gene Expression and β-Endorphin Secretion

It is well known that alcohol itself does not have any affinity for pre- or post-synaptic receptors in neurons of the brain (Myers, 1989). But the condensation products of alcohol metabolites and dopamine, the tetrahydroisoquinolines like salsolinol, show binding to dopamine receptor, as we demonstrated. In combination with the fact that salsolinol induced voluntary alcohol drinking (Myers, 1989) and the binding of salsolinol to dopamine receptors, after intracerebroventricular application in rats, as described above, a hypothesis was suggested that salsolinol is implicated in the production of a β-endorphin deficiency, reported in the literature after chronic ethanol treatment (Dave et al., 1986; Seizinger et al., 1984). Furthermore, the β-endorphin levels measured in the cerebrospinal fluid of alcoholics were significantly lower than those of controls, whereas the ACTH levels were five times higher than those of the control values (Genazzani et al., 1982).

β-Endorphin and adrenocorticotropin (ACTH) (Fig. 6) are the important elements of the hypothalamus-pituitary-adrenal stress axis, which is included in the regulation of the reward system and mental processes, like motivation or craving. β-Endorphin and ACTH are formed by limited proteolysis from their precursor peptide proopiomelanocortin (POMC), a peptide consisting of 265 amino acids. The first step in the biosynthesis of both β-endorphin and ACTH is the transcription (formation of a messenger RNA) of the POMC gene. The amount of formed mRNA is a measure of the biosynthesis of POMC, and by that of β-endorphin and ACTH. Our own experiments with voluntary alcohol drinking in rats showed that, in the anterior as well as in the neurointermediate lobe of the pituitary, the POMC gene expression was decreased after chronic alcohol exposure (Winkler et al., 1995). However, there were no reports about the effect of TIQs on POMC gene expression. Therefore, we investigated the influence of salsolinol on the POMC gene expression in a cellular model, the neuroendocrine anterior pituitary cell line AtT-20/D16v, which shows a highly reproducible POMC gene expression. Taking into account our cytotoxicological studies, a final salsolinol concentration of 1 μmol/l was used. The cells were treated for 4 h with salsolinol.

As shown in Fig. 7, the S(–)-enantiomer of salsolinol caused a significant decrease in

human β-endorphin (β-END)

H-Tyr-Gly-Gly-Phe-Met-Thr-Ser-Glu-Lys-Ser-Gln-Thr-Pro-Leu-Val-Thr-Leu-Phe-Lys-Asn-Ala-Ile-Ile-Lys-Asn-Ala-Tyr-Lys-Lys-Gly-Glu-OH

human ACTH (1-39)

H-Ser-Tyr-Ser-Met-Glu-His-Phe-Arg-Trp-Gly-Lys-Pro-Val-Gly-Lys-Lys-Arg-Arg-Pro-Val-Lys-Val-Tyr-Pro-Asn-Gly-Ala-Glu-Asp-Glu-Ser-Ala-Glu-Ala-Phe-Pro-Leu-Glu-Phe-OH

Fig. 6   Amino acid sequences of β-endorphin and adrenocorticotropin (ACTH).

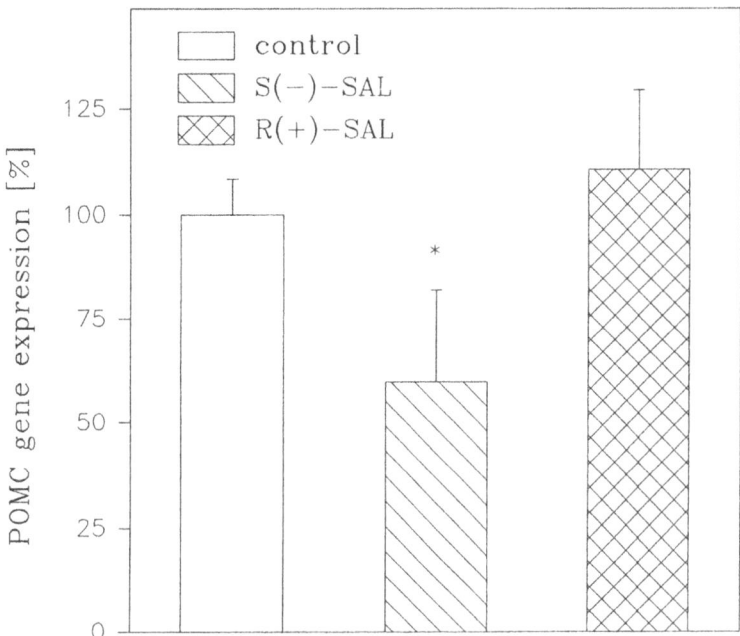

Fig. 7 Influence of R(+)- and S(–)-salsolinol on the POMC gene expression of AtT-20/D16v cells. The cells were incubated with the TIQs at a concentration of 1 μmol/l for 4 h. The values over the bars represent SD. * Significant difference between S(–)-salsolinol versus the control (p < 0.05).

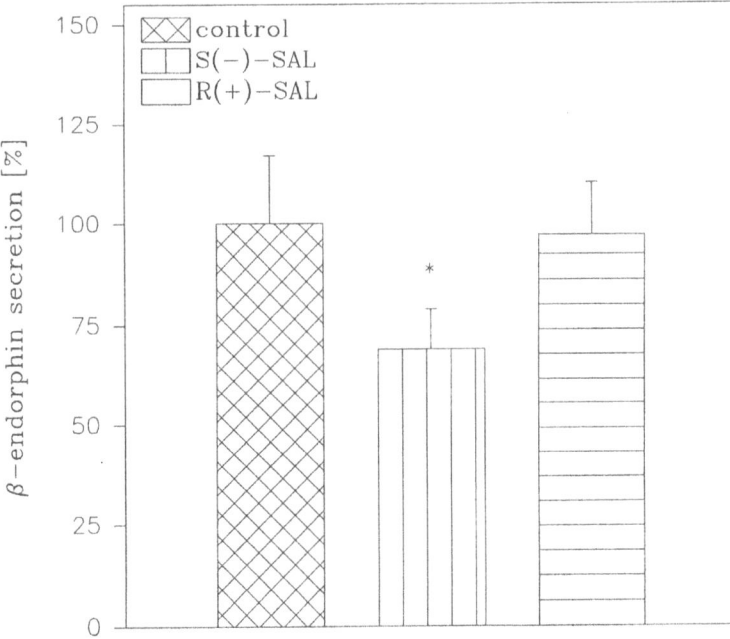

Fig. 8 Effect of R(+)- and S(–)-salsolinol on the β-endorphin secretion by AtT-20/D16v cells. The cells were incubated with the TIQs at a concentration of 1 μmol/l for 4 days, the medium plus fresh TIQs was changed daily. On day 5 the cells were incubated with fresh medium plus salsolinol, the β-endorphin secreted during 4 h in this medium was than estimated by RIA as described in materials and methods. The values over the bars represent SD. * Significant difference between S(–)-salsolinol versus the control (p < 0.05).

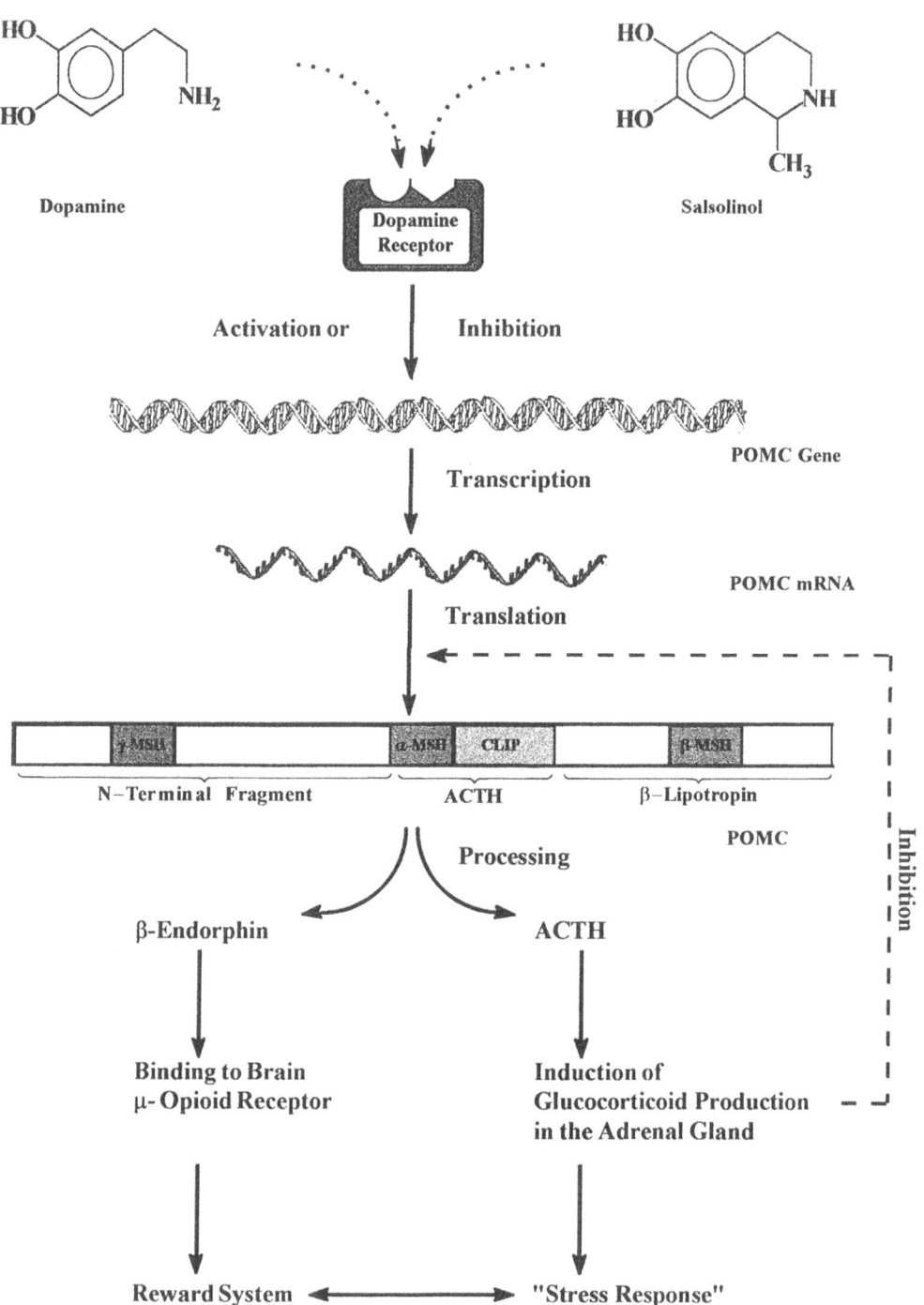

Fig. 9 Proposed model for the explanation of the biological effect of salsolinol *in vivo* via interaction with dopamine receptors, resulting in changes of the POMC gene expression and inhibited formation of β-endorphin. POMC = proopiomelanocortin, ACTH = adrenocorticotropin, MSH = melanocyte-stimulating hormone, CLIP = corticotropin-like intermediate peptide.

the POMC mRNA level, whereas no changes were detectable after incubation with the R(+)-salsolinol. The D_2 receptor-agonist bromocriptine also caused a decrease in the POMC gene expression in the intermediate lobe of the pituitary (Dyr et al., 1993). In accordance with these results, S(−)-salsolinol also inhibited the β-endorphin secretion of AtT-20 cells (Fig. 8), R(+)-salsolinol did not influence the cell system. In these experiments, the cells were treated for 4 days with the TIQ, and the medium was changed daily to fresh medium plus fresh salsolinol. By that the influence of a repeated salsolinol treatment was studied.

In previous experiments, without the daily change of the medium and in short-term experiments with only 4 h salsolinol incubation of the cells, no effect on β-endorphin secretion was observed. This demonstrates that only the intact salsolinol molecule and not a newly-formed oxidation product was able to inhibit the β-endorphin secretion, and that the secretion process itself was not affected by salsolinol, but rather the biosynthesis of β-endorphin via the POMC gene expression was. The enantioselectivity of the inhibition of POMC gene expression and β-endorphin secretion by S(−)-salsolinol and the specific binding of this enantiomer to dopamine receptors are strong indications of a link between the chronic effects of alcohol intake and this tetrahydroisoquinoline, which might be involved in the establishment of the opioid deficiency in alcoholics via inhibition of POMC gene expression, as summarized in Fig. 9. On the other hand, the stress response is modified via an impaired biosynthesis of ACTH. The changed interaction between the reward system and the stress response as a result of the action of salsolinol seems to be an important element for the explanation of pharmacological and toxicological effects induced by TIQs.

References

Ben-Sachar D., Zuk R., and Glinka Y. (1995) Dopamine neurotoxicity: Inhibition of mitochondrial respiration. J. Neurochem. 64:718–723.

Dave J.R., Lee E.E., Karanian J.W., and Eskay R.L. (1986) Ethanol exposure decreases pituitary corticotrophin-releasing factor binding, adenylate cyclase activity, proopiomelanocortin biosynthesis and plasma β-endorphin. Endocrinology 118:280–286.

Dostert P., Strolin Benedetti M., and Dordain G. (1988) Dopamine-derived alkaloids in alcoholism and in Parkinson's and Huntington's diseases. J. Neural. Transm. 74:61–74.

Dyr W., McBride J., Lumengt L., Li T.K., and Murphy J.M. (1993) Effects of D_1 and D_2 dopamine receptor agents on ethanol consumption in the high-alcohol-drinking (HAD) line of rats. Alcohol 10:207–212.

Fickel J., Savoly S., Vogel U., Furkert J., and Melzig M.F. (1994) The proopiomelanocortin (POMC) gene expression of AtT-20 mouse pituitary cells is dependent on cell culture conditions. Cell. Mol. Biol. 40:201–209.

Genazzani A.R., Nappi G., Facchinetti F., Mazella G.L., Parrini E., Sinforiani E., Petraglia F., and Sovaldi F. (1982) Central deficiency of β-endorphin in alcohol addicts. Clin. Endocrinol. Metab. 55:583–586.

Haber H., Henklein P., Georgi M., and Melzig M.F. (1995) Resolution of catecholic tetrahydroisoquinoline enantiomers and the determination of R- and S-salsolinol in biological samples by gas chromatography-mass spectrometry. J. Chromatogr. B 672: 179–187.

Haber H., Putscher I., Fickel J., Schümann M., and Melzig M.F. (1993) Easy preparation of R- and S-salsolinol of high optical purity. Pharmazie 48:700–702.

Kikuchi K., Nagatsu Y., Makino Y., Mashino T., Ohta S., and Hirobe M. (1991) Metabolism and penetration through the blood-brain-barrier of parkinsonism-related compounds: 1,2,3,4-tetrahydroisoquinoline and 1-methyl-1,2,3,4-tetrahydroisoquinoline. Drug Metab. Dispos. 19:257–262.

Makino Y., Ohta S., Tachikawa O., and Hirobe M. (1988) Presence of tetrahydroisoquinoline and 1-methyl-tetrahydroisoquinoline in foods: Compounds related to Parkinson's disease. Life Sci. 43:373–378.

Maruyama W., Takahashi T., Minami M., Takahashi A., Dostert P., Nagatsu T., and Naoi M. (1993) Cytotoxicity of dopamine-derived 6,7-dihydroxy-1,2,3,4-tetrahydroisoquinolines. Adv. Neurol. 60:224–230.

Maruyama W., Dostert P., Matsubara K., and Naoi M. (1995) N-methyl-(R)-salsolinol produces hydroxyl radicals: involvement to neurotoxicity. Free Radic. Biol. Med. 19:67–75.

McNaught K.S.P., Thull U., Carrupt P.A., Altomare C., Cellamare S., Carotti A., Testa B., Jenner P., and Marsden C.D. (1995) Inhibition of complex I by isoquinoline derivatives structurally related to 1-methyl-4-phenyl-1,2,3,6-tetrahydropyridine (MPTP). Biochem. Pharmacol. 50:1903–1911.

Melzig M., and Zipper J. (1993) Effect of salsolinol on cultivated endothelial cells. Neurochem. Res. 18:689–693.

Myers R.D. (1989) Isoquinolines, beta-carbolines and alcohol drinking: Involvement of opioid and dopaminergic mechanisms. Experientia 45:436–443.

Putscher I., Haber H., Winkler A., Fickel J., and Melzig M.F. (1995) Effect of S(–)- and R(+)-salsolinol on the POMC gene expression and ACTH release of an anterior pituitary cell line. Alcohol 12:447–452.

Seizinger R., Höllt V., and Herz A. (1984) Effects of chronic ethanol treatment on the *in vitro* biosynthesis of proopiomelanocortin and its posttranslational processing to β-endorphin in the intermediate lobe of the rat pituitary. J. Neurochem. 43:607–613.

Shamma M., and Moniot J.L., eds. (1978) Isoquinoline Alkaloids Research. Plenum, New York.

Sjöquist B. Perdahl E., and Winblad B. (1983) The effect of alcoholism on salsolinol and biogenic amines in human brain. Drug Alcohol Depend. 12:15–23.

Sjöquist B., Borg S., and Kvande H. (1981) Catecholamine derived compounds in urine and cerebrospinal fluid from alcoholics during and after long-standing intoxication. Subst. Alcohol Actions Misuse 2:73–77.

Suzuki K., Mizuno Y., and Yoshida M. (1990) Inhibition of mitochondrial respiration by 1,2,3,4-tetrahydroisoquinoline-like endogenous alkaloids in mouse brain. Neurochem. Res. 15:705–710.

Willets J.M., Lambert D.G., Lunec J., and Griffiths H.R. (1995) Studies on the neurotoxicity of 6,7-dihydroxy-1-methyl-1,2,3,4-tetrahydroisoquinoline (salsolinol) in SH-SY5Y cells. Eur. J. Pharmacol. 293:319–326.

Winkler A., Roske I., Furkert J., Fickel J., and Melzig M.F. (1995) Effects of voluntary ethanol ingestion on the POMC gene expression in the rat pituitary and on the plasma β-endorphin content. Alcohol Alcoholism 30:231–238.

Winkler A., Siems W.-E., Putscher I., and Melzig M.F. (1994) Evidence for the expression of the dopamine D_2 receptor in AtT-20 mouse pituitary tumor cells. Cell Biol. Intern. 18:We-16/ 487.

Index

The manufacturer's authorised representative in the EU is Springer
Nature Customer Service Centre GmbH, Europaplatz 3, 69115 Heidelberg,
Germany. If you have any concerns regarding our products, please
contact ProductSafety@springernature.com

Printed and bound by CPI Group (UK) Ltd, Croydon, CR0 4YY
29/04/2026
02099472-0018